# Evoked Brain Potentials and Behavior

# THE DOWNSTATE SERIES OF
# RESEARCH IN PSYCHIATRY AND PSYCHOLOGY

A Continuation Order Plan is available for this series. A continuation order will bring delivery of each new volume immediately upon publication. Volumes are billed only upon actual shipment. For further information please contact the publisher.

# Evoked Brain Potentials and Behavior

*Edited by*

**HENRI BEGLEITER**
*Downstate Medical Center*
*Brooklyn, New York*

PLENUM PRESS • NEW YORK AND LONDON

Library of Congress Cataloging in Publication Data

Conference on Evoked Brain Potentials and Behavior, Downstate Medical
   Center, State University of New York, 1977.
   Evoked brain potentials and behavior.

   (The Downstate series of research in psychiatry and psychology; v. 2)
   Includes index.
   1 Neuropsychology — Congresses. 2. Evoked potentials (Electrophysiology) — Congresses. 3. Human behavior — Congresses. 4. Electroencephalography — Congresses. I. Begleiter, Henri. II. Title. III. Series. [DNLM: 1.
Behavior — Congresses. 2. Evoked  potentials — Congresses. W1 SO 945
v.2/WL102 C7414 1977]
QP360.C66  1977                    616.8                    78-31448
ISBN 0-306-40145-2

Proceedings of a Conference on Evoked Brain Potentials and Behavior
held at the Downstate Medical Center, State University of New York,
Brooklyn, New York, May 19–21, 1977

© 1979 Plenum Press, New York
A Division of Plenum Publishing Corporation
227 West 17th Street, New York, N.Y. 10011

Printed in the United States of America

# Foreword

This volume is the second in "The Downstate Series of Research in Psychiatry." It is a series devoted to the presentation of significant research with relevance for both clinicians and researchers in the multiple subfields of psychiatry. This book focuses on the interactions between psychic phenomena and physical processes as studied by evoked brain potentials. It presents material concerned with physiological and psychological unifying processes, as well as research concerning technology and methods of obtaining meaningful measurements. As such it is representative of biological psychiatry at its best. Thus, it represents another step in new directions in psychiatric research but not an unanticipated direction.

Scientific investigation into the human psyche took an unexpected turn when Sigmund Freud in the last part of the 19th Century turned his attention from neurological concerns to those of psychology. His first attempts at explanations as noted in the "project," included a heavy emphasis on the biological substrate of behavior. As his researches into the functioning of the unconscious mind continued, he moved further and further from biological explanations, although he never overlooked the fundamental importance of these factors. His research into the psychology of the mind dominated the thinking of psychiatrists for the first part of the 20th Century, and the major advances in our knowledge of the human psyche came from psychological laboratories, clinical studies and models of the mind which, on the whole, excluded the findings of basic research on the actual functioning of the central nervous system.

Coincident with the above developments, biological studies continued as noted, for example, by Cannon's emergency theory involving affect and physiological responses. Such studies, however, did not represent the main thrust of psychiatry and Cannon did not work within the discipline of psychiatry or under the auspices of a department of psychiatry. Further, little attention was focused upon integrated studies of the physical functioning of that great reservoir of the mind, the unconscious or in later terminology the Id and the unconscious Ego.

Research once again took an unexpected turn when during the
French Indo-China conflict Thorazine was given wounded soldiers.
The French used Thorazine to lower the body temperature in these
wounded for transport to hospitals.  It was noted as a side-effect
that along with the lowering of the body temperature there was an
observable tranquilizing of the soldiers.  This observation led to
the use of the drug in psychiatric institutions to quiet the violent.
The results were so phenomenal that patient care was revolutionized
and psychopharmacology developed not only as a clinical tool but as
a special discipline along with other studies of the biochemistry of
the brain.  Other approaches towards unraveling the mysteries of the
mind-brain (psyche and soma) complex exist.  Among these is the one
concerned with the study of the electrical activity of the brain.

Researchers and clinicians have long been aware of the existence of bio-electric potentials in the body, and the electrocardio-
graph has long been an investigative tool for those studying the
heart.  Similarly, electroencephalography developed both as a clinical and research tool and much investigation was conducted on the
electrical activity of the brain.  We thus approach the subject with
which this volume is concerned.  Before the present papers could be
written, however, it was first necessary for computer technology to
emerge and develop to the point that computer extracted evoked potentials of the brain could be readily recorded and analyzed in an
attempt to elucidate the relationship between mind and brain.

In a way, we are swinging back to earlier days with newer and
more sophisticated attempts at integrating neurological approaches
with psychological insights.  Numerous types of psychological stimuli may now be studied in new ways by evoked brain potentials.  This
is an exciting research direction and will, in time, be of great
benefit.  Meanwhile, the pioneers work on and this volume is a tri-
bute to their dedication and a report of their efforts.

Dr. Begleiter has worked long and hard to produce this volume,
the second in our series.  He has brought together an outstanding
group of scientists and built a conference based on significant
concepts and their elucidation.  The results are here spelled out.
It is my hope that all who read this volume will not only be edified,
but that they will also enjoy the presentation.

Robert Dickes, M.D.
Professor and Chairman
Department of Psychiatry

# Preface

Although man has been the subject of scholarly pursuits for many centuries, as yet there is a paucity of factual information about the nature of human behavior. The behavior of man is caused by a myriad of complex biological, psychological and sociological processes. However because man is a biological being, it is intuitively obvious that a complete understanding of the nature and causes of behavior will necessitate that behavior be studied from a biological perspective.

For several centuries scholars concerned themselves with the "mind-brain dualism." However, in the last several years it has become more and more apparent that the mind does not appear to exist apart from the brain. The task of examining the relationship between brain and behavior, while no less compelling than in the past, has recently reached a point of extreme interest with the establishment of a new specialty called NEUROSCIENCE. Today neuroscientists are rapidly gaining a better understanding of how mental experiences and cognitive functions arise from physical processes in the brain.

Until quite recently, the prospect of examining the relationship between neurophysiological and psychological variables seemed unattainable because of the baffling complexity of the various brain signals, and the technical problems in neurobiological signal analysis. The advent of versatile computers for collecting evoked brain potentials associated with complex perceptual processes have provided the most exciting data on the relationship between brain and behavior in man.

For more than a decade, a number of investigators have demonstrated that specific components of the evoked brain potential are more related to the psychological demands of the situation than to the presentation of the evoking stimulus. It is now generally accepted that there exist basic neural processes which are intimately related to important cognitive processes.

This conference was organized to provide the most recent information on evoked brain potentials and behavior. The delineation

of coding of functional information by neuroelectric processes in
the brain is quite essential to an understanding of the ways in
which the human organism undergoes change with experience.  This
neuroelectric coding of sensory information is generally well reflected in the evoked potential.  If there is an attribute unique
to man, it is his capacity for conceptual processing which provides
a complex framework for classifying stimuli.  Because man has an
available conceptual classification system for stimuli and symbols
he is able to process information about the environment quite rapidly.  The advantage of more efficient processing of information is
that the organism can respond more readily and appropriately to the
environment.

The book has been divided in four sections to reflect the general topics addressed at the conference.  The papers in section I of
the book reflect the efforts of some investigators to study the
neural representation of stimulus meaning.  Papers in section II and
III represent the attempts of some investigators to utilize evoked
potential techniques for the delineation of various central nervous
system disorders and psychopathological processes.  Papers in section
IV were solicited by the editor in an attempt to illustrate some new
approaches to data analysis.  The first three sections consist of
groups of three data papers dealing with a specific topic, followed
by a discussion of those papers.

In general the papers reflect the growing interest in studying
the relationship between brain and behavior.  If we are to defeat the
psychological ills which so uniquely plague man, if we are to have an
approximate environment for man we must know more about man's psychobiological characteristics and requirements.

# Contents

Section II

BRAIN DYSFUNCTION AND EVOKED POTENTIALS

Section III

PSYCHOPATHOLOGY AND EVOKED POTENTIALS

Section IV

DATA ANALYSIS

Section I

# STIMULUS MEANING AND EVOKED POTENTIALS

# STIMULI WITH BIOLOGICAL SIGNIFICANCE

Victor S. Johnston

Department of Engineering Psychology

New Mexico State University

Life lives on negative entropy (6). It is only by the exploitation of the spatial and temporal orderliness in their environment that organisms can survive in a world governed by the Second Law of Thermodynamics. Lorenz (6) has eloquently stated that [a living system] "very much like a prairie fire greedily gathers energy and, in a positive feedback cycle, becomes able to gather more energy, and to do so the quicker, the more it has already acquired." Thus, the biological luxury of animal life can only exist at the expense of those heterotrophs who, until recently, were the only life forms to make efficient use of the virtually limitless and distributed energy source supplied by the sun.

The evolution and survival of the human brain attests to the effectiveness of its design. It is organized to seek out and store the temporal relationships between events and use this knowledge to enhance its energy acquiring capacity and maintain its own intricate complexity. Knowledge, in this context, refers to biologically significant information. The human brain acquires knowledge by storing the probabilistic temporal relationship between events (information) relevant to its survival (utility).

In recent years, technological advances have provided experimenters with a small window for examining the workings of a brain actively acquiring knowledge. This methodology, the recording of event locked potentials, has allowed a systematic investigation of the effects of information and utility on the bioelectric response of the human brain. The new insights, gleaned by this approach, suggest mechanisms whereby the neural tissue stores knowledge, as well as providing a tool for detecting abnormal brain functioning.

## INFORMATION AND THE STIMULUS LOCKED POTENTIAL

In the parlance of information theory, uncertainty refers to the degree of randomness or entropy in a set of events. It is a numerical quantity, measured in binary digits (BITS), and unrelated to the nature, significance or meaning of these events to an observer. The uncertainty in a set of independent events is related to the probability of occurrence of the individual elements included within that set, and its calculation is dependent upon the following assumptions concerning the probability distribution of the elements:

(a)   $0 \leq P(X) \leq 1$

(b)   $\Sigma \, P(Xi) = 1$

(c)   $P(X_1 \cup X_2 \cup \ldots X_n) = P(X_1) + P(X_2) \ldots + P(X_n)$.

When these assumptions are valid, then the individual uncertainty about the occurrence of one specific event $(X_1)$ within the set is equal to the logarithm, to the base 2, of the reciprocal of the probability of occurrence of that event.

(d)   $H(X_1) = -\log_2 P(X_1)$

(e)   $H(X_1/X_1) = -\log_2 (1) = 0$

When event $X_1$ occurs, its probability of occurrence is one, and the uncertainty is now zero (e). This reduction in uncertainty is a measure of the amount of information transmitted by event $X_1$.

Consider an observer who is predicting the outcome of a series of coin tosses. Since the probability of a head is equal to the probability of a tail, then one bit of information is transmitted by each event (equation d). However, a human observer does not treat each coin toss as an individual event, and, after four consecutive heads, he may express a high subjective probability in the occurrence of a tail on the next toss. The observer is treating the coin tosses as an nth order Markov process in which individual events are dependent upon prior events. In the absence of a precise understanding of the process by which the subjective probability distribution is formulated, we can still arrange to measure the amount of information transmitted by requiring the observer to express his subjective probabilities so that the assumptions of the probability distribution (equation a, b and c) are not violated. By predicting a tail, he is stating that his subjective probability concerning the occurrence of a tail is $> 0.5$ and his subjective probability concerning the occurrence of a head is $< 0.5$. Using these subjective probabilities in equation d, we can see that disconfirmation transmits more information than confirmation under these conditions.

The relationship between uncertainty reduction and late components of cerebral evoked potentials was first noted by Sutton (13). These studies revealed that a late positive component of stimulus locked potentials ($P_3$) was related both to the time and amount of uncertainty reduction. A large $P_3$ component was observed following the presentation of a low probability stimulus compared with the magnitude of this component elicited by a stimulus with a high probability of occurrence. Sutton further demonstrated that this late positive wave was independent of the nature, or even the occurrence (14) of a physical energy change in the environment, and that disconfirming events produced larger $P_3$ waves than confirming events even when the probabilities of these outcomes were equal. These experiments, indicating the endogenous nature and stimulus independence of the $P_3$ wave, together with its observed relationship to the magnitude and time of uncertainty reduction, suggest that this component of the stimulus locked potential reflects the amount of subjective information transmitted by an event.

In signal detection tasks, the final uncertainty after an event has occurred is not always zero. If the $P_3$ component reflects the subjective information transmitted by a stimulus then, given that the initial uncertainty is constant, the $P_3$ amplitude should decrease with increasing final uncertainty in the occurrence of that stimulus. Using a confidence rating as a measure of final uncertainty, Squires et al demonstrated this relationship using threshold stimuli (10). For both "hits" and "false alarms," these experiments revealed that $P_3$ amplitude decreased as subjects became less confident in their detection. In the same study, however, these authors reported larger $P_3$ components following superthreshold stimuli on "hit" trials than on "correct rejection" trials, despite "the similar frequencies of occurrence and percentage correct of the two types of decisions." According to the information theory analysis, the $P_3$ amplitude should be constant for "hits" and "correct rejections" when the frequency of stimulus presentation and omission are equal. It should be noted, however, that an examination of the relationship between "hits" and "correct rejections" involves comparing evoked responses to different physical events. The stimulus was presented on "hit" trials, but not on the "correct rejection" trials. Although Sutton has previously demonstated the independence of $P_3$ on the nature of physical energy occurrence, $P_3$ amplitude has not been shown to be unaffected by the presence or absence of a stimulus event. Indeed, an examination of the evoked waveform in the Squires study reveals that $P_3$ on "hit" trials is an inflection on the negative slope following $P_2$. Since $P_2$ is large following stimulus presentation, a baseline to peak measure of $P_3$ would be dependent upon the amplitude of $P_2$. In the absence of a Principal Components Analysis (1), which would allow

$P_3$ magnitude to be measured independent from $P_2$, the observed
result is open to alternative explanations.

An alternative hypothesis relating the magnitude of the $P_3$
component to outcome probability has been presented by Teuting
et al (15). These authors have demonstrated that when the sequential
probabilities between two equiprobable events are manipulated, then
$P_3$ appears to be a fuction of the outcome probability rather than
the sequential objective stimulus probability. However, from the
viewpoint of the uncertainty reduction hypothesis, it is necessary
to allow the subject to assert the subjective probability in his
prediction from trial to trial in order to determine the magnitude
of the uncertainty reduction to be correlated with $P_3$ amplitude.
The simplifying assumption that the predicted event reflects the
stimulus with the highest subjective probability is not always valid.
For example, a subject may predict a stimulus with a low subjective
probability if a large payoff is associated with confirmation of this
prediction. In order to evaluate the uncertainty reduction hypothesis,
it is necessary to record the prediction and allow the subject to
express his subjective probability in the occurrence of the predicted
event. In the Tueting et al study, it is probable that the high risk
guesses would be accompanied by low subjective probability estimates.
If this is the case, then the observed relationships could be incor-
porated within the framework of the information hypothesis. The
alternative outcome probability hypothesis presented by Tueting et al
fails to predict the large $P_3$ to disconfirmation noted by Sutton (13)
when the outcomes were equiprobable, and does not account for data
obtained using threshold level stimuli where $P_3$ amplitude "is mainly
a function of decision confidence, with outcome probability per se
playing little or no role, at least over a range of values. (10)"

Recently, Squires et al (11) have made a first attempt to define
the variables responsible for the fluctuation in subjective probability
from trial to trial. These authors have concluded that the "subject
forms a local subjective probability distribution that reflects event
frequency within a 'sliding' window." It appears that subjective
probability may be a function of the nature and sequence of as many as
four events in the prior stimulus sequence as well as the global
probabilities of those events. Hopefully, future research will clarify
these relationships and negate the necessity for obtaining subjective
probability estimates from the experimental subjects on a trial to
trial basis.

## UTILITY AND STIMULUS LOCKED POTENTIALS

Several authors (2, 12) have noted that "task relevance" is
a major variable determining the amplitude of the $P_3$ component of
cerebral evoked responses. As yet, there have been no attempts
to systematically manipulate this variable. It is the author's
position that stimulus utility may be a more appropriate description

of the psychological dimension involved in these studies. Utility may be modified, for an observer, by asserting that a stimulus has significance in the performance of a behavioral task. It is difficult, however, to manipulate the degree of task relevance, so a more appropriate procedure may be to use stimuli with well established, stable and quantifiable utilities, such as money.

## AN EXPERIMENTAL APPROACH

The following experiment was designed to investigate the effects of systematic variations in the quantity and quality (utility) of information on stimulus locked potentials, particularly the $P_3$ component. At this time, nine subjects have participated in this experiment which was advertized as a prediction task in which up to one hundred dollars could be won or lost! Subjects were informed that their task was to predict whether a high frequency or a low frequency tone would occur as these stimuli were presented in a "complex sequence." A total of 960 such predictions were involved in an experimental session. Seated in the experimental room, a subject registered his prediction, and his uncertainty in that prediction, by pressing one of five response buttons. A high certainty and a low certainty button were available for each prediction (high or low tone) and the fifth button corresponded to a no prediction option. Following any prediction response, a bet was displayed on a small viewing screen in front of the subject. The value of the bet could be 0¢, 20¢ or $2, selected at random on each trial. The subject was aware of the random nature of the bet selection. After a one second delay, a high tone or a low tone was presented, and the subject won or lost the bet according to his prediction. In the event of no prediction by the subject, the bet could be neither won nor lost. By employing a pseudo-random sequence for stimulus presentation and bet selection, the experimenters arranged for the probability of confirmation to be equal to the probability of disconfirmation following any prediction/utility combination. In this manner, after any prediction response by the subject, the experimenters could record evoked potentials to confirming or disconfirming events at all three utility levels, under conditions of equal outcome probabilities for confirmation and disconfirmation. At the end of the experiment, the subject was allowed to select any sequential block of one hundred trials on which to compute his wins and losses.

A PDP8/e computer controlled all the experimental contingencies, and collected the behavioral and electrophysiological data. On each trial, vertex evoked potentials, digitized at a rate of one point every six milliseconds, was collected during the 768 milliseconds immediately following the presentation of the high or low tone. Eye movements and blinks were also collected using vertical EOG electrodes, and evoked potentials were "tagged" if

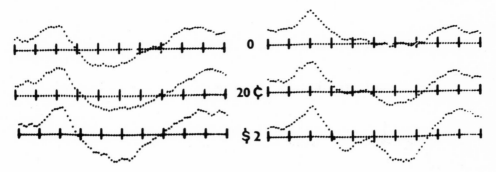

Figure 1.   Average Evoked Potentials for one subject showing the
            effects of Confirmation (left) and Disconfirmation (right)
            at three different bet levels.  All averages are equated
            for the nature of the eliciting stimulus and the outcome
            probability.  Negativity at the active electrode is an
            upward deflection, and the time marker indicates 50 milli-
            second epochs.

any EOG activity was detected during the collection period.  The
digitized waveforms, together with behavioral data indicating the
subject's prediction, the bet level, the outcome, and the EOG
tag were stored on magnetic tape during the intertrial interval.

    An examination of the behavioral data indicated that several
subjects had not made sufficient responses within one or more
of the response categories to ensure reliable data points under
these conditions.  In the following analysis therefore, only
high tone and low tone predictions will be considered and no
attempt will be made to distinguish between confidence levels.
The data from each subject was further examined to test the
hypothesis that the probability of confirmation was not significantly different from the probability of disconfirmation.  A
$Chi^2$ test revealed that there was no significant difference
between the probabilities of these outcomes at any level of
utility, in any subject ($\alpha = 0.05$).

    A computer program sorted the waveforms collected from each
subject and computed the average waveforms obtained under twelve
different conditions.  Only records collected in the absence
of eye movements or eye blinks were included in these averages.
The twelve conditions corresponded to confirmation and disconfirmation at each of the three bet levels when the presented stimulus
was a high tone or a low tone.  Fig. 1. shows the waveforms
recorded from one subject.  The high and low tone data has been
combined, so that the records in Fig. 1 represent average waveforms

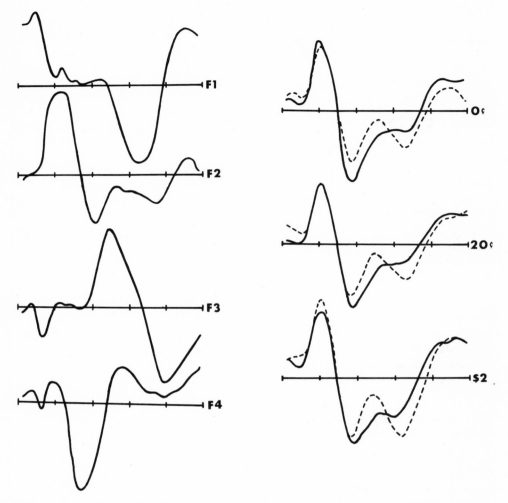

Figure 2.    Averaged Evoked Potentials (right) and Factor Loadings
            (left) for all experimental subjects.  Both Confirmed
            (———) and Disconfirmed (---) waveforms are shown at
            each bet level.  The time marker indicates 100
            millisecond epochs.

collected under equiprobable outcomes and stimulus conditions.  A
$P_3$ component is clearly present in all disconfirmed waveforms and
appears to increase in amplitude as a function of utility.   To
quantify these differences, and define the confirmation-disconfirmation effects,  the fifty-four waveforms collected from all of the

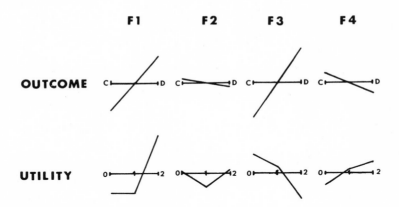

Figure 3.   Mean Factor Scores for all four factors as a function
            of Outcome and Utility. C-Confirmation; D-Disconfirma-
            tion; 0-0¢ Bet; 1-20¢ Bet; 2-$2 Bet.

experimental subjects were analyzed by a Principal Components Analysis and Varimax Rotation (1).   Each waveform used in this procedure
consisted of a 480 millisecond epoch reduced to forty digitized
values, which were corrected to a zero mean.

     Four factors accounted for 82% of the variance in the data.
The factor loadings, showing when each rotated factor was most
active, are plotted in Fig. 2.   The average evoked potentials,
averaged across all subjects under the six experimental conditions,
are also plotted for comparison.   There appears to be a close
correspondence between the time of maximum activity of the factors
and the components of the average evoked potentials.   The first
factor is active at the time of the $P_3$ component of the average
evoked response.   Factor 2 is most active during the $N_1$ component;
factor 4 corresponds to the $P_2$ component in the average waveforms.
Factor 3 is biphasic in nature with maximum and minimum activity
in the $N_2$ and 'late $P_3$' regions in the evoked response.   The factor
loadings of these factors also bear a close resemblance to factors
2, 3, 4 and 6 described by Squires et al (12).

     Factor scores were evaluated for each of the factors for each
of the fifty-four waveforms to determine if any factor was differentially loaded as a function of the independent variables.   This
data is summarized in Fig. 3.   The reliability of these effects was

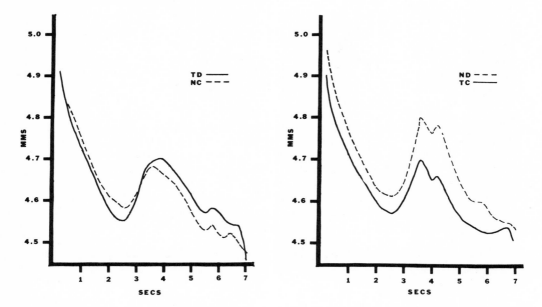

Figure 4.   Mean Pupillary Dilation (in mms) when a tone (right) or
            the absence of a tone (left) confirms or disconfirms a
            subjects' prediction.   The confirming or disconfirming
            event occurs 3 seconds after the prediction and pupillary
            dilation is measured from the minimum pre-stimulus peak
            to the maximum post-stimulus peak.   TD-Tone Predicted,
            Disconfirmed; NC-No Tone Predicted, Confirmed; ND-No
            Tone Predicted, Disconfirmed; TC-Tone Predicted, Confirmed.


evaluated by independent ANOVAs of the factor scores of each of
the factors.

Only $F_1$ and $F_3$ were sensitive to changes in information or
utility.   Factor 1 showed a significant increase in factor scores
( p <.01) in disconfirmed compared with confirmed waveforms.
Increasing utility from zero to two dollars also resulted in a
significant increase in $F_1$ scores (p <.05).   The interaction was
not significant.   Factor 3 was only sensitive to changes in information.   The factor scores for disconfirmed waveforms were significantly larger than confirmed ( p <.01) for this factor.   Again,
the interaction was not significant.

Neither $F_2$ nor $F_4$ varied as a function of the independent
variables in this experiment.   It was observed, however, that
$F_2$ scores discriminated between the subjects in the experiment.

That is, if a subject had a positive (or negative) $F_3$ factor score under one experimental condition, then there was a high probability ($p = .78$) that this subject would have positive (or negative) factor scores under the other five experimental conditions. There is no obvious psychological dimension (e.g. sex or task performance) which would indicate the nature of the individual differences which are reflected in $F_2$ scores.

The results of this experiment indicate that increases in the information or utility of a stimulus results in high $F_1$ scores. Since $F_1$ is most active in the $P_3$ region of the average evoked response, increases in information or utility produce large $P_3$ components in stimulus locked waveforms. This result supports the earlier report by Squires et al (12) who found a similar factor sensitive to changes in signal probability and task relevance. The current results also suggest that the $N_2$ component of the average evoked response may increase in amplitude with increases in information. This region of the waveform does appear to be affected by changes in utility.

## AROUSAL AND THE $P_3$ COMPONENT

The above experiment shows that $P_3$ amplitude is correlated with increases in information and utility. The significance of these findings is not clear at this time but several lines of evidence suggest that $P_3$ is a cerebral correlate of the orienting response. Perhaps the most direct evidence has been provided by Friedman et al (3), who examined the relationship between $P_3$ amplitude and subsequent pupil dilation. These investigators revealed that "$P_3$ amplitude and pupillary dilation are inverse monotonic functions of stimulus probability." We have conducted a parial replication of the Friedman et al study in our laboratory (4). In our investigation, two stimulus events a tone, and the absence of a tone were equiprobable. The subject was required to predict which event would occur on the next trial and three seconds later, as indicated by a sweeping clock, the tone would or would not occur. A Whittaker Corporation Series 1000 TV Pupillometer interfaced with a PDP 8/e computer monitored the pupil response for a 7-second period following the prediction. The experimental results are summarized in Fig. 4. It was found that the average pupil dilation following disconfirmation was significantly larger than the dilation following confirmation under both the stimulus present and stimulus absent conditions ($p < .005$, Wilcoxon). This experiment indicates that pupil dilation, like $P_3$, is elicited in the absence of a physical energy change in the environment and is time locked to the time of uncertainty reduction.

It has also been observed that both novel (high information) and reinforcing (high utility) stimuli produce surface negative steady potential shifts (8) and prolonged desynchrony of the EEG (9). Thus a close correlation exists between those events which enhance the $P_3$ component of the average evoked response and those events which produce a generalized arousal response. If $P_3$ is indeed a central correlate of the arousal response, it is the earliest physiological index of arousal that has been detected and may reflect a cognitive evaluation of the stimulus (7) leading to a generalized cortical arousal. Such an arousal, perhaps mediated by a partial depolarization of cortical neurons via the reticular activating system, would result in a prolongation of any cortical mode of oscillation in the neural tissue. This prolonged cortical activity is evidenced by the desynchrony following novel or reinforcing events. John (5) has proposed a mechanism whereby such prolonged modes of oscillation could initiate protein synthesis within the active neural circuits. In this manner, when a stimulus (or response), with no significance to the organism, is followed in close temporal contiguity by a novel or reinforcing event, then this conjoint mode of oscillation could become consolidated and the temporal relationship between these events permanently stored in the structure of neural networks. Knowledge has been gained, and a stimulus with no utility to the organism has now become a stimulus with biological significance.

## REFERENCES

1.  Donchin, E. A multivariate approach to the analysis of average evoked potentials. lEEE Transactions in Biomedical Engineering, 1966, 13, 131–139.

2.  Donchin, E., and Cohen, L. Average evoked potentials and intramodality selective attention. Electroencephalography and Clinical Neurophysiology, 1967, 19, 325–335.

3.  Friedman, D., Hakaren G., Sutton, S., and Fleiss, J.L. Effects of Stimulus Uncertainty on the Pupillary Dilation Response and the Vertex Evoked Potential. Electroencephalography and Clinical Neurophysiology, 1973, 34, 475–484.

4.  Haughney, G.V. Pupillary Responses as a Function of Prediction and Outcome. Unpublished Masters Thesis, New Mexico State University, September, 1975.

5.  John, E.R. Mechanisms of Memory. Academic Press, New York and London, 1967.

6.  Lorenz, K. Life as a Knowledge Process. In K.H. Pribram (Ed) On the Biology of Learning. Harcourt, Brace and World, Inc. New York: 1969.

7.  Ritter, W. and Vaughan, H.G.  Average Evoked Responses in
        Vigilance and Discrimination:  A Reassessment.  Science
        1969, 164, 326-328.

8.  Rowland, V.  Steady-Potential Phenomena of Cortex.  In Quarton,
        G.C., Melnechuk, T. and Schmitt, F.O. (Eds) The
        Neurosciences; a Study Program.  The Rockefeller University
        Press, New York:  1967.

9.  Sokolov, E.N.  Perception and the Conditioned Reflex.  Pergamon
        Press, New York: 1963.

10. Squires, K.C., Squires, N.K. and Hillyard, S.A.  Decision
        Related Cortical Potentials during an Auditory Signal
        Detection Task with Cued Observation Intervals.  Journal
        of Experimental Psychology:  Human Perception and
        Performance.  1975, 1(3), 268-279.

11. Squires, K.D., Wickens, C., Squires, N.K. and Donchin, E.  The
        Effects of Stimulus Sequence on the Waveform of the
        Cortical Event-Related Potential, Science 1976, 193
        1142-1145.

12. Squires, K.C., Donchin, E., Herning, R.I. and McCarthy, G.
        On the influence of Task Relevance and Stimulus Probability
        on Event-Related-Potential Components.  Electroencephalo-
        graphy and Clinical Neurophysiology, 1977, 42, 1-14.

13. Sutton, S., Braren, M., Zubin, J. and John, E.R. Evoked-Potential
        Correlates of Stimulus Uncertainty.  Science, 1965, 150,
        1187-1188.

14. Sutton, S., Tueting P., Zubin, J. and John, E.R.  Information
        Delivery and the Sensory Evoked Potential.  Sciences, 1967,
        155, 1436-1439.

15. Tueting, P., Sutton, S. and Zubin, J.  Quantitiative Evoked
        Potential Correlates of the Probability of Events.
        Psychophysiology, 1971, 7(3),  385-394.

# EVENT-RELATED BRAIN POTENTIALS:

# A TOOL IN THE STUDY OF HUMAN INFORMATION PROCESSING[1]

Emanuel Donchin

Cognitive Psychophysiology Laboratory
Department of Psychology, University of Illinois
Champaign, Illinois  61820

## INTRODUCTION

A cognitive psychologist of note who is not particularly impressed with event-related potentials (ERPs) commented recently, while reviewing a grant application, that studies of the behavioral correlates of ERPs can be described as studies in which "phenomena are in search of a theory." The intent was pejorative, but I found the statement complimentary. I was especially pleased because several years ago in a review of one of my own proposals another referee suggested that in the field of ERPs "one sees a technique futilely searching for phenomena!" We have, it would seem, made good progress in the last decade if we have found phenomena and are now searching for a theory. A detailed review of this progress is presented by Callaway, Tueting, and Koslow (in press).

---

[1] Preparation of this report was supported by DARPA through contract #N00014-76-C-0002 with the office of Naval Research. This same contract supported all of the studies conducted at the Cognitive Psychophysiology Laboratory described in this report. The somewhat informal nature of this chapter is due to the fact that it was first presented as a "minicourse on ERPs" before the 1977 convention of the Society for Psychophysiological Research in Philadelphia.  I am grateful to Don Fowles, the Program Committee chairman, for giving me this assignment. Gregory Chesney's help in the preparation of this manuscript is gratefully acknowledged, as are the comments of Connie Duncan-Johnson and Gregory McCarthy.

This chapter reviews one facet of the progress in ERP research during the past decade. This will be a parochial presentation focusing on studies conducted at the Cognitive[2] Psychophysiology Laboratory at the University of Illinois. The small province of ERP research covered is concerned with the extent to which the ERP indexes "complex psychological processes," more fashionably referred to as "human information processing." (For a more comprehensive review of this literature see Donchin, Ritter, & McCallum, in press; Picton, Campbell, Baribeau-Braun, & Proulx, in press).

## THE BIOCYBERNETIC PROGRAM

It may be easier to understand our studies within the framework of the challenge to which we have been responding. This challenge was presented by the "Biocybernetic" project, sponsored by the Defense Advanced Research Projects Agency. This project is an attempt to develop a psychophysiological communication link between humans and computers as they interact in systems in which a person and a computer are jointly assigned a task (often called "man-machine" systems). The success of such a joint effort depends on the appropriate distribution of responsibilities between its components and on the ability of the components to communicate.

The relation between man and machine in a system such as the automobile is generally fixed at design time and remains constant over the life of the system. More advanced systems are often "adaptive." That is, the operating characteristics of the system can be modified as circumstances change. An adaptive controller, to determine the distribution of labor between man and machine, often needs data on the state of the operator. There is, however, a gross asymmetry in the flow of data between man and the machine. The data stream flowing from computer to man is vast--virtually unlimited. Any number of display devices, dials, annunciators,

---

[2] The research program described in this chapter owes whatever success it has to the efforts of numerous collaborators. Professors C. Wickens and D. Gopher have been instrumental in guarding our Experimental Psychology flank. Drs. Nancy and Ken Squires contributed much during their stint as research associates in the lab. And, of course, nothing would have happened without the graduate students, whose roster included, at one time or another, Greg Chesney, Connie Duncan-Johnson, Earle Heffley, Ron Herning, Dick Horst, Jack Isreal, Skip Johnson, Marta Kutas, Greg McCarthy, and Moshe Yuchtman.

and such can be attached, at a price, to a computer. On the other hand the human's assortment of means for communicating with a machine is limited. In general, some overt skeletal movement must be executed. Operators push buttons, twiddle dials, or control joy sticks. Even communication in a natural language, or in a computer language generally requires the use of the collection of push buttons known as a keyboard.

The operator is particularly weak in communicating such crucial details as the specific manner in which he[3] allocates attention to tasks, the amount of his spare capacity, the degree to which he comprehends the instructions or the priority structure which he imposes on his tasks. Furthermore, the adaptive algorithms built into man-machine systems often assume knowledge of the probabilities and utilities which an operator maps on the environment (Sheridan & Ferrell, 1974). These are often poorly estimated (Becker & McClintock, 1967). Moreover, even if the operator can provide this information, having to provide it, on demand, might prove disruptive to his appointed tasks. The biocybernetic program addresses this problem by adding a data channel to the system. It assumes that a channel carrying psychophysiological data, acquired from an operator during task performance, can supply the adaptive controller with at least part of the required information. The program thus assumes that mental activities manifest themselves in a variety of physiological signals. It further assumes that it is possible to make strong inferences about mental activity from such signals.

## DIFFICULTIES AND SPECIAL REQUIREMENTS OF BIOCYBERNETICS

Unfortunately, the task is far from trivial. To serve as a biocybernetic channel the signals must satisfy several requirements. It is necessary that there be a well-defined vocabulary of physiological signals; that is, there must be a unique, reliable relationship between some physiological signal and specific aspects of mental activity. The messages conveyed over the channel must not be ambiguous. Furthermore, the messages must be capable of flowing in real time. A man-machine system cannot await the computation of signal averages to make its adaptive decisions. The vocabulary utilized by this biocybernetic channel must be comprehensible on-the-fly, as the human performs his tasks. Finally, one cannot claim success without demonstrating that the channel is, in fact, useable. Knowing that

---

[3] The words "he" and "his" are used in this paper in place of "he or she" and "his or her."

Chinese has a rather rich vocabulary is of no use to  someone  who does  not  speak  the language and who needs to communicate with a monolingual Chinese. Similarly, if the  computer  cannot  utilize the  biocybernetic  data,  the  data might as well not exist. The implication here is that information must be  about  things  which are in fact useful to the system. It would be particularly useful if the data do not duplicate  that  which  can  be  obtained  more easily, or more cheaply, by more traditional means. So, the order is for a well-defined vocabulary of  electrophysiological  signals that  provides,  in  real  time,  useful  and unique data about an operator's mental life. A tall order indeed.

In 1972 my associates and I  undertook  to  develop  such  a channel using the human ERP,[4] and in  particular  ERP  components, often  called  "endogenous,"  such  as the P300, or the contingent negative variation (CNV) (see Donchin et al., in press). In 1972, this  appeared  a  possible,  if unlikely, venture, as will appear from a review of the early history of ERP research.

## HISTORICAL REVIEW

The key to the study of the human ERP has  been  the  signal averager.  A  very  early version was described by Francis Galton (1878)  and  is  shown  in  Fig. 1.  Galton's  paper,  entitled "Composite  Portraits,"  was  the  forerunner of what seems to have been a fairly flourishing research endeavor in the last decade  of the  nineteenth  century  (Pearson, 1924). Galton wanted to study the correlation between physiognomy and character as  well  as  to develop  a  better  method for characterizing faces. His idea was simple. Assume, reasoned Galton, that there is a "criminal"  type with  characteristic  facial  features. Then all criminals should look alike and one could recognize a criminal with a glance. This clearly  is  not  the  case.  Perhaps  criminals' faces represent random deviations from a basic type.  To  identify  the  criminal face,  Galton  superimposed photographically a series of faces all belonging to known criminals. In the emerging composite face  the random  deviations  will cancel and the resultant "composite face" will be the "type" sought. The instrument shown  in  Fig. 1  did exactly  this.  It  allowed  Galton  to  photograph  on  the same negative eight different faces. The result is shown  in  Fig. 2.

---

[4] Ours was only one of several such efforts. While I review here the Illinois project,  other  studies  conducted  within  the framework of ARPA'S Biocybernetic program, especially by J. Vidal, C. Rebert, J. Beatty, and R. Champan, had  an  important  influence on our own program.

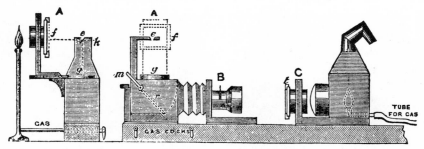

A  The body of the camera, which is fixed.
B  Lens on a carriage, which can be moved to and fro.
C  Frame for the transparency, on a carriage that also supports the lantern; the whole can be moved to and fro.
r  The reflector inside the camera.
m  The arm outside the camera attached to the axis of the reflector; by moving it, the reflector can be moved up or down.
g  A ground-glass screen on the roof, which receives the image when the reflector is turned down, as in the diagram.

e  The eye-hole through which the image is viewed on *g*; a thin piece of glass immediately below *e* reflects the illuminated fiducial lines in the transparency at *f*, and gives them the appearance of lying upon *g*—the distances *fk* and *gk* being made equal, the angle *fkg* being made a right angle, and the plane of the thin piece of glass being made to bisect *fkg*.
f  Framework, adjustable, holding the transparency with the fiducial lines on it.
t  Framework, adjustable, holding the transparency of the portrait.

Figure 1. Francis Galton's signal averager. This is an "advanced" version with which such composite faces, shown in Figure 2, were obtained. The original Galton averager consisted of a box camera mounted a fixed distance from a cross to which pictures of the faces were attached. (From Pearson, 1924)

Clearly, as Galton himself pointed out, the resulting composite face appears quite normal. As a typology, the technique failed. If it had any value it was in confirming that it is not possible to find the mind's construction in the face. While we are far removed from that particular blind alley, it does convey the central idea of signal averaging. Namely, that it is possible to extract, through numerical superimposition, or averaging, an estimate of a signal from instances in which a signal is mixed with random noise.[5]

That the ongoing EEG activity obscures specific responses to stimuli has, of course, been known, or assumed, since its discovery. Caton (1875) in his report to the British Medical Association describes a transient, evoked response, recorded from

---

[5] I am indebted to Douglas Medin for bringing this aspect of Galton's work to my attention.

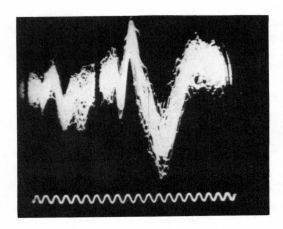

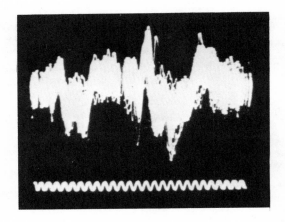

Figure 4. Evoked potentials obtained by Ciganek using the superimposition technique. Each of the traces is obtained by repeatedly photographing the face of an oscilloscope. This technique is reasonably effective for observing evoked potentials while the amplitude of the evoked potential relative to the ongoing EEG activity is large, as in the upper figure. Displays such as are presented in the bottom figure are more commonly obtained. (From Ciganek, 1964)

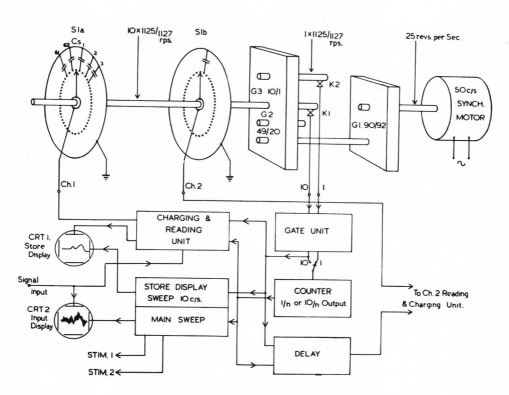

Figure 5.  An early Analog signal averager.  Averaging
is achieved by charging a bank of capacitors at Sla and
Slb.  (From Dawson, 1954)

His was an analog device, in which capacitors served to summate
the voltages. There were many other such devices, all ingenious,
but all bulky, and none of wide general use (Barlow, 1957; Dawson,
1951; Rosner, Allison, Swanson, & Goff, 1960). In 1959, Clynes
developed a digital signal averager, converting a device used in
nuclear physics to the Mnemotron Computer of Average Transients
(CAT) and the study of the ERP was launched (Clynes & Kohn, 1960).

## EVOKED POTENTIALS AND ATTENTION

I am concerned here only with those studies appearing soon
after Clynes' invention that dealt with the "relation between
evoked potentials and psychological processes." Many experiments
were reported, all sharing a similar design. Subjects were placed
in conditions in which "attention" was known to vary and the ERPs
were recorded; ERPs elicited by the same physical stimuli were
obtained while the subjects were "attending" or "not attending" to
the stimuli. Recall that in the 1950s and the 1960s attention was
a concept shunned by psychologists. For example, when revising
Woodworth's 1938 volume on experimental psychology, Woodworth and
Schlosberg (1954) eliminated the chapter on attention. To the
extent that attention was discussed it was viewed as a process
that modulates the excitability of cortical tissue (Lindsley,
1951). In this vein, stimuli attended-to were supposed to produce
large ERPs, reflecting increased cortical excitability, perhaps
modulated by the reticular activating system. This view was
consistent with the then-celebrated study of Hernandez-Peon,
Scherrer, and Jouvet (1956), which influenced much of the ERP work
conducted with humans in the early Sixties. In Fig. 6, for
example, are shown data published by Garcia-Austt and his
associates (Garcia-Austt, Vanzulli, Bogacz, & Rodriguez-Barrios,
1963). They were interested in the effects of habituation on
evoked-potential amplitude and, therefore, presented their
subjects with thousands of stimuli, evaluating the variation in
ERP amplitude over the stimulus series. They did observe changes
in ERP amplitude with "habituation," but these were small and hard
to interpret. Satterfield (1965) reported increases in the
amplitude of the evoked response with "attention."

Many of these early studies treated all stimuli presented
under the same instructional regime as if they were identical.
Thus, all ERPs elicited by stimuli to which the subject was
instructed to attend were averaged and this ERP was compared to
another averaged ERP obtained when the subject was told to ignore
the stimuli. But the subject's response may vary from trial to
trial. Identical stimuli presented under seemingly identical
conditions may well elicit different ERPs due to differences in
the subject's reaction to stimuli. It is important therefore to
obtain some behavioral measure of the subject's response to
stimuli. Averaging can then be guided by indices of the subject's
performance rather than by the experimenter's instructions.
Donchin and Lindsley (1966) used the subject's reaction time as an
index of the subject's attentiveness and sorted trials for
averaging according to the reaction time observed in the trial.
They demonstrated a negative correlation between reaction time and
the amplitude of the ERP; the faster the subject's response to a
stimulus, the larger the ERP elicited by the stimulus. These data

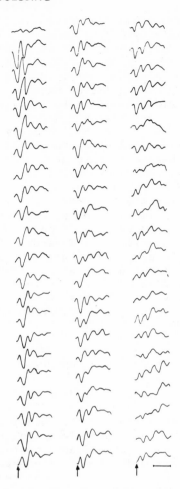

Figure 6. Average evoked potentials generated by a succession of stimuli. The waveforms show the fluctuations in the amplitude of the evoked response as the same stimuli are repeatedly presented to a subject. (From Garcia-Austt et al., 1963)

were interpreted as supporting the proposition that stimuli presented during heightened excitability elicit responses with shorter reaction times. Similar data were subsequently reported by Morrell and Morrell (1966) and others (Parasuraman & Davies, 1975; Picton, Hillyard, & Galambos, 1974; Ritter, Simson, & Vaughan, 1972).

An influential study was reported by Haider, Spong, and Lindsley (1964). Their subjects engaged in a vigilance task (Mackworth, 1950), and ERPs were elicited by the stimuli that the subjects were monitoring. Again, attention was indexed by the accuracy of the subject's performance. Haider et al. were able to demonstrate a negative correlation between the amplitude of the ERP and the number of signals missed by the subject. These (and similar) studies were notable because the behavioral and the electrophysiological data were recorded simultaneously. The results were suggestive and generated considerable interest and much research. The subsequent literature was, however, rather inconclusive. "Attention" was reported to cause increases in the amplitude of the ERP (Chapman & Bragdon, 1964; Debecker & Desmedt, 1966; Donchin & Lindsley, 1966; Ritter & Vaughan, 1969; Satterfield, 1965). Others reported no effects of attention on the ERP or decreases in ERP amplitude with attention (Hartley, 1970; Naatanen, 1967; Satterfield & Cheatum, 1964). It did not seem likely that a useful vocabulary of the ERPs would develop from so confused and tangled a literature. This indeed was very much the conventional wisdom during the late Sixties. Moray, for example, reflected the view of many when he stated that the psychophysiological studies have contributed very little to the study of attention (1969, pp. 158-179).

## THE STRUCTURE OF ERPs

The weakness of the early studies can be attributed, in part, to a tendency to treat the ERP as if it is a global representation of the state of cortical tissue. Many investigators felt it was sufficient to report the overall "amplitude" of the ERP as if it did not matter which particular feature of the wave was modulated by the experimental variables. Some even quantified the evoked response by measuring the length of the line traced by the ERP. It has proven, however, far more fruitful to consider the ERP a sequence of overlapping components, each possibly representing activity of different populations of nerve cells and each standing in different, often orthogonal, relations to experimental variables.

Fig. 7 provides a schematic view of the ERPs elicited by a click of moderate intensity. A series of voltage oscillations lasting at least 500 msec can be observed. In the first 10 msec of this epoch, seven wavelets can be seen (if thousands of trials are averaged). The provenance of these "bumps" is quite well established as the specific stations on the auditory pathway from the cochlea to the inferior colliculus. These waves are of value in clinical neurology (Jewett & Williston, 1971; Picton, Hillyard, Krausz, & Galambos, 1974).

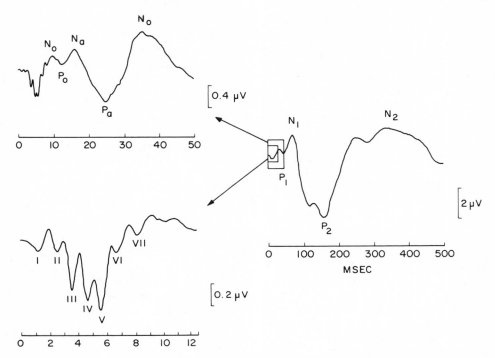

Figure 7. A schematic presentation of the configuration of the event-related potential elicited by a click of moderate intensity. Note the different time bases and different callibration signal in each of the three insets. Note also that different peak nomenclatures are used in the three cases and that component labellings for the data shown for the last 500 msec are different from those used in the rest of this chapter. (After Picton et al., 1974)

These "bumps" are followed by several components which can be observed over the first 50 msec following the click. Their origin is far less certain, though they have been attributed to thalamic activity; these components have found some use in audiometry (H. Davis, 1976). These early components are followed by a number of larger peaks and troughs. Almost invariably a negative peak appears about 100 msec after the click. It is followed by a positive peak at 160 msec. These are often called respectively N1 and P2 or, according to the convention used here, N100 and P160. The letter (N or P) indicates the polarity; the number, the modal latency of the peak (see Donchin, Callaway,

Cooper, Desmedt, Goff, Hillyard, & Sutton, 1977). These early components are obligatory responses to stimuli. By and large, if a subject is neither deaf nor dead, a click will elicit these early components. We refer to them as exogenous because they appear to be responses to external stimuli.

These are followed by a series of peaks and troughs which are not obligatory. Their amplitude depends on the psychological circumstances under which the stimuli were presented rather than on the physical nature of the stimulus. One can even record these late components in the absence of a stimulus (Klinke, Fruhstorfer, & Finkenzeller, 1968; Ruchkin & Sutton, 1973; Weinberg, Walter, & Crow, 1970). These "endogenous" components appear to represent activities invoked by the system rather than evoked by the stimuli.

The development of a lexicon of ERP components is contingent on the perception of the ERP as a sequence of overlapping components. Earlier attempts to develop a lexicon failed because instead of focusing on specific components and determining their relation to the underlying psychological activity, investigators homogenized the ERP, thereby losing sight of the crucial variables. Not until the mid- Sixties did it become clear that specific components of the ERP behave differently in response to "psychological" variables.

## THE P300 AND OTHER COMPONENTS

In 1963, in a symposium presented at a convention of the American Psychological Association in Los Angeles, Sutton and his collaborators reported that a component, which they called P3, appears in ERPs elicited by unpredictable stimuli that "reduce the subject's uncertainty" (Sutton, Tueting, Zubin, & John, 1965). A subsequent report, published in Science in 1967 and from which Fig. 8 is taken, has changed the field (Sutton, Tueting, Zubin, & John, 1967). Sutton and his co-workers were able to show that the waveform of ERPs elicited by identical physical stimuli varies as a function of the information conveyed by the stimulus. Another important aspect of Sutton's work was that the psychological variables were defined with some care. As noted above, too many studies that purported to study "attention" assumed that it is sufficient for the investigator to instruct the subject to "attend." As Sutton (1969) has aptly put it, the subjects can, and do, exercise their option to follow, or to ignore, the instructions. Their behavior must, therefore, be assessed. One must acquire specific measures of the subject's performance simultaneously with the electrophysiological measures. All assertions about the experimental conditions must be verified

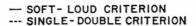

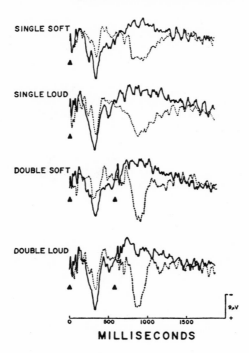

Figure 8. Event-related potentials elicited by single or paired tones which were either loud or soft. When a subject is categorizing tones by their intensity, only the first stimulus of a pair elicits a P300 component (solid lines). When the subject has to determine if one or two stimuli were presented on a given trial, both the presence of a second tone in the pair and the absence of a second tone following a single stimulus elicit a large P300 (dotted lines). These data provide strong evidence that P300 is an endogenous component which can be elicited in the absence of a physical stimulus. (From Sutton et al., 1967)

directly. The realization that this is so underlies, I think, much of the progress in ERP work in the last decade.

At that time Leon Cohen and I, at Stanford, were attempting to use ERPs in the study of binocular rivalry. We wanted to determine if stimuli presented to the "recessive" eye register an evoked response.  For this purpose, we asked subjects to monitor a binocular-rivalry display and indicate to us which eye was dominant and which recessive.  We also presented, at random, flashes to either eye.  Our intent was to study the response evoked by the flashes as a function of the eye's dominance.  To our chagrin, no ERPs were elicited by the stimuli.  The data we obtained are marked RIV in Fig. 9.  This was disconcerting because we knew that if you present a flash to a subject, it evokes a response.  To ascertain that the subject was seeing the flashes we instructed him to ignore the binocular rivalry target and to count the flashes.  When counted, the flashes generated large ERPs.  The major difference between the ERPs elicited by counted and uncounted stimuli was the appearance of a large positive component with a latency of about 250 msec, as can be seen in the ERPs marked FLASH in Fig. 9 (Donchin & Cohen, 1970).  We were replicating Sutton's result in a very different experimental

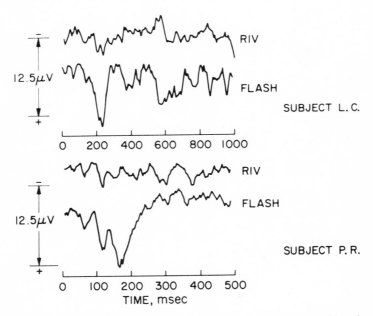

Figure 9.  Data from two subjects who were monitoring a binocular rivalry target.  The ERPs shown were elicited by brief flashes of light which were superimposed on the binocular rivalry target.  The ERPs marked <u>RIV</u> were recorded when the subject was monitoring the rivalry targets and indicating the dominant eye.  The ERPs marked <u>flash</u> were obtained when the subject was instructed to ignore the background rivalry targets and count light flashes.  (From Donchin and Cohen, 1970)

condition.  Again, a positive-going component appeared, or failed
to  appear,  depending on the task relevance of the data presented
to the subject.  This  incidental  observation  led  to  two  more
formal  studies  (Donchin & Cohen, 1967; Smith, Donchin, Cohen, &
Starr, 1970) both of which demonstrated that P300 is  elicited  by
task-relevant  stimuli.   Quite  early, then, it became clear that
the P300 depends upon some combination of  uncertainty  resolution
and task relevance.

        Yet another endogenous component was reported in  1964  when
Grey  Walter  and  his  associates  described the CNV.  Walter has
shown that a slow negative potential (see Fig. 10)  develops  over
the foreperiod of a reaction time (RT) trial, representing what he
chose at that time to call Expectancy (Walter,  Cooper,  Aldridge,
McCallum, & Winter, 1964).  Kornhuber and his associates  in  Ulm,
Germany,  were  the first to report that a similar event-preceding
negativity can be  seen  even  when  no  S1  is  presented.   They

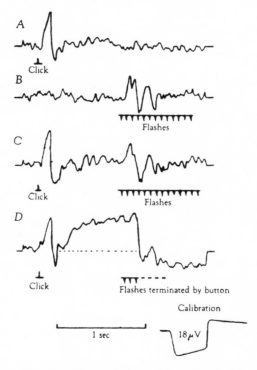

Figure  10.  The Contingent Negative Variation described
by  Grey  Walter  and  his  associates.   These  data
illustrate  the  dependence of the CNV on the assignment
of the task to the subject.  (From Grey Walter  et  al.,
1964)

described a series of movement-related potentials preceding and following a response (Kornhuber & Deecke, 1965); of particular interest to our discussion is a slow negative potential that begins as early as 800 msec prior to the movement and peaks just prior to the movement. This has been called the Readiness Potential (RP) by Kornhuber and his associates.

So, by the late Sixties, it was becoming clear that the ERP should not be viewed as a global index of the state of the brain, with "attention" a modulator of brain excitability. It appeared more useful to focus on specific relations between particular aspects of the waveform and their relationship to specific concomitants of mental activity. The question of interest is not "what is the 'state' of the brain," but rather "what are the specific information processing roles of the cell populations which are represented by the ERP?" It was this approach, I think, that enabled the development of an ERP lexicon. There remain, however, conceptual and methodological issues for discussion before proceeding to the ERP vocabulary.

## MANIFESTATIONS, NOT CORRELATES

Psychophysiology is often described as a search for the "physiological correlates of psychological processes." This view sometimes leads to a fallacy that takes the following form. A given psychophysiological measure is considered a "correlate" of some specific psychological process. This relation may be described by an assertion that response X (such as heart rate, galvanic skin response, or the amplitude of P300) is a correlate of process Y (such as attention, arousal or preparation). Attempts to validate such propositions require the demonstration of a correlation between a measure of response X and a measure of process Y. The processes are, of necessity, indexed by a measure of performance such as reaction time, or the number and type of errors committed by a subject. This is as it should be, but it is all too often forgotten that the behavioral measure is only an index of the internal process. Reaction time, for example, can be used as an index of attention, but reaction time is <u>not</u> attention (whatever attention is). Yet, the demand that a psychophysiological index be a correlate of a psychological process is all too often fallaciously translated into a demand that a correlation be demonstrated between the ERP component and some specific, arbitrarily chosen, overt index of behavior. When such a correlation is not found, investigators report with apparent glee a "dissociation" between the physiological and the psychological variable and conclude that "ERPs are full of sound

and fury, signifying nothing" (Clark, Butler, & Rosner, 1969;  see
also  subsequent  discussion  by  Clark,  Butler,  &  Rosner,  1970;
Donchin & Sutton, 1970; Paul & Sutton, 1973).

A typical case in point is the correlation between  the  CNV
and reaction time.  It is well established that within a series of
trials the amplitude of the CNV is only weakly related to reaction
time  (Hillyard,  1973; McCallum & Papakostopolous, 1973; Rebert &
Tecce, 1973; Tecce, 1972).  This can be viewed as disturbing,  for
if  the  CNV  is  an  index  of  preparation and the reaction time
depends on preparation, then a strong correlation between the  two
variables  can  be  expected.   But  this  expectation  implies  a
somewhat outdated model of human information  processing.   It  is
one I refer to in Fig. 11 as the S-R model.  The organism in  such
a model is considered to be essentially inert.  Stimuli activate a
sequence of information-processing stages,  modulated  perhaps  by
"arousal"  or  "attention,"  which  lead  to  an  overt  response.

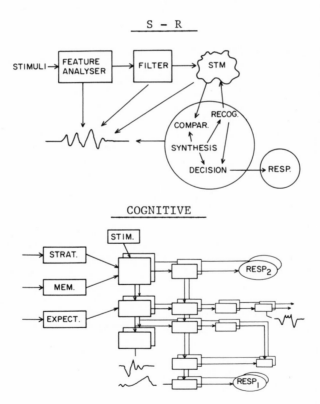

Figure  11.   Two conceptualizations of the events which
occur in an experimental trial.

Processing terminates when the overt response is emitted. Within
the context of such a model the ERP lexicon must specify the
stages of processing to which any given ERP component can be
associated. One assumes, given such a model, that all ERP
components that reflect information-processing activities on a
given trial must appear and terminate before the execution of the
response. Thus, the fact the subject can press a response lever
long before P300 is elicited suggests that there is no
relationship between P300 and information processing. Similarly,
the CNV must have its effect on response speed by modulating the
excitability of the brain during the foreperiod. If so, then a
large CNV must imply a fast reaction time. This view is not
consistent with the data I shall review below. The approach is
also inadequate on conceptual grounds. Consider, as an alternate,
the model labeled in Fig. 11 as "cognitive." In this view, the
subject brings into a trial expectancies, strategies, or plans.
He continues to process data delivered in the past. Memory is
being reordered. Old, unsolved problems are treated. Stimuli
presented on a trial impinge on this stream and invoke a variety
of parallel processes. Several of these processes might lead to
overt responses. Others will result in no overt response on the
specific trial, but will change a subject's strategies in ways
that will be manifested only on successive trials. Many
"processors" might be activated in parallel. If in the operation
of such a processor a population of neurons is synchronously
activated and this activity appears to scalp electrodes as a
voltage oscillation, an ERP component appears. The ERPs are
manifestations, at the scalp, of activities of cell populations.
Components of these potentials may be directly related to an overt
response. For example, movement-related potentials are associated
with an overt response. Other components might be related to
overt responses in a somewhat more complex way. For example,
Hillyard and his associates report that N100 changes in amplitude
with the direction of selective attention (Hillyard, Hink,
Schwent, & Picton, 1973; Schwent & Hillyard, 1975; Schwent,
Hillyard, & Galambos, 1976a, 1976b; Schwent, Snyder, & Hillyard,
1976). Other ERP components may be manifestations of cortical
processes which have no overt concomitant on any given trial, but
which strongly affect the subject's strategies. The important
point is that an ERP component is not a "correlate" of some
diffuse psychological state variable but is rather a
manifestation, at the scalp, of neural activity which plays a
certain role in the informational transactions of the brain. Our
task is to determine the functional role of the component rather
than to seek preconceived correlations between the component and
ill-defined psychological constructs. This is particularly true
for components that represent "strategic" information processing
(Donchin et al., in press). These are also the components of
interest for a biocybernetic channel because they index activities

that cannot be otherwise observed. I believe that this "cognitive" view is central to progress in the study of the ERP in humans.

## DEFINITION AND MEASUREMENT OF COMPONENTS

Now to a methodological digression. I have been discussing "components." The concept seems self-evident. Many investigators see a component in each peak or trough in the ERP which appears with some regularity at specific points in time. Thus, in order to study the components, we need to measure base-to-peak amplitudes or some other feature that characterizes the peaks and troughs, such as their area or magnitude. This, unfortunately, is not as simple as it sounds. The components tend to overlap. In particular, some slow components range over large parts of the epoch and tend to carry the shorter components. Consider, for example, Fig. 12. It shows ERPs recorded simultaneously at different electrode sites across the head in a rather complex experiment conducted by Heffley in our laboratory. The details are not important for this discussion. Assume that you wish to describe differences between the electrodes in the amplitude of the peak labeled A in Fig. 12. If you refer the amplitude to a "baseline" defined as the segment just preceding the first stimulus, the amplitudes will obviously be determined by the amplitude of negative potential preceding peak A. In other words,

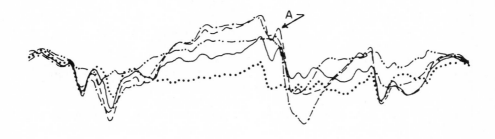

$F_{pz}$ ........
$F_z$ ————
$C_z$ — — — —
$P_z$ —.—.—.—
$O_z$ —..—..—

Figure 12. ERP waveforms obtained in a typical CNV experiment. These ERPs were recorded simultaneously from the electrode sites shown in the legend.

the baseline has changed and one cannot obtain a measure of peak A independent of the value of the baseline. Peak-to-peak amplitudes might be more apt in this case, but often the positive-going and the negative-going aspects of the wave are independently manipulated by experimental variables and the peak-to-peak measure might be misleading.

The problem of component overlap and the problem of baseline fluctuation make the definition, identification, and measurement of components somewhat problematic (see Donchin & Heffley, in press). I have preferred an approach that defines components in terms of the deviations of each ERP from the grand mean average of all the ERPs obtained in that experiment. Fig. 13 might clarify the concept. The line in the middle frame of Fig. 13 is the average of all the ERPs obtained at all electrode sites for all experimental conditions for all subjects in an experiment (McCarthy & Donchin, in press). Each ERP will deviate from this grand average. These deviations, in the usual logic of experimental analysis, can be attributed to the subject, to the experimental condition, to the electrode, and, of course, to random uncontrollable variation. Inspection of many of the ERPs obtained in this experiment (Fig. 13 bottom) reveals, of course, that there is variance between the waveforms. The analysis of the data is the process whereby we account for this variance. We would like to know how this variance is related to the different experimental variables, how much is accounted for by subject variables, how much by the experimental variables or by the electrodes. The variance can be partitioned not only across the experimental conditions but also along the epoch into different, orthogonal, components of variance. Each component can then be studied separately and its deviation from the grand mean partitioned among the sources of experimental variance. Principal component analysis (PCA) is a means for identifying orthogonal sources of variance, in which variance is referred to the grand mean waveform rather than to the mean value of the EEG in the epoch. The PCA provides measures for the orthogonal sources of variance. It is then possible to analyze the relationship between each of these components and the experimental variables using standard analyses of variance (Donchin, 1966, 1969).

A component is defined as an independent source of variance in the experiment. The analysis always proceeds in two phases. In the first phase, we analyze the variance using the PCA to identify the sources of variance. This yields a "loading plot" as shown in the top frame of Fig. 13. The display indicates that there are four or five components in this data set and that each of these happens to be active at a different segment of the epoch. The height of the loading curve represents the degree of association between the component and the data recorded over the

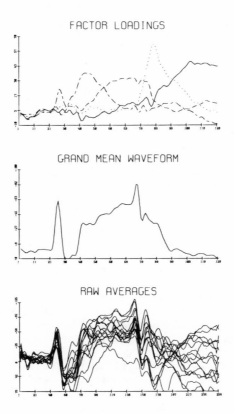

FACTOR LOADINGS

GRAND MEAN WAVEFORM

RAW AVERAGES

Figure 13. In the center graph is shown the grand
average ERP computed on the basis of the data obtained
from all subjects in all experimental conditions from
all electrodes in an experiment (McCarthy & Donchin, in
press). In the bottom panel, we superimposed some of
the ERPs obtained for a specific experimental condition
in this same experiment. Clearly, most of the ERPs
deviate from the grand mean waveform. There are
different degrees of variance at different segments of
the epoch. The PCA is a technique for determining the
extent to which the grand mean can be partitioned into
components. As the top panel shows, PCA of these data
identified five components. The segment of the epoch
over which each component is active is indicated by the
magnitude of the factor loading. (After McCarthy &
Donchin, in press)

epoch. For each of the components we compute a "component score" that measures the magnitude of the component in any given ERP. It is these component scores that are related to the experimental variables. The analysis of the component scores permits statements about the magnitude of components and the extent to which the magnitudes are significantly affected by the electrodes. This procedure clarifies the data analysis. It also allows rapid handling of massive data bases. (For a detailed review, and some caveats, see Donchin & Heffley, in press.)

So, our experimental plan in elucidating the ERP vocabulary is to conduct experiments in which aspects of human information processing are systematically manipulated so that the number of independent components can be identified and their functional significance outlined. A weak analogy to this process is presented in Fig. 14. Classical psychophysiological technique (if we accept the definition of psychophysiology as an endeavor in which behavioral variables are manipulated and physiological variables recorded) is analogous to the mapping of receptive fields of individual neurons in the sensory systems. The single-unit investigator begins with a neural element, a single neuron to be exact, whose electrical activity is monitored. Visual space is systematically sampled until that subset of visual space which affects the response of the element is identified. One does that by varying stimuli systematically, "listening" for increases or decreases in the activity of the neuron.

The general class of stimuli is first identified in a rather gross manner. One then continues with finer and finer manipulations of stimulus dimensions until the exact definition of the stimulus set which causes the response to occur is determined. That, then, is considered the receptive field of the neuron.

Analogously (rather weakly analogously), this is what we do when we try to determine the meaning of an ERP component. Here, again, we have neural elements. Not one, but a multitude. They happen to have a property of being simultaneously activated at certain critical points in the information-processing activity of the cortex. We try to map the receptive field of this cell population, in what may be called "cognitive space." This, of course, is a rather nebulous concept, and not as well defined as visual space. Cognitive space consists inter alia of the decisions, expectations, plans, strategies, associations, and memories that we can manipulate in the experimental psychology laboratory. We engage in systematic exploration of this space while observing the behavior of the ERP component. We try to identify the subset of cognitive space which modulates the

A WEAK ANALOGY
RECEPTIVE FIELD MAPPING

Visual Space

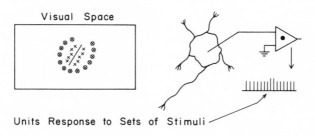

Units Response to Sets of Stimuli

Goal : Delineate the Subset of Space
and Map its Characteristics on the Response.

Cognitive Space

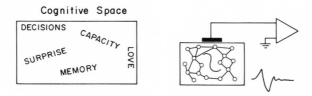

Figure 14.  The study of event-related potentials can be
viewed as a mapping of the receptive fields of neural
populations in cognitive space.

behavior of the component.  This subset, the receptive field of
the component, is the definition for our lexicon of ERP
components.

Note that there are at least four degrees of freedom to such
a definition.  The amplitude of the component might be modulated.
Its latency might be changed.  We can manipulate its scalp
distribution, and its relation to the behavioral variables, or
receptive field, might be modulated.  We normally allow at least
two of these variables to change freely.  Even if the amplitude
and the latency of an ERP component change we would still consider
it the same component.  On the other hand, the scalp distribution
and the receptive field must generally remain constant to define a
component.  For example, two components seem to have the same
cognitive receptive field, the P300 and the "Slow Wave" (Duncan-
Johnson & Donchin, 1977; K. Squires, Donchin, Herning, & McCarthy,
1977; N. Squires, K. Squires, & Hillyard, 1975).  They do,

however, show different scalp distributions. For this reason we consider them two different components. On the other hand, the P300 component might have widely different amplitudes and considerably different latencies, and yet, as long as a component has the scalp distribution typical of P300 and the cognitive receptive field of P300, we would consider it a P300. The defining characteristic seems to be scalp distribution. This makes sense because, if a component represents the activity of a distinct neuronal population, the effect of that population on different scalp electrodes can be expected to remain constant under all modulations of the component. I am assuming here that it is the scalp distribution that is directly related to the locus of the neuron population inside the head.

I shall illustrate our approach to the analysis of ERP components and its use in developing the ERP lexicon with two studies of event-preceding negativities. The first, a study of the readiness potential (RP), illustrates the importance of defining components in terms of experimental manipulations. The second illustrates the power of a proper componential analysis. I shall then describe in some detail the current lexical definition of the P300 component and illustrate how this definition can be utilized in the development of the biocybernetic communication channel.

## AN ANALYSIS OF MOVEMENT-RELATED POTENTIALS

Let us begin by considering the movement-related potential and its relation to the contingent negative variation. Much has been written on this issue (Deecke, Scheid, & Kornhuber, 1969; Donchin, Gerbrandt, Leifer, & Tucker, 1972, 1973; Gilden, Vaughan, & Costa, 1966; Kornhuber & Deecke, 1965; Low, Borda, Frost, & Kellaway, 1966; Vaughan, 1969). It has been suggested that the CNV is an RP that happens to be time-locked to the warning stimuli because an overt response is required following S2 (Kornhuber & Deecke, 1965). For this to be the case, it must be true that if the subject need not perform an overt response following the second stimulus, there ought not to be a readiness potential. This is not the case as shown by Donchin et al. (1972); see also Cohen, 1969; McAdam, 1974; McAdam & Rubin, 1971. Though there is some evidence that the CNV tends to be larger if an overt response follows S2 (Irwin, Knott, McAdam, & Rebert, 1966; Low et al., 1966).

Several investigators suggested that the CNV consists of at least two components, one appearing immediately after S1 reflecting an "orienting" process (Klorman & Bentsen, 1975; Loveless, 1975; Loveless & Sanford, 1974; Weerts & Lang, 1973);

the other, appearing at the end of the S1–S2 interval, has been considered a readiness potential (Rohrbaugh, Syndulko, & Lindsley, 1976; Syndulko & Lindsley, 1977). It has also been asserted that in order to observe the "early" component of the CNV one must use long interstimulus intervals. Typically, four-second intervals have been used. Rohrbaugh et al. (1976) have suggested that the CNVs recorded with shorter intervals consist of a mixture of these two components.

It is implied by this hypothesis that every movement is associated, in an obligatory fashion, with a preceding negative wave. Is this indeed the case? Kutas and Donchin (1977; in press; for details see Kutas, 1977) report a study that provides important data on movement-related potentials. The subjects squeezed a dynamometer with either the right or the left hand. The force with which a subject responded was monitored, as was the electromyographic activity in both hands. In some experimental conditions the subjects were required to squeeze the dynamometer at a self-paced rate, always with one hand or the other. In other conditions the subjects squeezed in response to a stimulus, using the right or left hand in an entire series. In yet other conditions the hand to be used was indicated by an imperative stimulus. In some conditions the imperative stimulus was preceded by a warning stimulus. The data are illustrated in Fig. 15. A negative-going potential appears in the central or frontal electrodes prior to the movement in several of the traces. Using traditional terminology some of these will be called CNVs, others will be called RPs. It is probably the case that both components are represented in these records. Kutas and Donchin (in press) attempted to disassociate the two components through experimental control. The characteristics of the response served as the independent variables. Specifically, the responding hand and the point in time at which the subject knew which hand he would have to use on a given trial were varied. In some conditions, the subject knew in advance the hand, but did not know the time of the response. In other conditions, he knew neither the hand nor the time to respond until the imperative stimulus was presented. It is reasonable to expect a movement-related potential to be larger over the hemisphere contralateral to the responding hand. This laterality should not be manifest until such time as the subject knows the responding hand. The RP can therefore be expected to be asymmetric (which, in fact, it is; see Kutas & Donchin, 1974; 1977). Furthermore, the direction of the asymmetry should reverse with the responding hand. Fig. 16 shows the potential difference between the right and the left central electrodes. When the potential is positive-going, the left hemisphere is more negative than the right and when it is negative-going, the right hemisphere is more negative than the left. Each of the pairs of traces represents the data obtained in one of the five experimental

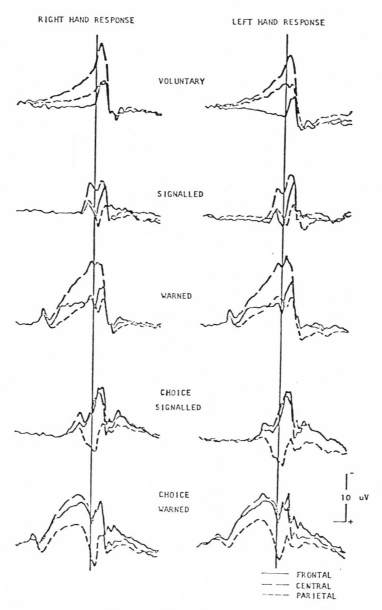

Figure 15. Movement-related potentials, recorded from three midline electrodes in five different experimental conditions. The conditions differed in the degree, and the manner, to which the subject could prepare the response. (From Kutas, 1977)

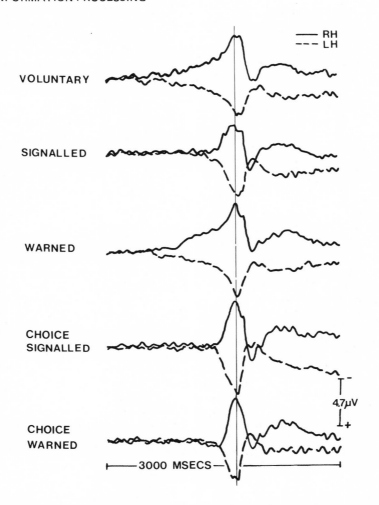

Figure 16. The ERPs in each pair represent the difference between the readiness potential recorded over the right and the left hemispheres in each of the five experimental conditions while the subjects were squeezing the dynamometers with either the right (RH) or the left (LH) hand. (After Kutas, 1977)

conditions--one trace for right-hand responses, the other for left-hand responses. Clearly, if the two traces in any pair are out of phase, then the potentials have reversed polarity with the responding hand. This did happen in each of the experimental conditions. The time at which this laterality appeared varied with the time at which the subject knew with which hand he would respond. These potentials satisfy the definition of an RP. Is this activity all there is of event-preceding negativity? The data of Fig. 17 show that the answer is no. These are data recorded at the right and left central electrodes referred to a common reference. Clearly there is an asymmetry that reverses with the responding hand; but if we subtract the asymmetric component there remains residual preparatory activity which is symmetric under all experimental conditions. It is plausible to consider this residual to be equivalent to the CNV. It appears that at least two components exist in the period preceding the response, two components defined by their differential response to experimental variables rather than by their waveform.

## MULTIPLE COMPONENTS DURING THE FOREPERIOD

We now examine the extent to which very long intervals must be used to dissociate the late from the early CNV. Relevant data are described by McCarthy and Donchin (in press). The subjects were presented with a series of slides, in each of which there were three drawings. Two of the objects drawn were structurally related. That is to say, they were similar in shape. Two other objects are functionally related. In one slide, for example, were shown an axe and a flag, which were drawn to be similar. The third object was a tree. The tree and the axe were functionally related. The subject on some trials was to report which of the two were structurally matched and, on other trials, which were functionally matched. Thus, one of the independent variables was the type of match the subject had to make.

The slides were always preceded by a warning tone which heralded their arrival. In some experimental series the tones were always the same and the subject performed the same match on all trials in the series. We called this a "fixed" presentation mode. In other series, the warning tone could be one of two tones. It indicated to the subject whether he was to make a structural or a functional match. This we called a "mixed" presentation mode. Thus the second independent variable was presentation mode. Examination of the reaction times shows that making a functional match took considerably longer than making a structural match. Subjects also made many more errors when attempting functional matches than when attempting structural matches. Interestingly, the mode of presentation had no effect on the subjects' reaction times or on their error rates. Thus, one independent variable had a strong effect on the subjects' performance. The other independent variable had no such effect on performance. The ERPs, shown in Fig. 18, present a different picture. It turns out that there is no difference between the

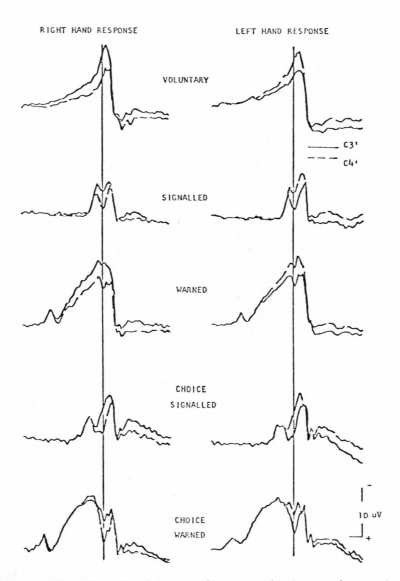

RIGHT HAND RESPONSE    LEFT HAND RESPONSE

VOLUNTARY

C3'
C4'

SIGNALLED

WARNED

CHOICE
SIGNALLED

CHOICE
WARNED

10 uV

Figure 17. ERPs in the same five conditions shown in Figure 15. The pairs of superimposed ERPs represented data recorded simultaneously over homologous, contralateral sites on the scalp. (From Kutas, 1977)

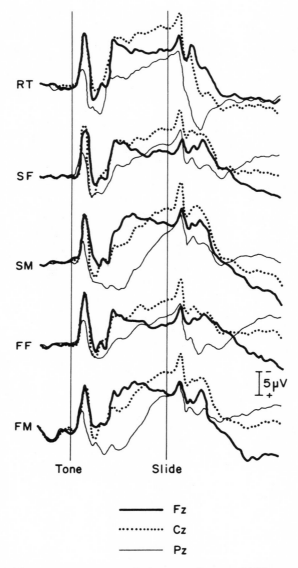

Figure 18. ERPs recorded at four different scalp locations in each of four experimental conditions which differed in the match the subject was required to make at S2 (functional and structural) and the degree to which S1 indicated the type of match. RT – reaction time; FF – fixed functional; FS – fixed structural; FM – mixed functional; SM – mixed structural. (From McCarthy and Donchin, in press)

ERPs elicited in association with the structural and the functional match. This, despite the fact that this task has been reported by Levy (1974) to strongly differentiate the functioning of the right and the left hemisphere in split-brain patients. On the other hand, the mode of presentation had a substantial effect on the waveform of the ERP. Different ERP waveforms were recorded at different electrodes in the different modes, especially in the early part of the epoch. There was an interaction between the electrode site and the mode of presentation. When the warning stimulus delivered information to the subject, a new component of the ERP appears in the early part of the epoch. A PCA of these data was used to measure their differences. The loading plots are those shown in Fig. 13. There are two distinct components in the interval between S1 and S2. The relation between these components and the experimental variables can be gleaned from an analysis of the component scores. The early component shows an interaction between the electrodes and the mode of presentation. There is no such relationship between the ERPs and the type of match (structural vs. functional). It is important to note that the PCA enabled us to demonstrate, using a one-second interval, the existence of two components in the epoch between the warning and imperative stimuli. Furthermore, an assessment of the relationship between these components and experimental variables shows that the early component depends upon the signal value of the first stimulus. One might even suggest that it is appropriate to consider this component part of the ERP elicited by S1 rather than an early component of the CNV. In many ways it behaves much like the component that has been called the "slow wave," by K. C. Squires et al. (1977).

This study presents yet another example of a "dissociation" between ERPs and behavior. The variables that manipulate performance fail to manipulate the waveforms. The variables that manipulate the waveforms fail to affect performance. The dilemma can be resolved if we consider the implications of the cognitive framework I presented above. The dissociation is disturbing only if we assume that the variance of the electrophysiological observations and the variance in performance represent an identical source of variance (this is what the term "correlates" implies). However, consider the possibility that the system is operated so as to maintain a fixed, optimal, performance output. The subject is always trying to respond as fast as he can with as few errors as he can make. This attempt to maintain a constant output must accommodate the continually changing circumstances. The variance in the response output may, thus, represent either changes in the desired output level or "noise" generated around this level. The variance in the electrophysiological observations, on the other hand, may represent adjustments, conscious or unconscious, in the subject's strategy under the changing circumstances. In other words--the subject's response is the final product of complex internal processes. The ERPs reflect aspects of the process, not necessarily the final product. An analogy used by McCarthy and Donchin (in press) is to the relationship between the depression of the accelerator lever in an automobile and the speed of the automobile. The correlation between these two variables is not 1.0. In fact, over the lifetime of an automobile it is probably much smaller. This is because the relationship between accelerator depression and the speed of the automobile depends on the terrain over which the car is traveling, the wind condition, the state of the car, the nature of the gasoline used, and the initial speed of the car. According to this "terrain hypothesis," the correlation between the CNV and reaction time, or the number of errors, or any other measure of the final "product" may be low because we do not take into consideration the terrain over which the system is operating. Note that, within the framework of the biocybernetic program, the terrain is a very important concept because it implies that, if true, the electrophysiological recordings might provide us with data that are not directly available while observing the subject's performance. The ERPs will allow us to infer the psychological terrain defined in terms of effort, allocation of attention, spare capacity or motivation. Data on these processes are generally not available through other means yet it is such data which are required by an adaptive man-machine system.

## EARLY STUDIES OF P300

In the remainder of this chapter I will focus on one component of the ERP, called here the P300. The assertions I shall make about P300 are well supported by work conducted at several different laboratories (Harter & Salmon, 1972; Hillyard, Squires, Bauer, & Lindsay, 1971; Ritter & Vaughan, 1969). All converge on the same general set of conclusions. I shall describe the work that my associates and I have conducted at the University of Illinois. For a more detailed review of the literature on P300 see Donchin et al. (in press) and Picton et al. (in press).

As I noted above, the P300 was discovered by Sutton and his co-workers. Their subjects were presented with series of tones. In some experimental conditions they knew well in advance which tone would be presented on each trial. On other occasions, the tones appeared in some random order. The subject had to predict prior to each trial which tone would be presented. Of course, when they knew the tones in advance the prediction was only pro forma. Tones that appeared in a random order "reduced the subject's uncertainty." It was the contention of the papers published by Sutton and his co-workers that stimuli which reduce

the subject's uncertainty elicit a large P300.   This  result  was
somewhat reminiscent of earlier work by Chapman and Bragdon (1964)
and by Davis (1964).  Donchin and Cohen (1967), as well as  Ritter
and  Vaughan  (1969)  and Hillyard (1969), successfully replicated
Sutton's work within different experimental contexts.   Here  then
was   a   component  of  the  ERP  whose  appearance  depended  on
situational demands rather than on the physical properties of  the
eliciting stimuli.

     For a while, however, more  interest  focused  on  the  CNV.
Soon  after  the  original  report  by Walter's group,  numerous
investigators proceeded to study the CNV.  A "CNV  group"  emerged
within  two  or three years.  It was not until the 1973 meeting of
that group that  a  substantial  portion  of  its  attention  was
directed  to  the  P300.   Among  the  initial reasons for greater
interest in the CNV was that it appeared possible to consider  the
P300  as a rather diffuse reaction to preparatory sets.  This view
took the form either of the assertion that it is possible that the
CNV and the P300 are "two sides of the same coin," as suggested by
Donchin and Smith (1970), who pointed out that the  positive-going
resolution  of  the CNV tends to have a latency of about 300 msec.
Donchin and Smith noted that one must be  aware  of  the  possible
contamination  of  P300  studies by concurrently elicited CNVs and
that it is important to determine  experimentally  the  extent  to
which  these  two  phenomena  are  related.   Others  have taken a
somewhat stronger point of view: Wilkinson (1976),  Karlin  (1970)
and Naatanen (1970, 1975) have all emphasized the possibility that
the P300 is "nothing but" a reactive response, or in a  sense--the
after discharge of the CNV.

     In 1973, in preparation for  the  Bristol  CNV  congress,  a
group  of  investigators  (Donchin, 1976) addressed this issue and
devised an experimental test to determine if the CNV and the  P300
are  the  same,  or different, components.  A specific experiment was
designed by the group  and  was  conducted  by  Donchin,  Tueting,
Ritter,  Kutas, and Heffley (1975).  The variables known to affect
the  CNV  and  the  variables  known  to  effect  the  P300   were
systematically  varied.   A  PCA of the data revealed two distinct
components of the variance, one of which could be identified  with
the  CNV,  the other with the P300.  When the relationship between
these components and the experimental variables was  assessed,  it
was  found  that  the  P300 was  associated  primarily  with  the
predictability  of  the  stimuli  and  was  not  affected  by  the
presentation of the warning stimulus.  The CNV, on the other hand,
was associated with the presentation of the warning stimulus.   It
was  also  shown  that the scalp distributions of the CNV and P300
were quite distinct.  The P300 is largest in parietal sites and is
quite  small  in  the  frontal  electrodes.  The CNV, on the other
hand, is largest at the central  electrodes.   The  issue  of  the

relation of the CNV and the P300 has not surfaced recently except for Wilkinson's suggestion that the results might have been confounded by a "resident CNV" which was not observable in the absence of a warning stimulus (Wilkinson, 1976; Wilkinson & Spence, 1973). However, until the existence of such a resident CNV is demonstrated, the issue remains moot.

Thus, a stimulus will or will not elicit a P300 as a function of its predictability whether or not it is preceded by a warning stimulus. The more unpredictable the stimulus, the more likely it is to elicit a P300. In the early studies, this was presented as a somewhat dichotomous effect in which stimuli either did, or did not, resolve the subject's uncertainty. It was fairly important to determine if gradations of predictability would be associated with gradations in the amplitude of the P300. An early and very fine study relating to this issue was conducted by Tueting et al. (1971). They were able to show that the amplitude of P300 increases as the probability associated with the eliciting stimulus decreases. In a study from our laboratory, similar results were obtained. We varied the complexity of the rule used to generate the sequences rather than the probability of the stimuli. Here again, the simpler the sequence-generating rule, the more predictable the stimulus or, in other words, the smaller the amplitude of P300 (Donchin, Kubovy, Kutas, Johnson, & Herning, 1973).

## P300 AND SUBJECTIVE PROBABILITY

As we began the biocybernetic project in 1973, we had reasonable confidence that the P300 was indeed a real component and that its receptive field was clearly associated in some fashion with the probability of stimuli. It was also recognized at the time that unpredictability is not sufficient to elicit a P300. The subjects must also "be paying attention" to stimuli or, as I prefer to state it, the stimulus must be "task relevant" if it is to elicit a P300. This point is illustrated by data reported by Duncan-Johnson and Donchin (1977). They utilized what has come to be called the "oddball" experimental paradigm. The subject is presented with a Bernoulli series of stimuli and is told to count the number of events of one kind in the series. In this case subjects heard a series of tones each having one of two different pitches. The subjects were instructed to count the higher of the two tones in all series except one in which they counted the lower tone. The independent variable in the experiment consisted of the probabilities of the two stimuli. Some of the data are shown in Fig. 19. It can be seen that the amplitude of the P300 varies monotonically with the probability of the stimulus. It does not matter much which of the two stimuli is

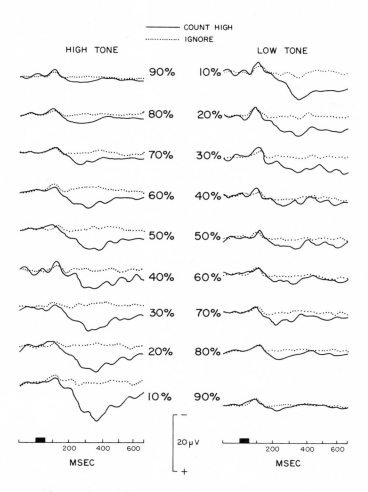

Figure 19. The ERPs elicited by high and low tones presented in a Bernoulli series with the probabilities as indicated. Data are shown for experimental conditions in which the subjects counted the high tones in each series (solid lines) and from a series in which the subject was instructed to solve a word puzzle while the tones were presented (dotted lines). (From Duncan-Johnson and Donchin, 1977)

being counted. As long as the subject is counting tones, then the
rarer  tone elicits a P300 component whose amplitude declines with
increasing  probability  of  the  stimulus,  and,  of  course,
correspondingly,  the  amplitude  of  the P300 elicited by the other
stimulus increases. For this to occur, it is absolutely essential
that the subject count one or the other tone. When the subject is
presented with the same  series  of  tones  while  performing  yet
another  task,  such as reading a book or solving a word puzzle, we
obtain the records shown in Fig. 19 by the dotted line in which an
N100-P160  can be discerned, but there is no P300. The importance
of task relevance in determining the amplitude of P300 is examined
by Johnson and Donchin (1978).

   Any attempt to utilize these  findings  in  a  biocybernetic
channel  assumes that it is possible to identify the existence and
measure the amplitude of a P300 in real time (that is, immediately
following  the presentation of a stimulus). Earlier work from our
laboratory suggested that stepwise  discriminant  analysis  (SWDA)
can  be  used  for this purpose (Donchin, 1969; Donchin & Herning,
1975). This was confirmed by K. C. Squires and  Donchin  (1976),
who reported that it is possible to detect P300s in single trials.
The classification was correct about 80% of the time. Of  course,
this  means  that  20% of the trials were misclassified. When the
trials on which the program "erred" were examined,  it  was  noted
that when the "rare" trials that were classified as "frequent" are
averaged, a P300 can be discerned in the average as shown in  Fig.
20. When frequent trials which were classified by  SWDA  as  rare
were  averaged,  they  do  show  a  small P300. Similar data were
reported by Donchin (1969). It is as if the subjects respond  to
some  frequent  stimuli  as  if  they  were rare, and to some rare
stimuli as if they were frequent. It was necessary  to  determine
if  there  is  a  rule  that  governs the variability of subjects'
responses to identical stimuli. We did indeed find  such  a  rule
and  it is described by K. C. Squires, Wickens, N. K. Squires, and
Donchin (1976). The rule emerged from a detailed  examination  of
the relationship between the amplitude of the P300 elicited by any
stimulus and the specific sequence of stimuli  that  preceded  it.
Consider  Fig.  21,  which  shows  data  collected  in the oddball
paradigm. The probability of the two stimuli was  equal  to  .50.
An  average  of all the high-tone trials is shown at the origin of
the tree. There is hardly any P300 in that average.  But  if  we
treat  separately high tones preceded by high tones and high tones
preceded by low tones, an interesting pattern appears.  It  turns
out  that when the eliciting stimulus is preceded by the alternate
stimulus it elicits a large P300. A small P300 is elicited  if  a
stimulus  repeats the immediately preceding stimulus. We examined
the effect of sequences up to five items in  length  as  shown  in
Fig. 21. A remarkably systematic relationship emerges between the
amplitude of P300 and the preceding  sequence  of  stimuli.   This

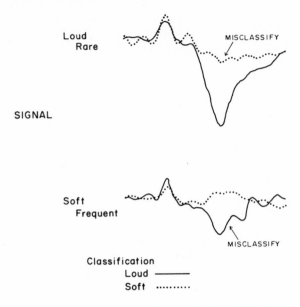

Figure 20.   The solid lines represent ERPs obtained by averaging trials which the Stepwise Discriminant Analysis program identified as the "rare loud" stimuli. The dotted line represents ERPs obtained by averaging trials which the program has identified as "soft frequent" stimuli.   Note that, in each case, the waveform of the ERP obtained from averaging the misclassified trials suggests that the program identified the correct waveforms.   (After Squires & Donchin, 1976)

pattern can be seen in what we call the "expectancy trees" shown in Fig. 22. Here, each ERP is represented by a number proportional to the amplitude of the P300 complex measured by a discriminant score. The measure includes contributions of N200 and the slow wave as well as a contribution of the P300 component. For simplicity we shall refer to it as P300. The magnitude measures are plotted against the order of the preceding sequence. If a high tone was preceded by an increasingly longer string of low tones, the amplitude of the P300 it elicits increases. If a high tone was preceded by a run of high tones, the amplitude of the P300 it elicits decreases. Thus, P300 amplitude does seem to vary from trial to trial depending on the sequential structure of the series.

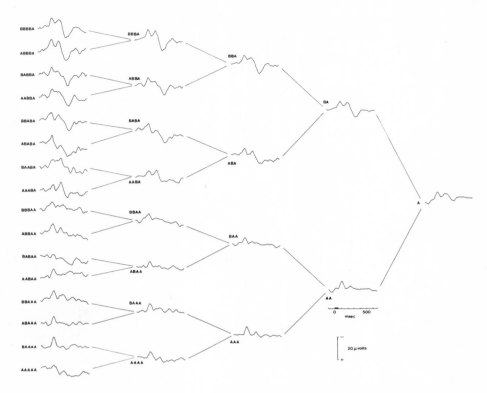

Figure 21. All the ERPs shown in this figure were
obtained by averaging trials elicited by an "A" stimulus
(a 1000-Hz tone). However, prior to averaging, the
trials were sorted depending upon the previous sequence
of stimuli. The effect of stimulus sequence on the
waveform of the ERPs was quite evident. (From Squires
et al., in press.)

        We proposed a model to account for this variability
(Duncan-Johnson & Donchin, 1977; K. C. Squires et al.,1976).
According to this model, P300 amplitude is proportional to the
subject's surprise at the occurrence of an event. The more
surprising an event, the larger the P300 it elicits. Surprise is,
of course, the reciprocal of expectancy. The more one expects
something to happen, the smaller the surprise when it does happen.
We postulated that the subject's expectancy for a stimulus depends
(when a series is entirely random) on the structure of the series
and that each stimulus presented affects the expectancy for all
succeeding stimuli. Stimuli whose expectancy is high when

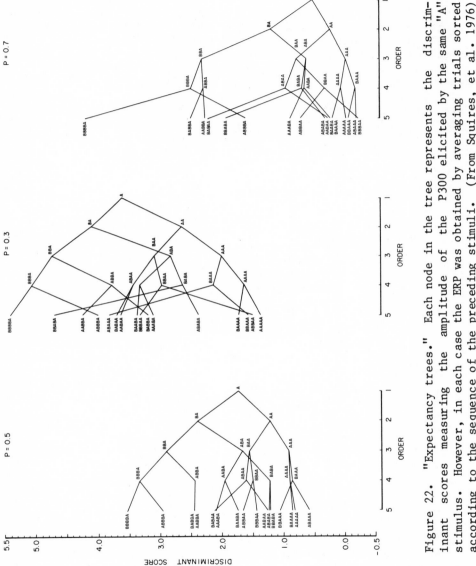

Figure 22. "Expectancy trees." Each node in the tree represents the discriminant scores measuring the amplitude of the P300 elicited by the same "A" stimulus. However, in each case the ERP was obtained by averaging trials sorted according to the sequence of the preceding stimuli. (From Squires, et al. 1976)

presented will elicit no P300; stimuli whose expectancy is low
will elicit a P300.

Our model draws heavily on models developed to explain
similar sequential trees recorded in reaction–time experiments
(Falmange, Cohen, & Dwivedi, 1975; Laming, 1969; Theios, 1973).
Computation of the expectancy for a given stimulus is illustrated
in Fig. 23. We make a simple assumption, namely, that when
confronted with a random sequence of events subjects expect events
to repeat rather than alternate. So, once a stimulus is
presented, the subject expects it to be repeated. The phrase "the
subject expects" should not be taken to imply that the subject is
aware of these expectations. We are describing the behavior of a
process of which the subject may, or may not, be conscious.
According to our model a stimulus, when presented, generates
expectancy for its repetition. This expectancy decays

EXPECTANCY MODEL

$E \subset M+P+A$

E = EXPECTANCY
M = "MEMORY" FACTOR
P = GLOBAL PROBABILITY
A = ALTERNATION FACTOR

$$M_{AN} = \sum_{i=N-I}^{N-m} \alpha^{N-i} S_i$$

where

$$S_i = \frac{0 \text{ for } (S = B)}{1 \text{ for } (S = A)}$$

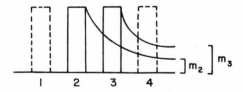

Figure 23. A model which attempts to account for
variation in the subject's expectancy that a given
stimulus will occur on a given trial as a function of
the specific sequence of stimuli which were presented on
the preceding trials. This model is described by
K. C. Squires et al. (1976).

exponentially. The rate of decay is one of the important parameters of the model that must be estimated for any set of data. Fig. 24 shows the state of affairs after a sequence of four stimuli. Preceding trial 5 the expectancy for a high tone is affected by the fact that a high tone was presented on trials 2 and 3. Due to the exponential decay, the high tone presented on trial 2 contributes only $M_2$ units to the expectancy of a high tone on trial 5. The high tone on trial 3 contributes $M_3$ units. Thus, according to the model, the expectancy of a high tone on trial 5 is equal to $M_2 + M_3$. An equivalent estimate of the expectancy for a low tone can be computed on the basis of the low tones presented on trials 1 and 4. This exponential decay element of the model attributes changes in ERP amplitude to what might be called a "short-term memory" for the structure of the series. Two other factors had to be included in the model. One is the a priori probability of the stimuli. A rare event elicits a larger P300 than a more frequent event. A third factor was required to account for the effects of a run of stimulus alternations (e.g., high-low-high-low--?).

This model accounted for approximately 78% of the variance in the magnitude of the P300 complex. It is important to note, however, that this is not a model about ERPs. It is a model for human information processing. The only assumption we make about ERPs is that there is an inverse relationship between expectancy and the magnitude of P300 or, if you will, a direct relationship between surprise and P300. This assertion is well supported by data (Duncan-Johnson & Donchin, 1977; K. C. Squires, Donchin, Herning, & McCarthy, 1977; K. C. Squires, Petuchowski, Wickens, & Donchin, 1977; Teuting, Sutton, & Zubin, 1971). The expectancy model proposes a rule whereby the subjective probabilities are associated with events when subjects are confronted with an entirely random series. Subjects seem to refuse to believe in randomness and impose a structure on the environment even when they "know" that no structure exists. This view of the world was well expressed by Ogden Nash in his poem, "Unfortunately, It Is the Only Game in Town," which begins as follows:

> "Often I think that this shoddy world would be more
>     nifty
> If all the ostensibly fifty-fifty propositions in it
>     were truly fifty-fifty.
> How unfortunate that the odds
> Are rigged by the gods.
> I do not wish to be impious,
> But I have observed that all human hazards that
>     mathematics would declare to be fifty-fifty are
>     actually at least fifty one-forty nine in favor of
>     Mount Olympius. . . ."

After giving several examples, he concludes:

"Why when quitting a taxi do I invariably down the door
       handle when it should be upped and up it when it
       should be downed?
By the cosmic shell game I am spellbound.
There is no escape; I am like an oyster, shellbound.
Yes, surely the gods operate according to the fiercest
       exhortation W. C. Fields ever spake:
Never give a sucker an even break."


Whether Ogden Nash is right or wrong, I do not know, but
that he describes a very common aspect of human performance is
indubitably true. Individuals do not behave as if things are, in
fact, fifty-fifty. The psychophysiological assertion we make is
that the amplitude of P300 is a function of the subjective
probability that individuals assign to events. An independent
assumption is that when events are random, the subjective
probabilities will be derived from the sequential structure of the
series. The amplitude variations of P300 reflect a structure
which the individual has imposed on the environment. If the
relation is reliable P300 can serve as a useful tool in the study
of human information processing by providing an objective measure
of subjective probability.

Several of our recent studies were designed to test the
assertion that the variation in P300 amplitude is, in fact, due to
"cognitive" factors rather than to receptor adaptation or to
habituation. These studies were needed because it is possible to
account for the data reported by Squires et al. (1976) by invoking
the well-established tendency for repeated stimuli to elicit
responses of decreasing magnitude, either because the receptors
adapt or because the system habituates. This view implies that
P300 amplitude is determined by the specific sequence of stimuli
regardless of instructions to the subject. The alternate view
predicts that the amplitude of P300 associated with a given
sequence of physical stimuli will be affected by instructions that
manipulate the subject's expectancy. I will review, very briefly,
some of the studies designed to test this hypothesis.

Johnson and Donchin (1978a) examined the extent to which the
sequential effects depend on the physical nature of the stimuli or
on the categories into which subjects may classify stimuli. In
this variant of the oddball experiment three stimuli were used, an
1800-Hz, a 1400-Hz, and a 1000-Hz tone. The subject was to count
only one of the three stimuli. The physical series contained
three distinct stimuli, each with an a priori probability of .33.
An alternate description of the series, more consistent with the

subject's task, is that there were two <u>categories</u> of stimuli,  one
with  an a priori probability of .33 containing the stimulus to be
counted, and the  other  category  containing  the  two  uncounted
stimuli.   The  ERPs  elicited by these stimuli could behave as if
elicited by a triplet of equiprobable events or as if elicited  by
a  Bernoulli  series  in  which two events and their probabilities
were determined by the  stimulus  categories.   The  results  were
unequivocal.   In  Fig. 24a are presented ERPs elicited by each of
two stimuli presented in the standard oddball task.  The trees are
similar  to those shown in Fig. 23.  These data can be compared to
the trees obtained from the same subjects, in the   three   stimulus
series shown in Fig. 24b.  The two uncounted stimuli  are  treated
by  the  subject  as  if  both had an a priori probability of .67.
Thus the repetition of stimuli from the same  category  even  when
they are physically distinct serves to depress P300 amplitude.  It
is hard to see how receptor adaptation, or habituation to specific
stimuli,  can  account  for  these  data.   It seems that the ERPs
manifest processes that occur <u>after</u> the subjects have  categorized
physical stimuli into classes determined by the tasks.

      K. C. Squires,  Petuchowski,  Wickens,  and  Donchin  (1977)
evaluated the degree to which the sequential effects are unique to
auditory stimuli.  The same subjects were presented with  auditory
and  visual Bernoulli series.  The data obtained with the auditory
series replicated in all details the results  of  Squires  et  al.
(1976).   The  data  obtained  with the visual series are shown in
Fig. 25.  The trees associated with the  visual  target  stimuli
(that is, the stimuli that were counted) could be described by the
model that was developed on the auditory series.   The  non-target
visual  stimuli show a somewhat attenuated sequential effect.  Yet
the expectancy tree for the non-target  visual  stimuli  could  be
described  by  the  same  model  with a change in parameters.  The
influence which a visual  non-target  has  on  the  expectancy  of
subsequent  stimuli decays more rapidly than does the influence of
a visual target.  Remarkably, the relation between  the  decay  in
short-term  memory  in  echoic  and in iconic memory, which can be
inferred from the existing literature (Eriksen  &  Johnson,  1964;
Massaro,  1970; Sperling, 1960) is very similar to the decay rates
implied by these data.

      Further  evidence  that  the  data  reflect  aspects  of
information  processing  rather  than  receptor  adaptations  is
presented by Duncan-Johnson  and  Donchin  (1978).   The  previous
studies  implied  that  when  subjects are presented with a random
series and they have no evidence that the world is other than  50-
50, they tend to develop probability estimates on the basis of the
structure of the series.  What if explicit information  about  the
probability of events is available?

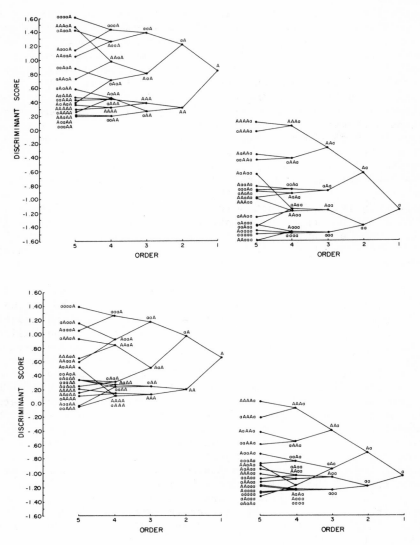

Figure 24. A. Expectancy trees elicited by a Bernoulli series of two stimuli--one presented with a probability of .33 and the other with a probability of .67. B. Expectancy trees obtained from the same subjects in the same manner, except that subjects were presented with a series of three equi-probable stimuli. The subjects were to count one of the three stimuli. For the creation of these trees, no distinction was made between the two uncounted stimuli. (From Johnson & Donchin, 1978a)

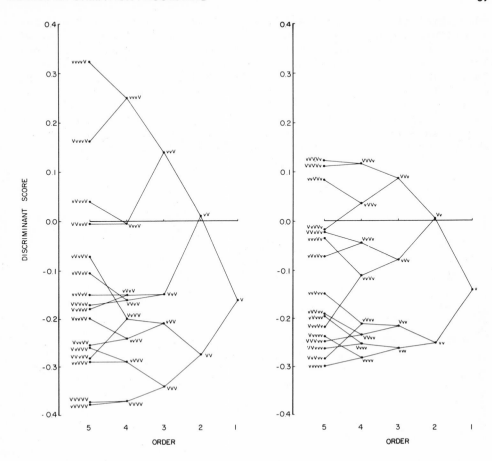

Figure 25. Expectancy trees obtained from a Bernoulli series of two visual stimuli. Note how a non-target, uncounted, visual stimulus is less afffected by the presentation of the preceding target stimuli than are either target visual stimuli, or auditory stimuli. (From Squires et al., 1977)

The subjects were presented with a series of paired tachistoscopic flashes separated by 400 msec. The second stimulus could be either the letter $\underline{H}$ or the letter $\underline{S}$. It was preceded by a star, by the letter $\underline{H}$, or by the letter $\underline{S}$. In one experimental condition, these three warning stimuli, which appeared with equal probability, bore no relationship to the S2 stimulus. Thus the series of $\underline{H}$s and $\underline{S}$s presented in the second position constituted a Bernoulli series. In these circumstances the amplitude of the

P300 elicited by either the H or the S depends very much on the
preceding sequence of Hs and Ss in the second position. This, of
course, replicates the data described above for Bernoulli series.
The expectancy trees in this control condition are shown in Fig.
26a. In the other experimental conditions, the a priori
probability that the second stimulus would be an H or an S was
indicated on each trial by the warning stimulus. For example, in
one condition an H indicated that the H was more probable than
the S, an S indicated that the S was more probable than the H,
while a star indicated that the probabilities of the H and the S

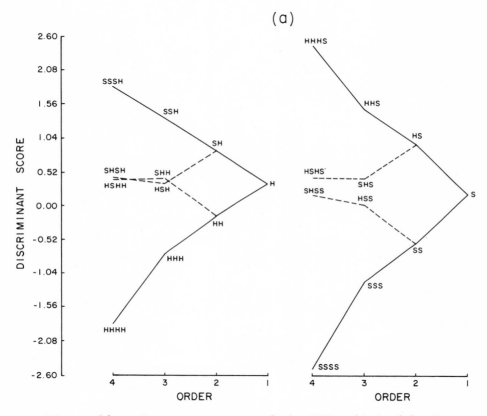

(a)

Figure 26a. Expectancy trees of the ERPs elicited by Hs
or Ss that were preceded by a warning stimulus that
provided the subject with no information on the
probability with which an H or an S will appear on that
trial. These trees are similar to those shown on the
previous figures. The amplitude of the P300 component
elicited by a stimulus is affected by the sequence of
stimuli presented on the preceding trials.

(b)

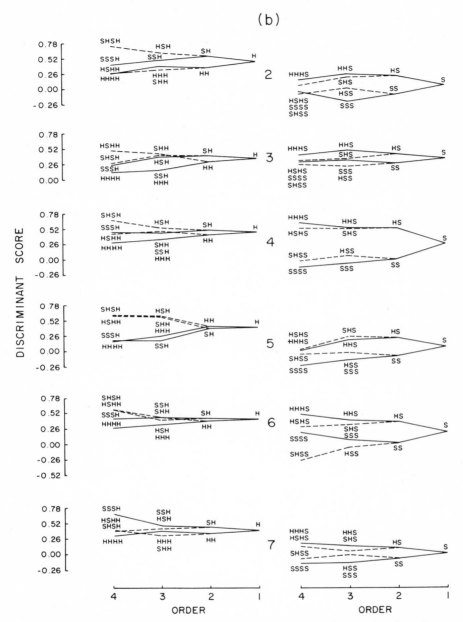

Figure 26b. Data from the six conditions in which the warning stimulus preceding each stimulus indicated the probability with which an H̲ or an S̲ will occur. Notice how the sequential effect virtually disappears when the subject no longer needs to derive estimates of the subjective probability from the past history of the sequence. (From Duncan-Johnson & Donchin, 1977)

were equal. In other words, the S1 was an explicit source of
information about the a priori probabilities of S2. In this case,
the effect of stimuli on the ERPs elicited by succeeding stimuli
is greatly diminished, as shown in Fig. 26b. The subject no
longer extracts information about the environment from the
sequential structure of the series. The amplitude of the P300
and, by inference, the subjective probability of the stimuli,
depend entirely on the a priori probability indicated by the
warning stimulus. This is illustrated in Fig. 27. The amplitude
of the P300 appears to depend on the information available to the
subject rather than on the physical properties of the series.
This is strong evidence that with P300 we are indeed tapping the
probability structure that the subject imposes on the environment
and that P300 amplitude can serve as a useful clue to a subject's

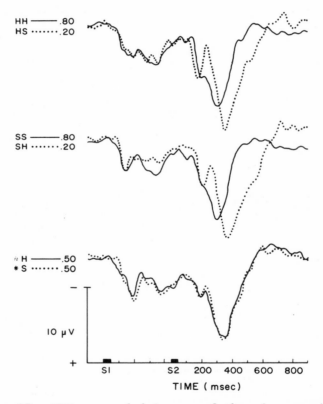

Figure 27. ERPs recorded in one of the six experimental
conditions in which an S1 informed the subject of the
probability of the impending S2. Notice that S2s whose
probability is indicated to be .20 elicit the larger
P300. (From Duncan-Johnson & Donchin, 1977)

expectancy.  For a detailed description of this study see  Duncan-
Johnson (1978).

A striking example is provided by data  which  Chesney  has
been  acquiring in our laboratory.  I will introduce this study by
making explicit an issue presented by our expectancy model.   The
assertion  that  subjects  expect stimuli to repeat is in conflict
with  the  common  view  that  the  "gambler's  fallacy"  governs
expectancy.   We  all  "know" that people tend to predict stimulus
change rather than stimulus repetition.  If the P300 is  an  index
of subjective probability, why isn't the subject more surprised by
a repeating sequence of five high tones than he is by a high  tone
appearing  after  four  low  tones?   There is, however, no direct
evidence that people always predict  what  they  actually  expect.
The  experimental  literature  is  replete  with  references  to a
dissociation between the perceived expectancy of an event and  the
predictions   declared   by   the   subject,  especially  when  the
consequences of different types of errors are  not  equal  (Beach,
Rose,  Sayeki,  Wise,  &  Carter,  1970;  Myers,  1976;  Neimark &
Shuford, 1959; Reber & Milward, 1968; Vlek,  1970).   However,  no
index,  other  than the subject's overt predictions, is available to
assess his expectancies, and so the existence of this dissociation
is  usually  inferred  from contradictions in the data rather than
from direct observables (see Messick & Rapoport,  1965).    Perhaps
P300  amplitude  might serve as an objective measure of subjective
probability.   Such an application depends on an  understanding  of
the relation between overt predictions and the P300.

Relevant data were obtained in an experiment  in  which  the
subjects  viewed  a computer display screen in the center of which
there could appear either a cross or a square, indicated  here  by
an  "X"  and  an  "O" respectively (character dimensions subtended
.233 by .500 degrees  of  visual  angle).   To  the  left  of  the
stimulus letter five other characters appeared.  In one condition,
these consisted of a filled rectangle.  In this case  the  subject
was  presented with a Bernoulli sequence of Xs and Os to the right
of a string of  filled  rectangles.   In  another  condition  the
subject's  memory  was  "aided."  The past history of the sequence
over the five most recent trials appeared  to  the  left  of  the
stimulus  figure so that if in the most recent trials the subjects
were shown O, O, X, X, O, this is precisely what appeared to  the
left  of  the  most  recently presented X or O.  The subjects were
assigned two tasks.  One required them to count one  of  the  two
items  as in the oddball studies.  In another series of trials the
subject had to predict prior to each stimulus if it would be an  X
or  an  O.   The P300 elicited during the  prediction  task  is
considerably larger than that elicited by the same stimuli  during
the  counting  task.   The ERPs elicited by each stimulus are
affected  by  previous  sequences  whether  the  subjects  were

predicting or counting, as shown in Fig. 28. It was also of
interest to note that the "memory aid" depressed the sequential
dependency effect, as shown by dashed lines in Fig. 29.

On every trial of the prediction paradigm the stimulus
either confirmed or disconfirmed the subject's prediction. There
have been several attempts, especially by Sutton and his
associates (Levit, Sutton, & Zubin, 1973; Sutton, Braren, Zubin, &
John, 1965; Tueting et al., 1971; see also Chesney, 1976), to
determine if confirming and disconfirming stimuli elicit different
ERPs. In general, no systematic relation was found. Similarly,
in this study, when the confirmations and the disconfirmations
were averaged, no difference could be observed between the two
ERPs (Fig. 29). These data appear inconsistent with the
assumption that P300 reflects surprise. A disconfirmation, one
might think, will be more surprising than a confirmation and
therefore should elicit a larger P300. But this view implies that
subjects' predictions faithfully reflect their expectations. Yet,
the subject can predict an X while expecting an O. If this is the

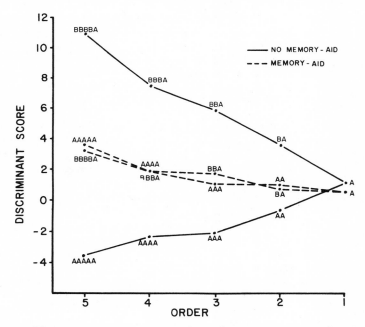

Figure 28. Expectancy trees based on a series of visual
stimuli appearing on the screen jointly with a mask
(solid line) and a tree obtained with the identical
stimuli, but with the past history of the sequence
presented simultaneously with each stimulus. (From
Chesney & Donchin, in preparation)

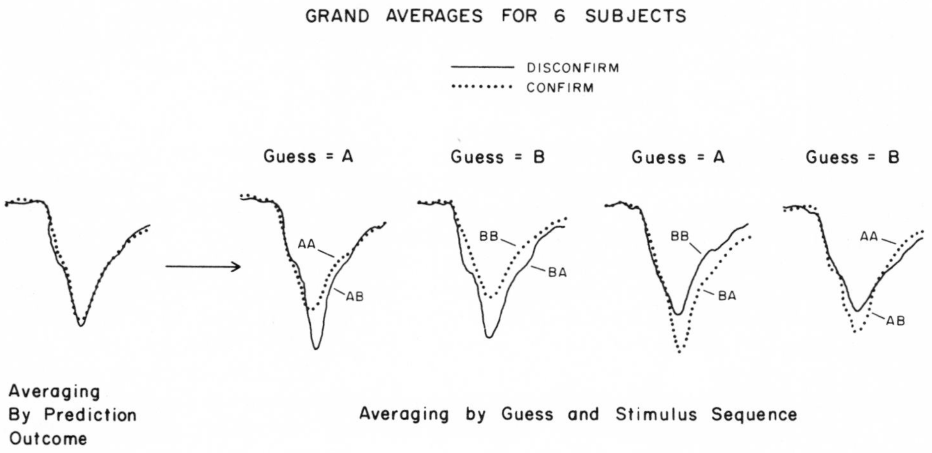

GRAND AVERAGES FOR 6 SUBJECTS

———— DISCONFIRM
········· CONFIRM

Guess = A          Guess = B          Guess = A          Guess = B

Averaging
By Prediction                    Averaging by Guess and Stimulus Sequence
Outcome

Figure 29. ERPs demonstrating that, while the amplitude
of the P300 component is the same whether   the stimulus
confirms  or disconfirms the subject's prediction, large
differences in amplitude obtain if the data  are  sorted
by  the  specific prediction made by the subject and the
degree to which  these  predictions  are  confirmed   or
disconfirmed.  (From Chesney & Donchin, in preparation )


case then some disconfirmations may be less surprising  than  some
confirmations.   If  the  subjective probabilities are governed by
our model of expectancy then subjects expect stimuli to repeat and
should be surprised when stimuli alternate.  The confirmation of a
repetition prediction should not, in this case, elicit a P300.  If
the  subject  predicts  an  alternation  and  this  prediction  is
confirmed, a large P300 should be  elicited.   Similarly,  if  the
subject  predicts  an  alternation  and is disconfirmed, a smaller
P300 should appear.  In other words, P300 amplitude would be large
in  association  with  alternations  and small in association with
repetitions.   Furthermore,   alternation   predictions,   when
confirmed,  would  elicit a large P300 and repetition predictions,
when  disconfirmed,  would  elicit  a  large  P300.   When   the
confirmations  and  disconfirmations were sorted according to this
rule and reaveraged we obtained the data in Fig. 29, which confirm
these predictions.  These data should be interpreted with caution.
Another way of describing  the  same  results  is  to  state  that
alternations  elicit  larger P300s than repetitions, no matter what
the subject predicted.  In current work we are  trying  to  decide
between  these two interpretations.  Yet, whichever is true, these
data account for previous failures to find a relation between  the
"confirmation,"   "disconfirmation,"   and   P300   amplitude.

Furthermore, these data show that a fuller picture of the
probability structure that the subject imposed on the environment
can be obtained by combining the information provided by P300 with
information derived from the subject's predictions.

Currently available data on the amplitude of P300 can be
summarized as follows. Task-relevant events are categorized by
subjects into classes which depend upon their tasks. Each class
is assigned some "subjective" probability. If an event in an
improbable class occurs, it will elicit a P300. The more
improbable the event, the larger the amplitude of the P300. This
will be true only if the events are task relevant. The problem of
task relevance has not been reviewed here. For more details see
Johnson and Donchin (1978b), and Donchin et al. (in press). The
functional significance of this component remains a matter of
controversy. Elsewhere (Donchin, 1975) I suggested that the
process manifested by P300 is invoked whenever data provided by a
stimulus call for a revision of hypotheses, or models, of the
environment held by the subject. This is analogous to the
"context updating" function postulated by Pribram and McGuinness
(1975) and is clearly consistent with Sokolov's model (1969).
Much of the recent data assembled in this laboratory is consistent
with this view (see, for example, Duncan-Johnson & Donchin, 1977;
Johnson & Donchin, 1978b; McCarthy & Donchin, 1976; K. C. Squires,
Donchin, Henning, & McCarthy, 1977). Stuss and Picton (in press)
have been led to the same view by their data, even though they
ascribe the context-updating function to a later component they
label P4. A detailed discussion of this issue is beyond the scope
of this review. The utility of P300 in the study of human
information processing does not derive from our understanding of
its functional significance. A demonstration of reliable,
systematic, relations between P300 and psychological processes
suffices. Needless to say, the elucidation of the functional
significance of P300 remains the most challenging problem
presented by this intriguing component.


THE LATENCY OF P300

In the preceding section, I used the label "P300" to refer
to the component of the ERP whose amplitude varies with the
subjective probability of task-relevant events. The label implies
that the component is elicited approximately 300 msec following
the occurrence of the event. Yet, the actual latency of this ERP
component is quite variable. The label P300 is applied in the
preceding sections to peaks whose latency ranged from 250 to 700
msec. This, of course, presents a problem. The latency of an ERP
component is defined as the interval, in msec, between the
occurrence of an eliciting event and the peak of the component.

For exogenous components, this definition suffices. The eliciting event is well anchored in time and one simply measures the time, relative to stimulus onset, at which the peak of the component appears. Endogenous components present a subtle problem. If the eliciting event is internal, that is to say, virtually unobservable, how is its onset to be measured? If P300 is a manifestation of the invocation of an internal processor which follows the recognition of the occurrence of an event whose subjective probability is low, then its latency should be measured from the instant this recognition occurs. But, how are we to know this instant? One strategy focuses on the endogenous events that are temporally related to external events. Either the endogenous event occurs at a fixed interval after a stimulus, or a synchronizing external stimulus is presented with the hope that it will coax the appearance of the internal event at the specified time. The assumption of a fixed internal latency inherent in these procedures is, however, questionable, especially as there is no ready procedure by which it can be validated. Nevertheless, this assumption has been made quite often and has led to some confusion. The confusion takes the form of considering as different components centro-parietal waves that behave like a P300 (Thatcher, 1977). It seems more reasonable to assume that the interval between a stimulus and the peak of P300 depends on the latency of the endogenous event, which, in turn, depends on the time required to recognize the stimulus and evaluate its relevance and subjective probability. Under these circumstances, P300 latency can be expected to vary quite widely, as widely as recognition time varies.

One difficulty presented by this interpretation is that it predicts a correlation between stimulus evaluation time and P300 latency; by implication it predicts a positive correlation between reaction time and P300. Here, the literature presents a mixed record (see review by Donchin et al., in press). Briefly summarized, it is the case that numerous studies have reported a positive correlation between P300 latency and reaction time (Bostock & Jarvis, 1970; Rohrbaugh, Donchin, & Eriksen, 1974; Roth, Kopell, Tinklenberg, Darley, Sikora, & Vesecky, 1975; Wilkinson & Morlock, 1967). Yet, a number of well-controlled studies report a dissociation between P300 latency and reaction time (Karlin & Martz, 1973; Karlin, Martz, Brauth, & Mordkoff, 1971; Karlin, Martz, & Morokoff, 1970). This state of affairs has led some to view the dissociation between P300 and reaction time as a major obstacle to the interpretation of P300 (see Tueting, in press, for a discussion of this problem).

The contradictions between different studies can be reconciled if one makes the simple, and plausible, assumption that P300 latency depends on stimulus-evaluation processes and is largely independent of response selection and execution time. This view is consistent with the conclusions drawn above from the analysis of P300 amplitude. If the component is invoked after a stimulus has been identified as surprising, identification must be completed before P300 is invoked. Thus, P300 latency will vary with stimulus-evaluation time. If the process manifested by P300 is related to contextual updating, with implications for the subject's future strategies rather than for his response to the specific stimulus on this specific trial, there is no need for a particular relationship between P300 latency and reaction time (Donchin et al., in press). The expectations that these two variables be positively and strongly correlated, as well as the expectation that P300 must precede reaction time, follow from the model described above as the S-R model. In that view, the subject's overt response is the terminal point of the information-processing activity invoked by a stimulus. However, if we assume, with the cognitive model, that the subject's overt response is only one of the many consequences of stimulus presentation, then it is plausible to expect P300 latency to be determined by one subset of the processes invoked by a stimulus, while reaction time is determined by others. The degree of correlation between the two will depend on the circumstances under which the subject operates. Evidence that P300 indeed depends on stimulus evaluation time has been presented by several investigators (Ford, Roth, Dirks, & Kopell, 1973; Gomer, Spicuzza, & O'Donnell, 1976; N. K. Squires, Donchin, K. C. Squires, & Grossberg, 1977). A detailed analysis of the relationship between P300 and reaction time has been presented by Kutas, McCarthy and Donchin (1977).

If P300 latency represents stimulus-evaluation time,[6] then its relation to reaction time should depend primarily on the extent to which the subject's reaction time depends on stimulus-evaluation. It is well known that subjects can trade speed for accuracy. Speed, in this case, implies that responses are emitted without waiting for full evaluation of the stimulus. It can be predicted, therefore, that the correlation between reaction time and P300 latency would depend on the subject's strategy. Kutas et al. (1977) tested this hypothesis by requiring subjects to discriminate between stimuli of varying degrees of complexity under both speed- and accuracy-maximizing regimes. They presented

---

[6] Note that the assumption that P300 latency is proportional to stimulus-evaluation time does not imply that the process manifested by P300 is a stimulus-evaluation process. The only implication is that stimulus-evaluation is complete before P300 is invoked.

subjects with series of words on a screen. In different series, the words were varied. In one series the names "Nancy" and "David" were presented on 20% and 80% of the trials respectively. In a second series, several female names, comprising 20% of the trials, and several male names comprising the remaining trials were presented. In the third series, synonyms of the word "prod" were presented 20% of the time against a background of other, unrelated, words. The ERPs elicited by the rare events in the series are shown on the left column of Fig. 30. It can be seen that whether subjects counted rare events, responded to them under accuracy instructions, or responded to them under speed instructions, the latency of the P300 was shortest for the fixed names and longest for synonyms. The waveforms presented in the left column of Fig. 30 seem to indicate that the amplitudes elicited in the different experimental conditions differed. However, these amplitude differences may reflect changes in the variability of P300 latency across the experimental conditions (Brazier, 1964). An interpretation of these amplitude differences was contingent, therefore, on the availability of a procedure for assessing the latency of P300 on each trial of the experiment. For this purpose we adopted a technique described originally by Woody for detecting ERP components whose onset time is unknown (Woody, 1967; see also Ruchkin & Sutton, in press). This technique yields an estimate of the latency of P300 on each trial. With such estimates available, it is possible to align all the individual trials at the same latency and thus obtain an estimate of P300 amplitude which is independent of latency jitter. The averages obtained after latency adjustment are shown on the right in Fig. 30. The latency differences between the ERPs obtained with the three series remain. The amplitude differences are diminished and no significant relation between P300 amplitude and the experimental condition could be found.

The latency adjustment procedure also provides a latency measure for each trial which can be compared to the reaction time recorded on that same trial. Scattergrams of P300 and the reaction time in the speed and the accuracy regimes for all subjects and all experimental conditions are presented in Fig. 31. This analysis confirmed the previous conclusions. The correlation between reaction time and P300 was lower (.257) during the speed regime than during the accuracy regime (.617). We concluded from these data that at least two processes are initiated by a stimulus. The first, a response selection and execution process, is indexed by the overt response. The second, a stimulus-evaluation process, is indexed by the P300 component. Under accuracy instructions response selection is contingent on stimulus-evaluation, the two processes are tightly coupled and reaction time is frequently longer than P300 latency. When subjects operated under speed instructions, stimulus evaluation

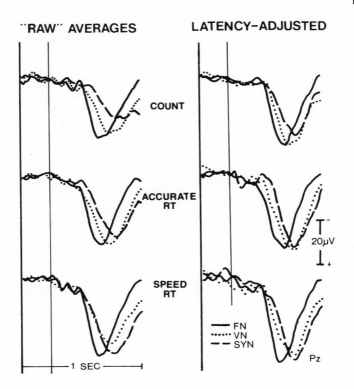

Figure 30. ERPs elicited by names presented on the PLATO screen, under three different instruction sets and for three different series of stimuli. The stimuli were as follows: FN, the name Nancy; VN, a group of different girls' names and SYN, a group of synonyms of the word prod. In each series the relevant stimulus category was presented on 20% of the trials while a different set of stimuli was presented on the rest of the trials. (From Kutas et al., 1977)

was more loosely coupled with response selection. Responses may be generated before the stimulus has been fully evaluated. The thrust of the data is clear. The correlation, or lack thereof, between reaction time and P300 latency cannot be interpreted without reference to the specific tasks the subjects are performing and the strategies they adopt. The theoretical difficulties which Tueting (in press) summarizes disappear if proper consideration is given to the different processes that

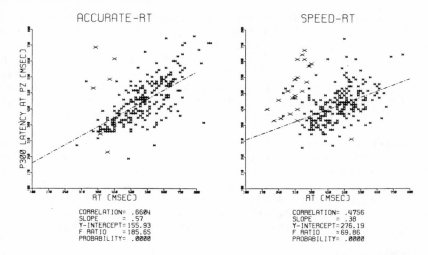

Figure 31. The relationship between the latency of P300 and reaction time when subjects are trying to be fast and when they are trying to be accurate. (From Kutas et al., 1977)

underlie reaction time. At present, it would be opportune to view changes in P300 latency as reflecting changes in stimulus-evaluation time.

## BIOCYBERNETIC CLOSED-LOOP APPLICATION

The purpose of the research program described above has been to lead to the incorporation of P300 measurements into a functioning man-machine loop so as to enhance the overall performance of the man-machine systems. For more details concerning our attempts to develop such biocybernetic loops, see Donchin (1976). To illustrate the approach I shall use an example described in detail by McCarthy, Kutas, and Donchin (in preparation). It is an attempt to break the speed-accuracy barrier. This study derives from the data presented by Kutas et al. (1977).

Consider an operator presented with a series of items which he must classify as belonging to one of two categories. The large majority of the items with which he is presented are not important. However, randomly interspersed within this series of neutral items are important items which must be properly classified. One can imagine a number of such examples, ranging

from the detection of defects in prescription pills on a
production line through the identification of enemy aircraft from
amongst other signals on a radar screen. In the example I shall
describe, the operators were presented on the cathode-ray tube
screen of a computer terminal with a series of names, 80% of which
were female names, 20% male names. Their task was to press a
button with one hand on the appearance of a male name, and with
the other hand on the appearance of a female name.

The subjects were either instructed to assure that their
classifications were correct; that is, they were abjured from
misidentifying female names as male and male names as female.
Under this regime reaction times to all stimuli were long. Mean
reaction time (over ten subjects) was 536 msec for correctly
identified female names, 632 msec for correctly identified male
names, and 461 msec for the incorrectly classified male names.
When subjects were instructed to be as fast as they possibly
could, regardless of the errors they made, reaction times
decreased to 389, 537, and 338, respectively. This reduction in
reaction time was purchased at the cost of many errors in
classification. The errors were probably due to response bias,
because the subjects rarely, if ever, classified a neutral item as
important. Whenever they pressed the "male" button, they were
almost invariably correct. However, 40% of the important items
were misclassified. This increase in errors with the increase in
speed is the "speed-accuracy tradeoff," presumed to be an
unshakable limit on performance (see, for example, Wood &
Jennings, 1976). One can be either fast or accurate, but rarely
both.

It occurred to us that it may be possible to incorporate a
biocybernetic error-correction algorithm in a system that would
allow subjects to respond as fast as they wished while allowing
the computer to correct for errors using an algorithm based on
P300. That this was feasible was suggested by some of the data
presented in Fig. 31. Note the Xs in the scatter diagrams. These
are trials in which subjects erred; the rare items were responded
to as if they were frequent. In every case, the reaction time was
shorter than the latency of P300. In other words, whenever the
subject acted before "thinking," he tended to err. Whenever
"thought" preceded action (as it presumably does whenever P300
latency is shorter than reaction time), the subject tended to be
correct. This interpretation of the data suggests that it should
be possible to identify the trials in which the subject erred by
evaluating the difference between reaction time and the P300
latency. McCarthy, Kutas, and Donchin (in preparation) developed
such an error-correcting biocybernetic algorithm and applied it to
the data obtained from the ten subjects that were assigned the
task of discriminating between male and female names. Briefly,

this decision-aiding procedure operated as follows. Whenever the subject gave an "important" response, the item was accepted as "important." If the subjects made a "neutral" response, the EEG was examined for the presence or absence of the P300. If P300 was absent, the trial was accepted as neutral. Those trials on which the subjects responded "frequent," but which were identified as containing a P300 by the first tier of the analysis, were subjected to further analysis in which the latency of the P300 was compared to the reaction time obtained on that trial. If reaction time was longer than P300 latency, the trial was accepted as neutral. That is, the subject's response was accepted as valid. However, if reaction time was shorter than P300 latency, the trial was considered to be a candidate for a misclassified "important" item. A third analysis was then conducted which utilized information about differences in waveform between correctly and incorrectly classified rare trials. Following this third tier of the analysis, some trials were considered to be definitely "important" and the rest were accepted as neutral.

The efficacy of this procedure can be evaluated as follows. Its benefits consist of all the important trials that were classified by the subject's response as neutral but were reclassified by the biocybernetic algorithm as important. Those are, in fact, the errors corrected by the biocybernetic algorithm. The cost consists of neutral trials which were classified correctly by the subject, but which the algorithm now considers important. The results obtained for the ten subjects show a very substantial benefit. In fact, most of the errors committed by the subjects were retrieved by the algorithm, albeit at the cost of increased errors in classifying the frequent items. Of course, in any such procedure, the costs and benefits must be evaluated in relation to the specific task. The absolute number of misclassified "frequents" following the algorithm is very large. The absolute number of retrieved "important" items is relatively small. If, however, it is the case, and we believe it often is, that in such tasks the operator's main responsibility is to avoid misclassifying the important items, then the cost-benefit analysis performed suggests that a substantial improvement in the system's performance is gained by the incorporation of the biocybernetic error-correcting code.

We do not suggest that operators engaged in classification, or managers of production lines, should hasten to purchase small, hand-held error-correcting biocybernetic gadgetry. This work is in early, developmental, stages and it may well be the case that no valid, practical application would appear for this particular example. Its importance is only in demonstrating the feasibility of utilizing electrophysiological data recorded from a subject's

scalp in complementing the data provided by the overt responses of
the subject utilizing more traditional response devices. This was
the mission of the biocybernetic program.

It appears, therefore, that through a detailed analysis of
the factors which govern the amplitude and the latency of the P300
component, it is possible to enhance interactions between human
and machine. It is possible that these data will provide an
additional and unique tool for the analysis of human information
processing. The collection of tools available for this purpose is
insufficiently rich and varied that we can afford to ignore any
such tool. I hope that this review provided evidence in support
of the assertion that the endogenous components of the human ERP
are a tool of great potential utility in the study of human
information processing.

Permission to reproduce figures was granted by authors and/or
publishers and full acknowledgement of sources appears in the
References. Specific copyright acknowledgements required by
publishers follow:

Figure 3: Cruikshank, R. M., Journal of Experimental Psychology.
   Copyright 1937 by the American Psychological Association.
   Reprinted by permission.
Figure 8: Sutton, S., et al., "Information delivery and the
   sensory evoked potential," Science, Vol. 155, pp. 1436-1439,
   1967. Copyright 1967 by the American Association for the
   Advancement of Science.
Figures 19, 26a, 26b, 27: Copyright (c) 1977, The Society for
   Psychophysiological Research. Reprinted with permission of the
   publisher from: "On Quantifying Surprise: The Variation of
   Event-Related Potentials with Subjective Probability," by C. C.
   Duncan-Johnson and E. Donchin, Psychophysiology, 1977, 14, 456-
   467.
Figure 22: Squires, K. C., et al., "Effect of stimulus sequence
   on the waveform of the cortical event-related potential,"
   Science, Vol. 193, pp. 1142-1146, 1976. Copyright 1976 by the
   American Association for the Advancement of Science.
Figure 24: Copyright 1976, The Society for Psychophysiological
   Research. Reprinted with permission of the publisher from:
   "Does P300 amplitude depend on the expectancy for physical
   stimuli or for stimulus categories?" Johnson, R. E., Jr. &
   Donchin, E. Psychophysiology, 1976, 15, 262.
Figures 30, 31: Kutas, M., et al., "Augmenting Mental
   Chronometry: The P300 as a Measure of Stimulus Evaluation
   Time," Science, Vol. 197, pp. 792-795, 1977. Copyright 1977 by
   the American Association for the Advancement of Science.
Poem excerpt from: Everyone but Thee and Me, by Ogden Nash.
   Reprinted by permission of Little Brown and Co. Copyright (c)
   by Ogden Nash. Originally appeared in The New Yorker.

REFERENCES

Barlow, J. S.  An electronic method for detecting evoked responses of the brain and for reproducing their average waveforms, Electroencephalography & Clinical Neurophysiology, 1957, 9, 340-343.

Beach, L. R., Rose, R. M., Sayeki, Y., Wise, J. A., & Carter, W. B.  Probability learning:  Response proportions and verbal estimates.  Journal of Experimental Psychology, 1970, 86, 165-170.

Becker, G. M., & McClintock, C. G.  Value:  Behavioral decision theory.  In P. R. Farnsworth, O. McNemar, & Q. McNemar (Eds.), Annual Review of Psychology, 1967, 18, 139-287.

Bostock, H., & Jarvis, M. J.  Changes in the form of the cerebral evoked response related to the speed of simple reaction time. Electroencephalography & Clinical Neurophysiology, 1970, 29, 137-145.

Brazier, M. A. B.  Evoked responses recorded from the depths of the human brain.  Annals of the New York Academy of Science, 1964, 112, 35-59.

Callaway, E., Tueting, P., & Koslow, S. (Eds.), Brain Event-Related Potentials in Man, Academic Press (in press).

Caton, R.  The electric current of the brain.  British Medical Journal, 1875, w, 278.

Chapman, R. M., & Bragdon, H. R.  Evoked responses to numerical and non-numerical visual stimuli while problem solving.  Nature, 1964, 203, 1155-1157.

Chesney, G. L.  The effects of prior expectancy and prediction outcome on the P300 component of the human average evoked potential.  Unpublished master's thesis, New Mexico State University, 1976.

Chesney, G. L. and Donchin, E.  Predictions, their confirmation, and the P300 component.  In preparation.

Ciganek, L.  Excitability cycle of the visual cortex in man. Annals of the New York Academy of Science, 1964, 112, 241-253.

Clark, D. L., Butler, R. A., & Rosner, B. S.  Dissociation of sensation and evoked responses by a general anesthetic in man. Journal of Comparative Physiological Psychology, 1969, 68, 315-319.

Clark, D. L., Butler, R. A., & Rosner, B. S.  Are evoked responses necessary?  A reply to Donchin and Sutton. Communications in Behavioral Biology, 1970, 5, 105-110.

Clynes, M., & Kohn, M.  The use of the Mnemotron for biological data storage, reproduction, and for an average transient computer. Abstracts of 4th annual meeting of the Biophysics Society:  1960, 23, Philadelphia, Pennsylvania.

Cohen, J.  Very slow brain potentials relating to expectancy:  The CNV.  In E. Donchin & D. B. Lindsley (Eds.), Average evoked potentials: Methods, results and evaluations. Washington, D.C.: U.S. Goverment Printing Office, 1969.

Cruikshank, R. M.  Human occipital brain potentials.  Journal of Experimental Psychology, 1937, 21, 625-641.

Davis, H.  Enhancement of evoked cortical potentials in humans related to a task requiring a decision. Science, 1964, 145, 182-183.

Davis, H.  Principles of electric response audiometry. The annals of otology, rhinology, and laryngology, 1976, Suppl. 28, 85, No. 3, Part 3.

Davis, P. A.  Effects of sound stimulation of the waking human brain.  Journal of Neurophysiology, 1939, 2, 494-499.

Dawson, G. D.  Cerebral responses to electrical stimulation of peripheral nerve in man. Journal of Neurology, Neurosurgery and Psychiatry, 1947, 10, 134-140.

Dawson, G. D.  A summation technique for detecting small signals in a large irregular background. Journal of Physiology, 1951, 115, 2-3.

Dawson, G. D.  A summation technique for the detection of small evoked potentials. Electroencephalography & Clinical Neurophysiology, 1954, 6, 65-84.

Debecker, J., & Desmedt, J. E.  Rate of intermodality switching disclosed by sensory evoked potentials averaged during signal detection tests. Journal of Physiology, 1966, 185, 52-53.

Deecke, L., Scheid, P., & Kornhuber, H. H. Distribution of readiness potential, pre-motion positivity, and motor potential of the human cerebral cortex preceding voluntary finger movements. Experimental Brain Research, 1969, 7, 158-168.

Donchin, E. A multivariate approach to the analysis of average evoked potentials. IEEE Transactions on Bio-Medical Engineering, 1966, BME-13, 131-139.

Donchin, E. Data analysis techniques in average evoked potential research. In E. Donchin & D. B. Lindsley (Eds.), Average evoked potentials: Methods, results and evaluations. Washington, D.C.: U.S. Goverment Printing Office, 1969.

Donchin, E. Brain electrical correlates of pattern recognition. In G. F. Inbar (Ed.), Signal Analysis and Pattern Recognition in Biomedical Engineering. New York: John Wiley, 1975.

Donchin, E. The relationship between P300 and the CNV (a correspondence). In W. C. McCallum & John R. Knott (Eds.), The responsive brain. Bristol: John Wright, 1976, pp. 222-234.

Donchin, E., Callaway, E., Cooper, R., Desmedt, J. E., Goff, W. R., Hillyard, S. A., & Sutton, S. Publication criteria for studies of evoked potentials (EP) in man. In J. E. Desmedt (Ed.), Attention, Voluntary Contraction and Event-Related Cerebral Potentials. Prog. clin. Neurophysiology, Vol. 1, Basel: Karger, 1977, pp. 1-11.

Donchin, E., & Cohen, L. Average evoked potentials and intramodality selective attention. Electroencephalography & Clinical Neurophysiology, 1967, 22, 537-546.

Donchin, E., & Cohen, L. Evoked potentials to stimuli presented to the suppressed eye in a binocular rivalry experiment. Vision Research, 1970, 10, 103-106.

Donchin, E., Gerbrandt, L. K., Leifer, L., & Tucker, L. Is the contingent negative variation contingent on a motor response? Psychophysiology, 1972, 9, 178-188.

Donchin, E., Gerbrandt, L. K., Leifer, L., & Tucker, L. R. Contingent negative variations and motor response. In W. C. McCallum & J. R. Knott (Eds.), Event-related slow potentials of the brain: Their relations to behavior. Proceedings of the 2nd International CNV Congress, Vancouver, 1971. Amsterdam: Elsevier Scientific Publishing Co., 1973.

Donchin, E., & Heffley, E.  Linear combinations in the analysis of ERPs.  In D. A. Otto (Ed.), Multidisciplinary perspectives in event-related brain potential research.  EPA-600/9-77-043, U.S. Government Printing Office, Washington, D.C.

Donchin, E., & Herning, R. I.  A simulation study of the efficacy of stepwise discriminant analysis in the detection and comparison of event-related potentials.  Electroencephalography & Clinical Neurophysiology, 1975, 38, 51-68.

Donchin, E., Kubovy, M., Kutas, M., Johnson, R., Jr., & Herning, R. I.  Graded changes in evoked response (P300) amplitude as a function of cognitive activity.  Perception & Psychophysics, 1973, 14, 319-324.

Donchin, E., & Lindsley, D. B.  Average evoked potentials and reaction times to visual stimuli.  Electroencephalography & Clinical Neurophysiology, 1966, 20, 217-223.

Donchin, E., Ritter, W., & McCallum, C.  Cognitive psychophysiology: The endogenous components of the ERP.  In E. Callaway, P. Tueting, & S. Koslow (Eds.) Brain event-related potentials in man, in press.

Donchin, E., & Smith, D. B. D.  The contingent negative variation and the late positive wave of the average evoked potential.  Electroencephalography & Clinical Neurophysiology, 1970, 29, 201-203.

Donchin, E., & Sutton, S.  The "psychological significance" of evoked responses: A comment on Clark, Butler, and Rosner.  Communications in Behavioral Biology, 1970, 5, 111-114.

Donchin, E., Tueting, P., Ritter, W., Kutas, M., & Heffley, E.  On the independence of the CNV and the P300 components of the human averaged evoked potential.  Electroencephalography & Clinical Neurophysiology, 1975, 38, 449-461.

Duncan-Johnson, C. C., & Donchin, E.  On quantifying surprise: The variation in event-related potentials with subjective probability.  Psychophysiology, 1977, 14, 456-467.

Duncan-Johnson, C. C., & Donchin, E.  Series-based vs. trial-based determinants of expectancy and P300 amplitude.  Psychophysiology, 1978, 15, 262.

Eriksen, C., & Johnson, H.  Storage and decay characteristics of nonattended auditory stimuli.  Journal of Experimental Psychology, 1964, 48, 28-36.

Falmange, J. C., Cohen, S. P., & Dwivedi, A. Two-choice reactions as an ordered memory-scanning process. In P. M. A. Rabbitt & S. Dornic (Eds.), *Attention and performance*, *V*. London: Academic Press, 1975.

Ford, J. M., Roth, W. T., Dirks, S. J., & Kopell, B. S. Evoked potential correlates of signal recognition between and within modalities. *Science*, 1973, *181*, 465-466.

Galton, F. Composite portraits. *Journal of the Anthropological Institute*, 1878, *8*, 132-142.

Garcia-Austt, E., Vanzulli, A., Bogacz, J., & Rodriguez-Barrios, R. Influence of the occular muscles upon photic habituation in man. *Electroencephalography & Clinical Neurophysiology*, 1963, *15*, 281-286.

Gilden, L., Vaughan, H. G., & Costa, L. D. Summated human EEG potentials associated with voluntary movement. *Electroencephalography & Clinical Neurophysiology*, 1966, *20*, 433-438.

Gomer, F. E., Spicuzza, R. J., & O'Donnell, R. D. Evoked potential correlates of visual item recognition during memory-scanning tasks. *Physiological Psychology*, 1976, *4*, 61-65.

Haider, M., Spong, P., & Lindsley, D. B. Attention, vigilance, and cortical evoked-potentials in humans. *Science*, 1964, *145*, 180-182.

Harter, M. R., & Salmon, L. E. Intra-modality selective attention and evoked cortical potentials to randomly presented patterns. *Electroencephalography & Clinical Neurophysiology*, 1972, *32*, 605-613.

Hartley, L. R. The effects of stimulus relevance on the cortical evoked potentials. *Quarterly Journal of Experimental Psychology*, 1970, *22*, 531-546.

Hernandez-Peon, R., Scherrer, H., & Jouvet, M. Modification of electrical activity in cochlear nucleus during "attention" in unanesthetized cats. *Science*, 1956, *123*, 331-332.

Hillyard, S. A. The CNV and the vertex evoked potential during signal detection: a preliminary report. In E. Donchin and D. B. Lindsley (Eds.), *Average Evoked Potentials: Methods, Results, and Evaluations*. Washington, D.C.: U.S. Government Printing Office, 1969.

Hillyard, S. A. The CNV and human behavior. A review. In W. C. McCallum & J. R. Knott (Eds.), Event-related slow potentials of the brain: Their relations to behavior. Proceedings of the 2nd International CNV Congress, Vancouver, 1971. Amsterdam: Elsevier Scientific Publishing Co., 1973.

Hillyard, S. A., Hink, R. F., Schwent, V. L., & Picton, T. W. Electrical signs of selective attention in the human brain. Science, 1973, 182, 177-180.

Hillyard, S. A., Squires, K. C., Bauer, J. W., & Lindsay, P. H. Evoked potential correlates of auditory signal detection. Science, 1971, 172, 1357-1360.

Irwin, D. A., Knott, J. R., McAdam, D. W., & Rebert, C. S. Motivational determinants of the "contingent negative variation." Electroencephalography & Clinical Neurophysiology, 1966, 21, 538-543.

Jewett, D. L., & Williston, J. S. Auditory evoked far fields averaged from the scalp of humans. Brain, 1971, 94, 681-696.

Johnson, R. E., Jr., & Donchin, E. Does P300 amplitude depend on the expectancy for physical stimuli or for stimulus categories? Psychophysiology, 1978, 15, 262.

Johnson, R. E., Jr. & Donchin, E. On how P300 amplitude varies with the utility of the eliciting stimuli. Electroencephalography & Clinical Neurophysiology, 1978b, 44, 424-437.

Karlin, L. Cognition, preparation, and sensory-evoked potentials. Psychological Bulletin, 1970, 73, 122-136.

Karlin, L., & Martz, M. J., Jr. Response probability and sensory-evoked potentials. In S. Kornblum (Ed.), Attention and performance, IV. New York: Academic Press, 1973.

Karlin, L., Martz, M. J., Brauth, S. E., & Mordkoff, A. M. Auditory evoked potentials, motor potentials and reaction time. Electroencephalography & Clinical Neurophysiology, 1971, 31, 129-136.

Karlin, L., Martz, M. J., & Mordkoff, A. M. Motor performance and sensory-evoked potentials. Electroencephalography & Clinical Neurophysiology, 1970, 28, 307-313.

Klinke, R., Fruhstorfer, H., & Finkenzeller, P. Evoked responses as a function of external and stored information. Electroencephalography & Clinical Neurophysiology, 1968, 25, 119-

Klorman, R., & Bentsen, E. Effects of warning-signal intensity on the early and late components of the contingent negative variation. Biological Psychology, 1975, 3, 163-175.

Kornhuber, H. H., & Deecke, L. Hirnpotentialanderungen bei willkurbewegungen und passiven bewegungen des menschen: Bereitsschaftpotential und reafferente potentiale. Pflugers Archiv fur die gesamte Physiologie des Menschen und der Tiere, 1965, 284, 1-17.

Kutas, M. Preparation to respond as manifested by movement-related brain potentials. Unpublished doctoral dissertation, University of Illinois at Urbana-Champaign, 1977.

Kutas, M., & Donchin, E. Studies of squeezing: Handedness, responding hand, response force, and asymmetry of readiness potential. Science, 1974, 186, 545-548.

Kutas, M., & Donchin, E. The effect of handedness, the responding hand, and response force on the contralateral dominance of the readiness potential. In J. Desmedt (Ed.), Attention, voluntary contraction and event-related cerebral potentials Vol. 1. Basel: Karger, 1977.

Kutas, M., & Donchin, E. The effects of subject strategies on the lateralization of movement related potentials, Proceedings of American EEG Society, Miami Beach, Florida, 1977. Electroencephalography & Clinical Neurophysiology, (in press).

Kutas, M., McCarthy, G., & Donchin, E. Augmenting mental chronometry: The P300 as a measure of stimulus evaluation time. Science, 1977, 197, 792-795.

Laming, D. R. J. Subjective probability in choice-reaction experiments. Journal of Mathematical Psychology, 1969, 6, 81-120.

Levit, R. A., Sutton, S., & Zubin, J. Evoked potential correlates of information processing in psychiatric patients. Psychological Medicine, 1973, 3, 487-494.

Levy, J. Psychobiological implications of bilateral asymmetry. In S. J. Dimond and J. G. Beaumont (Eds.), Hemispheric function in the human brain. London: Paul Elek, 1974.

Lindsley, D. B. Emotion. In S. S. Stevens (Ed.), Handbook of Experimental Psychology. New York: John Wiley, 1951.

Loveless, N. E. The effect of warning interval on signal detection and event-related slow potentials of the brain. Perception & Psychophysics, 1975, 17, 565-570.

Loveless, N. E., & Sanford, A. J. Slow potentials correlates of preparatory sets. Biological Psychology, 1974, 1, 303-314.

Low, M. D., Borda, R. P., Frost, J. D., Jr., and Kellaway, P. Surface-negative slow-potential shift associated with conditioning in man. Neurology (Minneapolis), 1966, 16, 771-782.

Mackworth, N. H. Researches on the measurement of human performance. Medical research council special reports, Series No. 268. London: H.M.S.O., 1950.

Massaro, D. Retroactive interference in short-term recognition memory for pitch. Journal of Experimental Psychology, 1970, 83, 32-39.

McAdam, D. W. The contingent negative variations. In R. F. Thompson & M. M. Patterson (Eds.), Bioelectric recording techniques: Part B Electroencephalography and human brain potentials. New York: Academic Press, 1974.

McAdam, D. W., & Rubin, E. H. Readiness potential, vertex positive wave, contingent negative variation and accuracy of perception. Electroencephalography & Clinical Neurophysiology, 1971, 30, 511-517.

McCallum, W. C., & Papakostopoulos, D. The CNV and reaction time in situations of increasing complexity. In W. C. McCallum & J. R. Knott (Eds.), Event-related slow potentials of the brain: Their relations to behavior. Proceedings of the 2nd International CNV Congress, Vancouver, 1971. Amsterdam: Elsevier Scientific Publishing Co., 1973.

McCarthy, G., & Donchin, E. The effects of temporal and event uncertainty in determining the waveforms of the auditory event related potential (ERP). Psychophysiology, 1976, 13, 581-590.

McCarthy, G., & Donchin, E. Brain potentials associated with structural and functional visual matching. Neuropsychologia, in press.

McCarthy, G., Kutas, M., & Donchin, E. Breaking the speed-accuracy barrier: Detection of errors in a choice reaction time paradigm using P300 latency. Manuscript in preparation.

Messick, D. M., & Rapoport, A.  A comparison of two payoff functions on multiple-choice decision behavior.  Journal of Experimental Psychology, 1965, 69, 75-83.

Moray, N.  Attention, selective processes in vision and hearing. London: Hutchinson, 1969.

Morrell, L. & Morrell, F.  Evoked potentials and reaction times: A study of intra-individual variability.  Electroencephalography & Clinical Neurophysiology, 1966, 20, 567-575.

Myers, J. L.  Probability learning and sequence learning.  In W. K. Estes  (Ed.),  Handbook of learning and cognitive processes, Vol. 3.  Hillsdale, N.J.: Lawrence Erlbaum Associates, 1976.

Naatanen, R.  Selective attention and evoked potentials.  Annales Academiae Scientiarum Fennicae, 1967, 151, 1-226.

Naatanen, R.  Evoked potential, EEG, and slow potential correlates of selective attention.  Acta Psychologica, 1970, 33, 178-192.

Naatanen, R.  Selective attention and evoked potentials in humans--a critical review.  Behavioral Biology, 1975, 2, 237-307.

Neimark, E. D., & Shuford, E. H.  Comparision of predictions and estimates in a probability-learning situation.  Journal of Experimental Psychology, 1959, 57, 294-298.

Parasuraman, R., & Davies, D. R.  Response and evoked potential latencies associated with commission errors in visual monitoring. Perception and Psychophysics, 1975, 17, 465-468.

Paul, D. D., & Sutton, S.  Evoked potential correlates of psycho-physical judgments: The threshold problem.  A new reply to Clark, Butler, and Rosner.  Behavioral Biology, 1973, 9, 421-433.

Pearson, K.  The life, letters, and labours of Francis Galton. Vol. 2, Researches of Middle Life.  Cambridge, Eng.: Cambridge University Press, 1924.

Picton, T. W., Campbell, K. B., Baribeau-Braun, J., & Proulx, G. B.  The neurophysiology of human attention: A tutorial review.  In J. Requin (Ed.), Attention and Performance, VII, in press.

Picton, T. W., Hillyard, S. A., & Galambos, R.  Cortical evoked responses to omitted stimuli.  Major problems of brain electrophysiology, Moscow: USSR Academy of Sciences, 1974.

Picton, T. W., Hillyard, S. A., Krausz, H. T., & Galambos, R. Human auditory evoked potentials, I: evaluation of components. Electroencephalography & Clinical Neurophysiology, 1974, 36, 179-190.

Pribram, K. H., & McGuinness, D. Arousal, activation, and effort in the control of attention. Psychological Review, 1975, 82, 116-149.

Reber, A. S., & Millward, R. B. Event observation in probability learning. Journal of Experimental Psychology, 1968, 77, 317-327.

Rebert, C. S., & Tecce, J. J. A summary of CNV and reaction time. In W. C. McCallum & J. R. Knott (Eds.), Event-related slow potentials of the brain: Their relations to behavior. Proceedings of the 2nd International CNV Congress, Vancouver, 1971. Amsterdam: Elsevier Scientific Publishing Company, 1973, 173-178.

Ritter, W., Simson, R., & Vaughan, H. G., Jr. Association cortex potentials and reaction time in auditory discrimination. Electroencephalography & Clinical Neurophysiology, 1972, 33, 547-555.

Ritter, W., & Vaughan, H. G., Jr. Averaged evoked responses in vigilance and discrimination: A reassessment. Science, 1969, 164, 326-328.

Rohrbaugh, J. W., Donchin, E., & Eriksen, C. W. Decision making and the P300 component of the cortical evoked response. Perception & Psychophysics, 1974, 15, 368-374.

Rohrbaugh, J. W., Syndulko, K., & Lindsley, D. B. Brain wave components of the contingent negative variation in humans. Science, 1976, 191, 1055-1057.

Rosner, B. S., Allison, T., Swanson, E., & Goff, R. W. A new instrument for the summation of evoked responses from the nervous system. Electroencephalography & Clinical Neurophysiology, 1960, 12, 532-545.

Roth, W. T., Ford, J. M., Lewis, S. J., & Kopell, B. S. Effects of stimulus probability and task-relevance on event-related potentials. Psychophysiology, 1976, 13, 311-317.

Roth, W. T., Kopell, B. S., Tinklenberg, J. R., Darley, C. F., Sikora, R., & Vesecky, T. B. The contingent negative variation during a memory retrieval task. Electroencephalography & Clinical Neurophysiology, 1975, 38, 171-174.

Ruchkin, D. S., & Sutton, S. Visual evoked and emitted potentials and stimulus significance. Psychonomic Society Bulletin, 1973, 2, 144-146.

Ruchkin, D. S., & Sutton, S. Emitted P300 potentials and temporal uncertainties. Electroencephalography & Clinical Neurophysiology, in press.

Satterfield, J. H. Evoked cortical response enhancement and attention in man. A study of responses to auditory and shock stimuli. Electroencephalography & Clinical Neurophysiology, 1965, 19, 470-475.

Satterfield, J. H. & Cheatum, D. Evoked cortical potential correlates of attention in human subjects. Electroencephalography & Clinical Neurophysiology, 1964, 17, 456.

Schwent, V. L., & Hillyard, S. A. Evoked potential correlates of selective attention with multiple-channel auditory inputs. Electroencephalography & Clinical Neurophysiology, 1975, 38, 131-138.

Schwent, V. L., Hillyard, S. A., & Galambos, R. Selective attention and the auditory vertex potential. I. Effects of stimulus delivery rate. Electroencephalography & Clinical Neurophysiology, 1976, 40, 604-614. (a)

Schwent, V. L., Hillyard, S. A., & Galambos, R. Selective attention and the auditory vertex potential. II. Effects of signal intensity and masking noise. Electroencephalography & Clinical Neurophysiology, 1976, 40, 615-622. (b)

Schwent, V. L., Snyder, E., & Hillyard, S. A. Auditory evoked potentials during multichannel selective listening: Role of pitch and localization cues. Journal of Experimental Psychology: Human Perception & Performance, 1976, 2, 313-325.

Sheridan, T. B., & Ferrell, W. R. Man-machine systems: Information, control, and decision models of human performance, Cambridge, Mass.: MIT Press, 1974.

Smith, D. B. D., Donchin, E., Cohen, L., & Starr, A. Auditory averaged evoked potentials in man during selective binaural listening. Electroencephalography & Clinical Neurophysiology, 1970, 28, 146-152.

Sokolov, E. N. In Maltzman, I. & Cole, K. (Eds.), Handbook of Contemporary Soviet Psychology. New York: Basic Books, 1969.

Sperling, G.   The information   available   in   brief   visual
presentations.   Psychological Monographs, 1960, 11 (Whole No.
498).

Squires, K. C., & Donchin, E.   Beyond averaging:   The use of
discriminant functions to recognize event related potentials
elicited by single auditory stimuli.   Electroencephalography &
Clinical Neurophysiology, 1976, 41, 449-459.

Squires, K. C., Donchin, E., Herning, R. I., & McCarthy, G.   On
the influence of task relevance and stimulus probability on
event-related potential components.   Electroencephalography &
Clinical Neurophysiology, 1977, 42, 1-14.

Squires, K., Petuchowski, S., Wickens, C., & Donchin, E.   The
effects of stimulus sequence on event related potentials: A
comparison of visual and auditory sequences.   Perception &
Psychophysics, 1977, 22, 31-40.

Squires, K. C., Wickens, C., Squires, N. K., & Donchin, E.   The
effect of stimulus sequence on the waveform of the cortical
event-related potential.   Science, 1976, 193, 1142-1146.

Squires, K. C., Wickens, C., Squires, N. K., & Donchin, E.
Sequential dependencies of the waveform of the event-related
potential:   a   preliminary   report.   In   D. A. Otto   (Ed.),
Multidisciplinary perspectives in event-related brain potential
research.   EPA-6001-9-77-043, U.S. Government Printing Office,
Washington, D.C., in press.

Squires, N. K., Donchin, E., Squires, K. C., & Grossberg, S.
Bisensory stimulation: Inferring decision-related processes from
the P300 component.   Journal of Experimental Psychology: Human
Perception & Performance, 1977, 3, 299-315.

Squires, N. K., Squires, K. C., & Hillyard, S. A.   Two varieties
of long-latency positive waves evoked by unpredictable auditory
stimuli   in   man.   Electroencephalography   &   Clinical
Neurophysiology, 1975, 38, 387-401.

Stuss, D. T., & Picton, T. W.   Neurophysiological correlates of
human concept learning.   Behavioral Biology, in press.

Sutton, S. The specification of psychological variables in an
average evoked potential experiment.   In   E.   Donchin & D. B.
Lindsley (Eds.), Average evoked potentials: Methods, results and
evaluations.   Washington, D.C.: U.S. Goverment Printing Office,
1969.

Sutton, S., Braren, M., Zubin, J., & John, E. R.   Evoked-potential correlates of stimulus uncertainty.   Science, 1965, 150, 1187–1188.

Sutton, S., Tueting, P., Zubin, J., & John, E. R.   Information delivery and the sensory evoked potential.   Science, 1967, 155, 1436–1439.

Syndulko, K., & Lindsley, D. B.   Motor and sensory determinants of cortical slow potential shifts in man.   In J. E. Desmedt (Ed.), Attention, voluntary contraction and event-related cerebral potentials, Vol. 1.   Basel:   Karger, 1977, 97–131.

Tecce, J. J.   Contingent negative variation (CNV) and psychological processes in man.   Psychological Bulletin, 1972, 77, 73–108.

Thatcher, R.   Evoked potential correlates of hemispheric lateralization during semantic information processing.   In S. Harnad, R. W. Doty, L. Goldstein, J. Jaynes, & G. Krauthamer (Eds.), Lateralization in the Nervous System.   New York:   Academic Press, 1977.

Theios, J.   Reaction time measurements in the study of memory processes:   Theory and data.   In G. H. Bower (Ed.), The psychology of learning and motivation:   Advances in research and theory, 7.   New York, Academic Press, 1973.

Tueting, P.   Event-related potentials, cognitive events, and information processing.   In D. Otto (Ed.), Multidisciplinary Perspectives in Event-Related Brain Potential Research.   Washington, D.C.:   EPA-600/9-77-043, U.S. Government Printing Office, in press.

Tueting, P., Sutton, S., & Zubin, J.   Quantitative evoked potential correlates of the probability of events.   Psychophysiology, 1970, 7, 385–394.

Vaughan, H. G., Jr.   The relationship of brain activity to scalp recordings of event-related potentials.   In E. Donchin & D. B. Lindsley (Eds.), Average evoked potentials:   Methods, results and evaluations.   Washington, D.C.:   U.S. Goverment Printing Office, 1969.

Vlek, C. A. J.   Multiple probability learning.   In A. F. Sanders (Ed.), Attention and performance, III.   Amsterdam:   North Holland Publishing Co., 1970.

Walter, W. G., Cooper, R., Aldridge, V. J., McCallum, W. C., & Winter, A. L. Contingent negative variation: An electric sign of sensorimotor association and expectancy in the human brain. Nature (London), 1964, 203, 380-384.

Weerts, T. C., & Lang, P. J. The effects of eye fixation and stimulus and response location on the contingent negative variation (CNV). Biological Psychology, 1973, 1, 1-19.

Weinberg, H., Walter, W. G., & Crow, H. J. Intracerebral events in humans related to real and imaginary stimuli. Electroencephalography & Clinical Neurophysiology, 1970, 29, 1-9.

Wilkinson, R. T. Relationship between CNV, its resolution, and the evoked response. In McCallum, W. C. & Knott, T. R. (Eds.), The Responsive Brain. Bristol, England, 1973. Bristol: John Wright, 1976.

Wilkinson, R. T., & Morlock, H. C., Jr. Auditory evoked response and reaction time. Electroencephalography & Clinical Neurophysiology, 1967, 23, 50-56.

Wilkinson, R. T., & Spence, M. T. Determinants of the post-stimulus resolution of the contingent negative variation (CNV). Electroencephalography & Clinical Neurophysiology, 1973, 35, 503-509.

Wood, C. C., & Jennings, R. Speed-accuracy tradeoff functions in choice reaction time: Experimental designs and computational procedures. Perception and Psychophysics, 1976, Vol. 19(1), 92-101.

Woodworth, R. S. & Schlosberg, H. Experimental Psychology, Henry Holt & Co., New York, 1954.

Woody, C. D. Characterization of an adaptive filter for the analysis of variable latency neuroelectric signals. Medical & Biological Engineering, 1967, 5, 539-553.

# NEUROELECTRICAL CORRELATES OF SEMANTIC PROCESSES

Dennis L. Molfese, Andrew Papanicolaou, Thomas M. Hess
& Victoria J. Molfese

Department of Psychology, Southern Illinois University

at Carbondale, Carbondale, Il. 62901

In recent years averaged evoked response (AER) techniques have been used with increasing frequency in attempts to study the possible relationships between brain responses and linguistic processes (Waner, Teyler, & Thompson, 1977). Researchers have succeed in demonstrating that certain major components of the AER are sensitive to acoustic and phonological changes such as inflection and phoneme category membership (Wood, Goff, & Day, 1971; Wood, 1975), voicing (Molfese a, in press) formant structure and consonant transitions (Molfese, Nunez, Seibert, & Ramanaiah, 1976; Molfese b, in press). In addition, AER components sensitive to syntactic and semantic factors have also been identified (Begleiter & Platz, 1969; Brown, Marsh, & Smith, 1973, 1976; Chapman, McCrary, Chapman & Bragdon, in press; Shelburne, 1972, 1973; Thatcher a, in press; Thatcher b, in press). Such research strongly suggests that various linguistic processes can be successfully assessed with AER techniques. However, few studies have attempted to investigate how the various linguistic elements such as phonology and semantics interact to produce differences in the AER. Chomsky & Halle (1968) have proposed a serial processing model which suggests that the language listener must first encode each phonological element in the order of its appearance and then, only after all such elements have been encoded, proceed to the semantic and syntactic processing levels. Others (Liberman, Cooper, Shankweiler & Studdert-Kennedy, 1967) have argued in favor of a parallel processing model in which certain acoustic elements such as consonant transition provide cues for identifying both the consonant and the subsequent vowel sounds. While the serial model holds that semantic processing would only begin after all phonological processing has been completed, the parallel model predicts that such processing would be completed prior to the actual presentation of

all phonological elements.  Semantic processing would then begin
prior to perception of the entire stimulus.

The majority of AER studies of linguistic processes have
employed standard AER analyses based on amplitude and latency
measures of major AER components.  Recently, however, a number
of researchers have employed multivariate analysis procedures in
attempts to identify more basic components that underly various
portions of the AER (Chapman, McCrary, Bragdon & Chapman, 1977;
Chapman et al, in press; Molfese et al, 1976, Molfese a, in press;
Molfese b, in press).

These analysis procedures were employed in the experiments
to be outlined in this chapter.  Although the findings from such
studies have identified some AER components which appear to relate
to general EP components such as P300 and CNV (Chapman et al,
1977), a number of components have been isolated which have not
been previously identified with traditional amplitude and latency
measures.  Since few studies employing the principal components
analysis techniques outlined by Chapman et al (1977) have been
published and these studies have generally involved quite different stimulus and task variables, there has been little opportunity to assess the reliability of such factors.  The stimulus
selection and construction for experiment 1 provided an initial
opportunity to assess the reliability of certain effects across
studies involving the principal components analysis.

The first study involved 10 right handed adults who listened
to a randomly ordered series of four meaningful and four nonsense consonant-vowel-consonant (CVC) syllables.  Each stimulus
was 350 msec in length.  The meaningful stimuli consisted of the
words /kaeb, paek, gaep, baek/ while the nonsense CVCs included
the items /kaek, paeb, gaek, baep/.  These two groups of CVCs
were matched in terms of voicing and place of articulation for
the initial and final consonants.  The middle vowel was the same
for all stimuli.  All subjects were instructed to press one telegraph key after a two second delay if they heard a word or a
second key if they heard a nonsense syllable.  Auditory evoked
potentials (AEPs) were recorded from $T_3$ and $T_4$ (Jasper, 1958) referred to linked ear lobes.

The AEPs were digitized at 5 msec intervals for a 550 msec
period (110 points) and averaged off line.  The 160 averages
from the group which were based on 16 repetitions of each stimulus
were submitted to a principal components analysis (BMD08M) after
Chapman, McCrary, Bradgon & Chapman  (1977) and Molfese et al
(1976).  The input data matrix consisted of the 110 time points
for each average which were treated as variables and the 160
averaged evoked potentials which were treated as cases.  The
principal components analysis identified 10 factors which accounted

for 93.16% of the total variance when the Eigen = 1.0 criterion
was used.  These factors were then rotated using the varimax
method.  Subsequently, the factor scores for each factor were
treated as dependent measures in independent Hemisphere (2) X
Meaning (2) X Voice of Initial Consonant (2) X Place of Articulation of Initial Consonant (2) Analyses of Variance in an attempt
to identify any relationships that might exist between the extracted factors and specific levels of the independent variables.
Intriguingly, several factors were found to vary systematically
as a function of stimulus meaning.  A main effect for meaning
(F = 11.67, df = 1, 9, p < .01) was found for Factor 1.  The
major component of this factor occurred during completion of the
final consonant sound between 320 msec and 440 msec following
stimulus onset.  A main effect for meaning was also found for
Factor 7 (F = 8.78, df = 1, 9, p < .05).  This factor was characterized by a major component that peaked between 6 and 60 msec
after onset.  The initial consonant burst and the beginnings of
the first consonant-vowel transition occurred at this time.  Factor
10 was the third factor that was sensitive to meaning differences
(F = 8.11, df = 1, 9, p < .05).  The major component of this last
factor occurred between 240 and 280 msec and overlapped in time
the end of the vowel sound.  The group evoked potentials for the
meaning and nonsense conditions are presented in Figure 1.
Positive polarity is up in this and in all subsequent figures.
Here, the three factors that reflected meaning differences are
indicated in the original waveforms.  Note that initial portion
of the component labeled "7" was the only one to be characterized
by larger positive amplitude in the nonsense condition.  The
negative going portion of this component, although apparently
larger in the meaning condition, was characterized by a great
deal of variability across subjects and was not found to be a
reliable indicator of meaning differences.  The other two factors
reflected larger amplitudes in the meaning condition.  The presence
of such differences in amplitude indicates that amplitude alone
can not be interpreted as an uniquivocal indicator of linguistic
processing.  Rather such differences could reflect a variety of
different multidimensional operations that might be involved in
such tasks.  The meaningful and nonsense stimulus groups were
matched on the basis of articulatory and acoustic features.  The
only difference between these two groups was due to stimulus
meaning.  The subject, it should be recalled, had to attend to
the final consonant in order to determine if the stimulus was
meaningful.  Factors 1 and 10 both contained major components that
overlapped in time the final portions of the stimulus.  In both
cases, changes in these components occurred either as the subject
heard the final consonant sound (more specifically, the transition
from the vowel to the final consonant) or just after completion
of the final sound.  A serial processing model of speech perception
would suggest that subjects would store  each sound in memory as
it occurred in order to identify the stimulus after receiving the

final consonant. However, the major component for Factor 7 occurred during the initial consonant burst, long before the presentation of the final consonant necessary to differentiate words
from nonsense syllables. Consequently, parallel processing of
speech cues must have been involved (Liberman et al, 1967). Some
aspect of the initial consonant burst had to contain information
concerning later sounds. Such notions are in line with research
conducted over the last two decades which focused on coarticulated
speech cues (Daniloff & Moll, 1968; Ali, Gallagher, Goldstein &
Daniloff, 1971). Coarticulation refers to the notion that the
production of speech sounds are influenced by adjacent speech
sounds. Daniloff & Moll (1968), for example, were able to demonstrate with cineflurograph techniques that lip rounding began
during closure of an initial consonant even though this feature
only characterized a vowel sound that occurred four consonants
later in that utterance. Other researchers have been able to
demonstrate that listeners attend to such coarticulated cues
and can use them effectively to identify later speech sounds.
Ali et al (1971) removed the final consonant or vowel-consonant
series from CVC and CVVC syllables. The abreviated syllables
were then presented to a group of subjects who were to indicate
whether the final consonant was nasal or non nasal. Responses
of all subjects were well above chance levels. In light of these
studies and the findings from the present study it would seem
likely that some information concerning the final consonant sound
is contained in the initial consonant burst and that language
listeners can make use of such early cues. However, there is a
second point that should be noted in light of Factor 7. The
latencies for the major component of this factor ranged from 6 to
60 msec after stimulus onset. Such early latencies have generally
been thought to reflect subcortical processing (Jewitt, Romano &
Williston, 1970). If this is indeed the case, then some semantic
processing must occur at that level. Such processes would involve
not only the identification of meaningful materials, but also
perhaps the mechanisms responsible for recognizing various acoustic
cues that carry necessary information for the identification of
such materials. The findings outlined in the present study would
appear to be the first indications of such mechanisms although
there have been a number of studies on subcortical language mechanisms (Ojemann, 1975; Brown, 1975).

The present study also offerred an opportunity to assess the
consistency of factors identified by the principal components
analysis across studies. Factor 3 was sensitive to changes in
voicing of the initial consonant (F = 14.6, df = 1,9 p < .01).
This factor differentiated the voiced consonants /g, b/ from
the unvoiced consonants /k, p/. The latencies for the major
component of this factor occurred between 65 msec and 140 msec
following stimulu onset. This factor is presented on the right
in Figure 2 (study 1). The latencies for the major component

**MEANING** **NONSENSE**

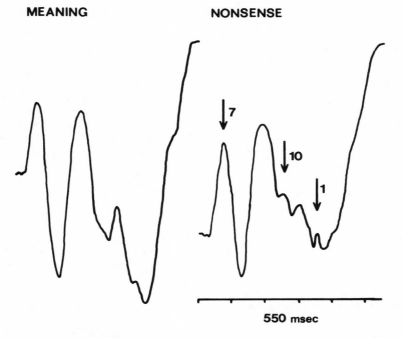

Figure 1. Group AEPs for the meaning and nonsense conditions.

**VOT STUDY** **STUDY 1**

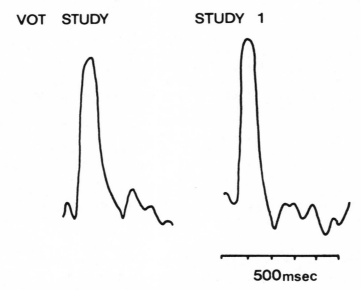

Figure 2. Factor loading for the AEP components sensitive to voiced/voiceless distinctions for two experiments.

of Factor 4 from an earlier study that involved only the manipulation of voicing - voice onset time (VOT)-were identical to
those for Factor 3 of the present study.  This factor (VOT study)
is also presented graphically in Figure 2.  The group averaged
evoked potentials for the voiced and not voiced stimuli are
presented in Figure 3 for both studies.  In both cases, the $P_1$,
$N_1$ and $P_2$ components were larger for the voiced condition
than for not voiced condition.  Even though the two studies involved different stimuli (the VOT study involved the CV syllables
/ba/ and /pa/), different number of stimuli, different tasks and
different subject populations, the factors from the two studies
that were sensitive to voicing changes were essentially the same
in terms of both amplitude and latency.  Such comparisons across
studies suggest that the factors identified by the principal
components analyses are reliable.

     In light of the success of the first study in identifying
portions of the evoked potential that appeared to reflect general
semantic processes, a second study was conducted in an attempt to
identify portions of the brain's electrical responses that might
reflect more specific semantic processes.  This study involved
presenting the word ball to subjects who were cued beforehand to
image or think of the name for two different concepts of ball--an
object (baseball, football) or a dance (fireman's ball, masquerade
ball).  In all cases, AEPs were recorded only to the word ball
and then the different conditions analyzed in an attempt to identify portions of the AEP that might be sensitive to conceptual
differences.

     Eight right handed adults, four males and four females with
a mean age of 25.6 years (range - 21.4 to 30.3 years), listened to
a stimulus tape that contained 64 repetitions of the word "ball".
The stimulus was 350 msec in duration and was produced by a native
American English speaker with a general American dialect.  The
testing procedures were identical to those employed in experiment
1 with the exception that four 5" x 7" cue cards were also used.
These consisted of a drawing of a baseball, a football, a fireman's hat and a face mask.  The S was shown one of these cue
cards approximately 10 to 15 seconds prior to stimulus onset.  The
card was then removed approximately 5 seconds before the auditory
stimulus was presented.  The stimulus tape was presented twice to
all Ss.  During the first presentation of the tape, half of the Ss
were instructed to image the object represented by the cue card
until they saw the next cue.  The Ss were instructed to image a
baseball or football when shown those cues.  The card with the
fireman's hat was a cue to image a ballroom dance (Fireman's Ball)
in which the dancers wore formal evening dress and the card with
the mask was a cue to image a Masquerade Ball dance.  The other
half of the Ss were instructed to think of the name of the cue
until they saw the next cue.  Half of the subjects were instructed

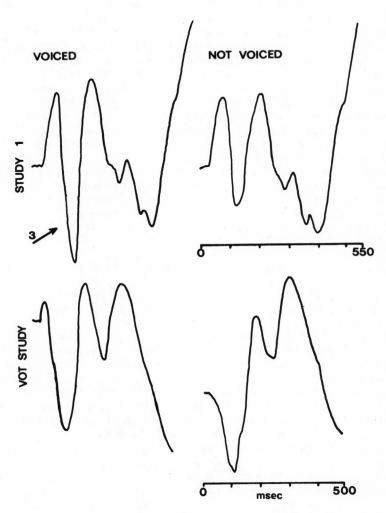

Figure 3.    Group AEPs for voiced and not voiced conditions for 2 experiments.

to image first while the other half of the subjects were instructed to think of the name of the cue. For the second task
the instructions were reversed for the two groups. Analyses performed were similar to those described for experiment 1. One
hundred twenty-eight averages were obtained from the 16 repetitions
of each stimulus for each of the two tasks (imaging, naming) for
each hemisphere, for the two sexes, for the four kinds of ball
for each of the eight subjects. A 100 (time point variables) x
128 (averaged evoked potential cases) input data matrix was then
constructed. Intercorrelations between the 100 variables were
then submitted to a principal components analysis. Using the
Eigen = 1.0 criterion, ten factors accounting for 93.86% of the
total variance were obtained and rotated using the varimax method
(Mulaik, 1972) with the BMDO8M computer program (Dixon, 1972).
The centroid and the ten factors obtained by the principal components analysis are plotted in Figure 4. The factor scores for each
factor were then treated as the dependent variable in an analysis
of variance (Myers, 1972) using the BMDO8V program (Dixon, 1972).
These Hemisphere (2) X Sex (2) X Task (2) X Meaning (4) analyses
of variance were performed in order to determine if any relationships existed between the factors and specific levels of the
independent variables.

One component, Factor 10, did appear to reflect conceptual
differences in the AEPs to the word "ball". The latencies of
the major components for this factor occurred between 385 and
435 msec. Planned comparisons of the Hemisphere x Meaning interaction indicated that LH responded differentially to the two concepts. This effect is presented graphically in Figure 5. The
factor scores plotted along the ordinate in this graph are the
means for the dependent measures in the analysis of variance.
These means reflect the weights for Factor 10. The LH apparently
responded similarly in the Baseball and Football conditions
(Stimuli A and B). It also failed to differentiate between the
Fireman's Ball and the Masquerade Ball conditions (Stimuli C and
D). However, only the LH distinguished between these two concepts
of ball---Object (A,B) versus Dance (C,D). The group averaged
evoked potentials for the Object and Dance conditions are compared
in Figure 6. Factor 10 corresponds to the late negative component
in both waveforms. This component is noticeably larger in the
Object than in the Dance condition. An additional component also
characterized the Dance concept. Given that only one auditory
stimulus was used for all conditions, these differences in the
AEP had to reflect some internal processing differences. In
addition, given that this factor was not characterized by a Task
effect or a Meaning X Task interaction, the conceptual component
tapped by this factor was the same regardless of whether subjects
were asked to image or think of the two concepts.

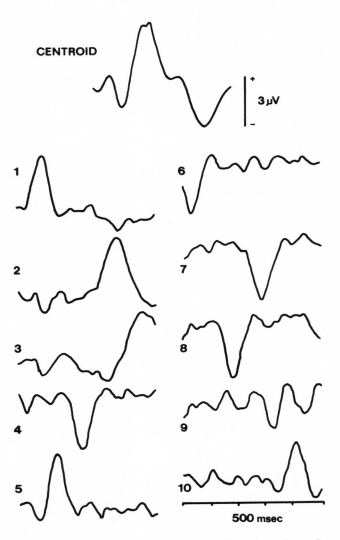

Figure 4.   The centroid and the 10 factors for the second experiment.

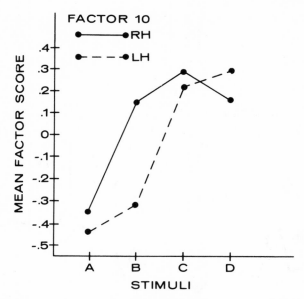

Figure 5.   Mean factor scores for the left and right hemispheres for the four stimulus conditions.

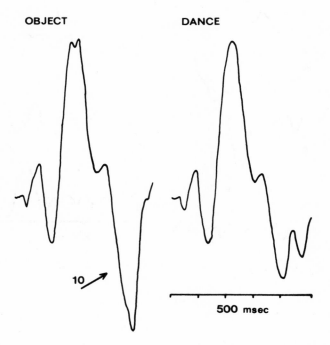

Figure 6.   Group AEPs for the two stimulus concepts.

Other components of the AER were sensitive to task variables. A main effect for Task was found for Factor 5 (F = 7.69, df = 1, 6, p < .05). Reliable differences occurred in the major components between 110 msec and 185 msec following stimulus onset when subjects were involved in the imagery task. The group averaged evoked potentials elicited during the Imagery and Verbal Tasks are presented in Figure 7. As indicated in the figure, the portion of the AER between points a and b was the area sensitive to task differences. In this case, the $P_1$ - $N_2$ and the $N_2$ - $P_3$ components were larger for the Image condition than for the Verbal condition. A Main effect for Task was also found for Factor 7 (F = 8.05, df = 1, 6, p < .05). This effect was due to the Task X Sex interaction (F = 6.01, df = 1, 6, p < .05) in which the males responded differently to the two tasks while the females did not. This effect is illustrated in Figure 8. Such sex effects have been noted by other researchers and have been theorized to reflect fundamental differences in cortical organization between males and females (Witelson, 1977). Such effects have not been previously found in AER studies involving acoustic rather than semantic processes even though those studies employed similar analyses (Molfese b, in press). Consequently, the findings of the present study could reflect differences in higher cortical function associated with cognitive processes rather than subcortical neural processes.

Significant Main effects were also found for Hemispheres (Factors 2, 3, 4, 6, 7, and 8). Although all these factors were sensitive to such differences, they did not behave uniformlly. These factors differed from each other in latency and in polarity (cf Figure 4). The major components for Factors 2 and 3 were negative in polarity for the LH and positive for the RH. These polarity differences were reversed for the two hemispheres for Factors 4, 6, 7 and 8. Such differences indicate that the two hemispheres were responding to the stimuli in different ways. Such effects have been noted previously across both acoustic and semantic studies (Molfese a, in press; Molfese b, in press; Molfese, Freeman & Palermo, 1975; Molfese et al, 1976). It should be noted that such differences in polarity reflect differences in the normalized distribution of the factor scores. As such, a positive weighting can be considered to be larger numerically than a negative one. Consequently, one could interpret Factors 2 and 3 to reflect more LH than RH processing while Factors 4, 6, 7 and 8 would reflect more RH than LH processing. The RH was apparently more involved in the earlier portions of the AER while the LH was dominant during the final portions.

A Sex X Hemisphere interaction (F = 16.22, df = 1, 6 p < .01) was found for Factor 1. A post hoc scheffe analysis indicated that this interaction was due to differences in LH responding between the males and females (p < .01). This effect is presented graphically in Figure 9. A Sex X Hemisphere interaction was also

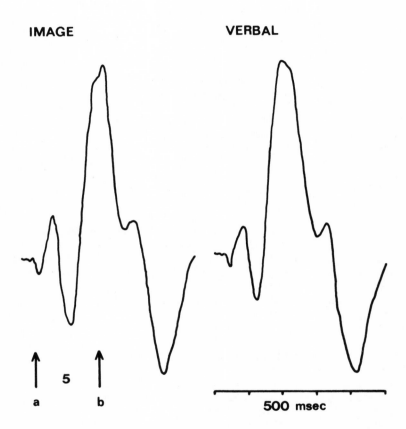

Figure 7.    Group AEPs for the two task conditions.

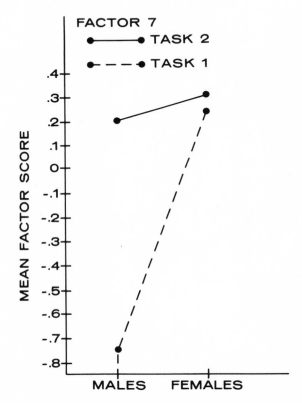

Figure 8.   Mean factor scores for males in the two task conditions.

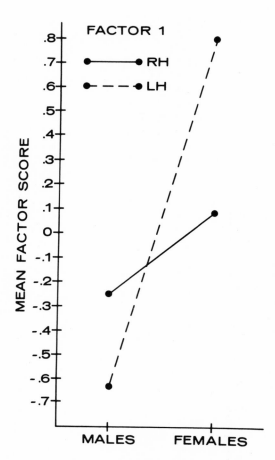

Figure 9.   Mean factor scores for the two hemispheric responses of males and females.

found for Factor 9 ($F = 20.25$, df = 1, 6, $p < .01$).  This effect, however, was due to RH differences between the two groups ($p < .01$). Such sex related effects are similar to those reported earlier with infants and preschool children.  As was the case with the Task X Sex interaction, such effects had not previously been found with adults in studies involving only acoustic tasks.  Again, such effects could reflect cortical differences in cognitive linguistic processes which do not appear in tasks which perhaps minimally tap such skills.

In summary, it appears that both experiments did lead to the identification of components of the AER which were sensitive to semantic and conceptual processes.  The findings from experiment 1 can be used to support the notion that there is a perceptual correlate of coarticulation.  Certain cues appear to be present in the initial consonant burst which provide information concerning later speech sounds.  Furthermore, given the early latencies of one AER component (as reflected in Factor 7), it appears that some subcortical region is able to utilize this information for semantic processing.  Experiment 1 also provided the basis for assessing the reliability of factors identified by the principal components analysis across studies.  Molfese (a, in press) identified one component that was sensitive to VOT changes in a phoneme identification task.  A component with similar latencies that also discriminated VOT was identified in experiment 1 even though subjects were involved in a quite different task and exposed to different stimuli than those employed by Molfese (a, in press).  Such findings appear to further support the reliability of multivariate analyses with AER data.

In experiment 2, one portion of the AER waveform (Factor 10) was found to be sensitive to the different concepts of Ball that subjects were instructed to either verbally think of or image.  In all cases, the AERs were elicited by exactly the same stimulus, the word "ball".  Consequently, the differences identified by means of the principal components analysis had to be due to some difference in the subjects' internal processing.  Such findings when placed in the perspective of the present volume suggests that the ambitious goals of deciphering the neural code as outlined by the work of such pioneers as Begleiter & Platz (1969) and Chapman et al (1977) may be realized in the not too distant future.

References

Ali, L.  Gallagher, T., Goldstein, J. & Daniloff, R.  Perception
    of coarticulated nasality.  Journal of the Acoustical Society
    of America, 1971, 49, 538-540.

Begleiter, H. & Platz, H.  Cortical evoked potentials of semantic
    stimuli.  Psychophysiology, 1969, 6, 91-100.

Brown, J. W.  On the neural organization of language:  thalamic
    and cortical relationships.  Brain & Language, 1975, 2, 18-30.

Brown, W. S., Marsh, J. T., & Smith, J. C.  Contextual meaning
    effects on speech evoked potentials.  Behavioral Biology,
    1973, 9, 755-761.

Brown, W. S., Marsh, J. T. & Smith, J. C.  Evoked potential wave-
    form differences produced by the perception of different
    meanings of an ambiguous phrase.  Journal of Electroencephalo-
    graphy & Clinical Neurophysiology, 1976, 41, 113-123.

Chapman, R. M., J. W. McCrary, H. R.  Bragoon, & J. A.  Chapman.
    In press.  Latent components of evoked potentials functionally
    related to information processing.  In J. E.  Desmedt (Ed.),
    Language and hemispheric specialization in man:  Cerebral
    event related potentials.  Basel: Karger, 1977.

Chapman, R. M., McCrary, J. W., Chapman, J. A., & Bragdon, H. R.
    Brain responses related to semantic meaning.  Brain & Language,
    in press.

Chomsky, N. & Halle, M.  Sound patterns of English.  New York: John
    Wiley & Sons, 1968.

Daniloff, R. G., & Moll, K. L.  Coarticulation of lip rounding.
    Journal of Speech & Hearing Research, 1968, 11, 707-721.

Dixon, W. J.  BMD Biomedical Computer Program: X-series supplement.
    Berkeley:  University of California Press, 1972.

Jasper, H. H.  The ten-twenty electrode system of the international
    federation of societies for electroencephalography:  Appendix
    to report of the committee on methods of clinical examination
    in electroencephalography.  The Journal of Electroencephalo-
    graphy and Clinical Neurophysiology, 1958, 10, 371.

Jewett, D. L., Romano, M. N. & Williston, J. S.  Human auditory
    evoked potentials: possible brain stem components detected on
    the scalp.  Science, 1970, 167, 1517-1518.

Liberman, A. M., Cooper, F. S., Shankweiler, D., & Studdert-Kennedy, M. Perception of the Speech Code. Psychological Review, 1967, 74, 431-461.

Molfese, D. L. Electrocortical correlates of speech perception in infants and adults. In R. Thatcher (Ed.), Neurometrics of Human Development and Cognition. New York: Academic Press, in press.

Molfese, D. L. Neuroelectrical correlates of categorical speech perception in adults. Brain & Language, in press.

Molfese, D. L., Freeman, R. B., & Palermo, D. S. The ontogeny of brain lateralization for speech and nonspeech stimuli. Brain & Language, 1975, 2, 356-368.

Molfese, D. L., Nunez, V., Seibert, S. M., & Ramanaiah, N. V. 1976. Cerebral Asymmetry: changes in factor affecting its development. Annals of the New York Academy of Sciences, 1976, 280, 821-833.

Mulaika, S. A. The Foundation of Factor Analysis. New York: McGraw-Hill, 1972.

Myers, J. L. Fundamentals of Experimental Design. 2nd Ed. Boston Allyn & Bacon, 1972.

Ojemann, G. A. Language and the Thalamus: object naming and recall during and after thalamic stimulation. Brain & Language, 1975, 2, 101-120.

Shelburne, S. A. Visual evoked responses to language stimuli in normal children. Journal of Electroencephalography & Clinical Neurophysiology, 1973, 34, 135-143.

Shelburne, S. A. Visual evoked responses to word and nonsense syllable stimuli. Journal of Electroencephalography & Clinical Neurophysiology, 1972, 32, 17-25.

Thatcher, R. Evoked potential correlates of delayed letter matching. Behavioral Biology, in press, b.

Thatcher, R. Evoked potential correlates of hemispheric lateralization during semantic information processing. In S. Harnad (Ed.), Lateralization in the Nervous System. New York: Academic Press, in press, a.

Waner, El, Teyler, T. J., & Thompson, R. F.   The Psychobiology
     of speech and language: an overview.   In J. Desmedt (Ed.),
     Language and hemispheric specialization in man: cerebral
     event related potentials.   Progress in clinical Neurophysiology,
     Vol. 3.   Basel: Karger, 1977.

Witelson, S.   Developmental dyslexia: two right hemispheres and
     none left.   Science, 1977, 195, 309-311.

Wood, C. C.   Auditory and phonetic levels of processing in speech
     perception: neurophysiological and information - processing
     analyses.   Journal of Experimental Psychology:   Human Percep-
     tion & Performance, 1975, 104, 3-20.

Wood, C. C., Goff, W. R. & Day, R. S.   Auditory evoked potentials
     during speech perception, Science, 1971, 173, 1248-1251.

# P300 -- THIRTEEN YEARS LATER

Samuel Sutton

Department of Psychophysiology

New York State Psychiatric Institute, New York, N.Y.

It was 13 years ago, almost to the day, in the spring of 1964 that we first observed P300.[1] The size of the component impressed us a great deal. Over the years, we were even more impressed with its reliability. In hundreds of experiments with normal subjects, using many variations of the original design, P300 was always found to be larger the greater the amount of uncertainty resolved.

However, as P300 has reached its bar mitzvah enormous changes have happened in the field of event related potentials as a whole. Not only have there been many new findings for P300 in a number of laboratories, but for a range of other components as well. Even with respect to diagnostic application, significant strides have been made in several areas.

Over the intervening years, many laboratories have searched for, and found, systematic relationships between psychological formulations and ERP variables, not only for P300, but also for other components. However, recently one hears murmurs of discontent among ERP researchers with an approach that is limited to

---

[1] P300 is so large and clear in guessing designs that unlike most scientific advances which tend to evolve, P300 was actually discovered on a particular day, May 20, 1964, which was the first day we ever looked at evoked potentials in a guessing paradigm. (The paper on which this chapter is based was presented on May 19, 1977.) Although up to that point we had been involved in a completely different set of ERP experiments, we were so startled by P300 that we dropped the other experiments immediately and turned our attention to P300.

seeking increasingly more elegant correlations between available
psychological formulations and ERP data. As I interpret this
phenomenon, the source of the malaise is the feeling that correlations of this sort, no matter how elegant, do not advance our knowledge enough. Partly, this kind of mood is generated by our growing confidence in the ERP tool. Such confidence leads researchers
to want to give a certain amount of priority to ERP data. When a
correlation between psychological formulations and ERP data does
not work out quite right, we are now a little more prone to examine
the psychological constructs than to look askance at our ERP methodology.

Donchin develops this point of view systematically in his chapter. He concludes that "the important point is that an ERP component...is rather a manifestation, at the scalp, of neural activity which plays a role in the information transactions of the brain.
Our task is to determine the functional role of the component rather
than to seek preconceived correlations between the component and
ill-defined psychological constructs." What is striking about this
formulation is that there is no longer any hint that the importance
of ERP components must be demonstrated by the fact that they fit
known psychological constructs. Rather it puts the shoe on the
other foot. The ERP components are taken as given, as being in a
sense the independent variables. The problem is what are their
psychological functional roles.

## RARENESS WITHOUT UNCERTAINTY

It is in this spirit that I wish to emphasize and to reinter-
pret some data collected some years ago which did not fit our psychological formulations. In an early experiment (Sutton, Braren,
Zubin, & John, 1965), we had found that P300 was much larger when
the subject guessed which of two stimuli would be presented -- we
called this the uncertain condition -- than when the subject was
told prior to each stimulus which of the two stimuli would be presented -- we called this the certain condition. Tueting at our
laboratory undertook to use an information theory formulation in
designing an experiment relating the amplitude of P300 to the degree
of uncertainty (Tueting, Sutton, & Zubin, 1970). In this experiment, she manipulated the relative frequency of occurrence of the
two stimuli. The stimuli were a high-pitched click and a low-
pitched click. Each stimulus occurred, in a given block of trials,
either at 20% probability, 40% probability, 60% probability, or 80%
probability (with the other stimulus at the complementary probability for that block of trials). In another experimental condition
she manipulated these probabilities as sequential probabilities.
In this condition, although the relative frequency of occurrence of
the two stimuli was 50:50, in different blocks of trials a given

stimulus followed the other at the different experimental probabilities.   As a result she generated an alternation probability
curve running from 20% to 80%, and a repetition probability curve
running from 20% to 80%.

   All experimental probabilities were run in both the uncertain
condition and the certain condition.  In the uncertain condition
the subject guessed prior to each trial which of the two stimuli
would be presented, and the occurrence of the high- or low-pitched
click to which the evoked potential was recorded confirmed or disconfirmed the subject's guess.  In the certain condition, the subject was told by the experimenter prior to each trial which of the
two stimuli would be presented.  The findings are presented in Fig.
1.

   On the right, the findings in the uncertain condition are presented.   Note that since some of the subject's guesses were right
and some were wrong, these data are presented as proportions of
hits and misses.  All six curves in the uncertain condition (relative frequency, alternation probability, repetition probability --
separately for right guesses and for wrong guesses) show a monotonic relationship between P300 amplitude and these proportions.
Thus the data in the uncertain condition fit within an information
theory framework.   These data have been in the literature for some

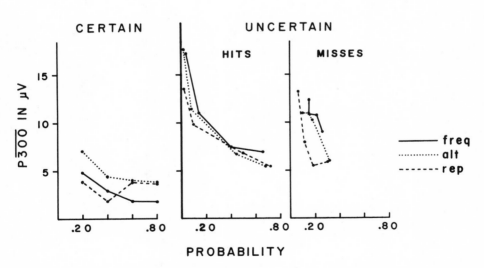

Fig. 1   Average amplitude of P300 for 4 subjects under conditions
of certainty and uncertainty as a function of relative frequency,
alternation probability and repetition probability (adapted from
Tueting et al., 1970).

time and I will not discuss them further.

Consider the curves on the left in the certain condition.
These are obtained in an experimental condition in which the subject is verbally told prior to each stimulus whether a high-pitched
click or a low-pitched click will be presented.  The subject cannot
be right or wrong, and the abscissa here is the experimenter-
manipulated probability.  In information theory terms, the information content of the stimulus in this condition is zero.  Yet two
of the three curves (left panel), the relative frequency (solid
line), and the alternation curve (dotted line), yield significant
slopes. The findings for these four subjects were replicated in
another experiment in our laboratory by Friedman (Friedman, Hakerem,
Sutton, & Fleiss, 1973).  Friedman only used the relative frequency
condition.  In Fig. 2 are shown the average data for 8 subjects
also run in the certain condition (left panel).  This curve also
has a statistically significant slope between P300 amplitude and

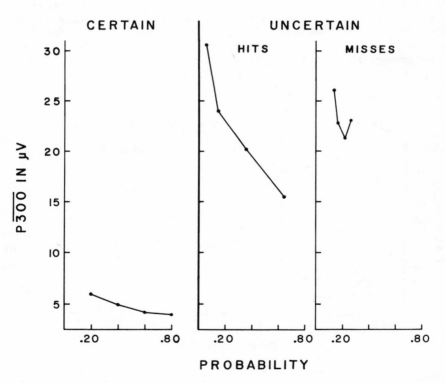

Fig. 2  Average amplitude of P300 for 8 subjects under conditions
of certainty and uncertainty as a function of relative frequency
(adapted from Friedman et al., 1973).

relative frequency.[2]

Here then we have a clear example of apparently systematic and
replicated ERP data which are clearly out of line with the information theory formulation which led to the experimental design.
An experimental condition which carried zero information should
have yielded no relationship between P300 amplitude and experi-
menter-manipulated probability.  From that point of view, it is
only the <u>absence</u> of a relationship for the repetition curve
(dashed line, left panel in Fig. 1) which "follows" the information theory prediction.  I will return to the question of the repetition curve below.

Given the monotonic findings for P300 for the relative frequency and alternation manipulations, there are two directions in
which to go.  One is to assume that some experimental artifact has
crept into these designs and has produced these findings in the
certain condition.[3]  The other is to boldly assume that information

---

[2]One aspect of the two studies which has never been commented on
is the large amplitude difference in the uncertain condition between the two studies, both of which were done in our laboratories.
While this might be dismissed as due to intersubject variability
or to trivial variation in experimental conditions, a P300 amplitude which is 2 to 2-1/2 times as large in one study as in another
which it was intended to replicate, deserves some comment.  One
factor may have been the fact that the number of trials in the
Friedman et al. study was less than in the Tueting et al. study.
While Tueting and Levit (1978) did not find a systematic trend for
P300 to decrease under roughly comparable experimental conditions
within a single 1-1/2 hour session, the studies being compared
here had a 4 to 1 ratio of trials and there may have been smaller
average P300s in the Tueting et al. study than in the Friedman et
al. study due to a habituation factor.  Another possible source of
difference is the recovery time of P300.  Friedman was doing pupil-
lography concomitantly and needed 10 to 14 seconds between trials
as compared to Tueting's 5 to 7 seconds.  While there are no existing data on the recovery time of P300, there is evidence that recovery time is longer the later the component.  For example, it
takes as much as 10 seconds for P200 to recover to full amplitude.

[3]A particularly subtle sort of artifact could have entered into
the Tueting et al. study since the certain and uncertain blocks
were to some extent interdigitated.  It would be conceivable that
the subjects' uncertainty during the blocks in the uncertain condition at a given probability somehow "crept into" or influenced
the blocks of trials in the certain condition.  However, in the
Friedman et al. study, for each probability the certain condition
blocks were completed before the uncertain condition was run.

theory as classically formulated is not providing a sufficient
guide to how the nervous system is contructed, and to use these
data to modify the formulation.

One interpretation of the findings in the certain condition
that can be dismissed with ease is that they represent some aspect
of sensory habituation.  It should be noted that the time scale is
all wrong for such an effect to be prominent in the data.  The
time interval between stimuli was 5 to 7 seconds in the Tueting et
al. study and 10 to 14 in the Friedman et al. study.  Several
events occur between successive stimuli in both studies.  In the
Tueting et al. study intervening events included the verbal identification of the next stimulus by the experimenter, the verbal
repetition of the information by the subject, fixation during part
of the trial, and rest for blinking and movement.  In the Friedman
et al. study, there were an even more complex series of events
between stimuli:  the fixation light brightened and this was followed by the subject's positioning his teeth in a bite board; the
experimenter verbally told the subject the identity of the next
stimulus, which the subject subsequently confirmed by pressing one
of two choice buttons; and several seconds after delivery of the
stimulus, the fixation light dimmed, the subject came out of the
bite board and verbally repeated the identity of the stimulus.

One clarification should be made with respect to the degree of
familiarity of the subjects with the experimental probabilities.
Prior to each block of trials in both studies the subject was told
the operative probabilities in that block.  Furthermore, particularly in the Tueting et al. study, subjects had a great deal of
exposure to each experimental probability.  In that study there
were 800 trials in the certain condition at each experimental probability.  For example, for the 20/80 relative frequency program,
each subject responded to 80 low-pitched clicks and 320 high-
pitched clicks in one subprogram, and to 80 high-pitched clicks
and 320 low-pitched clicks in the other subprogram.  In the Friedman et al. study there were fewer trials, one-fourth the number
used in the Tueting et al. study.

The possible relevance of the degree of familiarity, or the
prima facie obviousness of the experimental conditions to the findings was demonstrated in an experiment by Donchin, Kubovy, Kutas,
Johnson, and Herning (1973).  They compared two conditions in which
the subject always had prior knowledge of the stimulus, which
therefore carried zero information.  In one condition, the two
stimuli always occurred in simple alternation; in the other, the
sequence of the two stimuli was a recurring arbitrary pattern 9
stimuli long which the subject learned prior to evoked potential
recording.  P300 was smaller in the simple alternation condition.

Taking the ERP findings as our starting point leads me to

propose the following formulation:

(1) The nervous system is interested in rareness per se: the
<u>monotonic</u> trends in the data from both the certain and the uncer-
tain conditions are reflecting the relative degree of rareness,
rather than the degree of information or uncertainty.

(2) <u>However</u>, unpredictable events are more important to the
nervous system than predictable events.  The effect of unpredictability is to raise the level of P300 as reflected in the upward
shift of these curves from the certain condition to the uncertain
condition.  The amplitude of the curves on the right of Figs. 1
and 2 is greater than for the curves on the left.

(3) Even when stimuli are known in advance not all forms of
such prior knowledge are equivalent.  Different forms of prior
knowledge appear to have different import for the nervous system.
Two aspects:

   a) Novel change is more critical for the nervous system
   than novel repetition -- in fact, the phrase novel repetition
   may be a little bit difficult to swallow.  As defined in this
   experiment, two different clicks alternated rather frequently
   and what was novel was when one of them was repeated:  e.g.,
   high, low; high, low; high, low; high, low; high, low; high,
   low; high, low; high, low; <u>low</u>.  (This is a little exaggerated
   for clarity.)  This proviso is invoked to account for the failure to find a relationship for the repetition curve in the certain condition.  This peculiar behavior of novel repetition is
   foreshadowed by earlier data.  There are reaction time data
   going back to the 1940s which indicate that reaction times do
   not increase for novel repetitions, whereas they do increase
   for novel alternations (Mowrer, 1941; Mowrer, Rayman, & Bliss,
   1940).

   b) The nervous system is less responsive to more redundant
   events.  For example, simple alternation seems to have greater
   redundancy than a learned, less obvious sequence.

One aspect of the interpretation of the data in the certain
condition that requires additional experimentation for its clarification is that in the previous experiments the information provided to the subject as to the identity of the next stimulus was
always in the verbal form.  Control experiments should be performed
which rely on other modes of information transmission.

In the prior experiments, the subject should have had no difficulty at the level of knowledge involving which verbal label is
associated with which stimulus.  Certainly the subject had no
difficulty in identifying the two stimuli; they were highly

discriminable.  Furthermore, in the Tueting et al. study, across
the whole experiment, each subject heard and identified the high-
pitched click 7600 times and the low-pitched click 7600 times.
It should also be remembered that in both experiments the subject
repeated the verbal label after the occurrence of each stimulus
(and in Friedman et al.'s experiment there was an additional motoric identification).  However, there is a residual step which is
not clearly taken care of, that is the decoding step, which trans-
lates between the verbal and sensory forms of information.  The
verbally formulated certainty that a high-pitched click will occur
may not translate into equivalent certainty with respect to the
phenomenal experience.  It is conceivable that it is this decoding
step which leaves some residue of uncertainty which somehow gets
reflected in the monotonic relationship between experimenter-
manipulated probability and P300.  That a decoding step may be a
relevant issue is given support by the Donchin et al. (1973) finding that when stimuli were presented in simple alternation, P300
amplitude was increased by the addition of a fast and accurate
choice reaction time requirement.  This result may be interpreted
to reflect the additional decoding step necessary to translate the
stimuli to the proper motoric performance.

Control experiments would be desirable in which predictable
sequences are used to generate relative frequency programs in the
certain condition.  For example the 20/80 relative frequency condition can be generated by having repeated sequences of 4 high-
pitched clicks followed by a low-pitched click.  This might be
contrasted with the type of programs used by Tueting and Friedman
in which, except for the experimental probabilities, there were
essentially no other constraints on randomness.  If a predictable
sequence were to eliminate the relationship between relative frequency and P300, then it would cast into question the formulation
I have attempted with respect to the role of rareness per se.  On
the other hand, if it did eliminate the effect, it might put an
interesting tool into our hands for measuring informational properties in encoding situations.

## EQUIVOCATION AND P300

Within the context of an historical review, Donchin has described the broad scope of his laboratory's sophisticated work.
He has also presented a general formulation for P300 in terms of
the concepts of _expectancy_ and _surprise_.  While I believe that an
uncertainty resolution formulation is more adequate than expectancy and surprise for dealing with the same sets of data, I don't
think the experimental operations are currently available for
establishing the priority of one formulation over the other.

I would rather like to discuss here one issue that Donchin

left out of his formulation and this is the relationship that
Ruchkin and I proposed of P300 to equivocation. The term equivocation refers to the information theory concept of the information
loss due to the subject's a posteriori uncertainty of having correctly perceived an event (Ruchkin & Sutton, in press, b). In his
chapter, Donchin has reviewed the evidence for a somewhat related
concept, that of stimulus evaluation time (Kutas, McCarthy, &
Donchin, 1977) Donchin has shown that P300 latency is increased as
a function of the complexity of the cognitive processing involved
in the task.

Ruchkin and I were struck by the fact that P300 amplitude was
dependent on the immediacy and ease with which uncertainty about
an event could be resolved (Ruchkin & Sutton, in press, b). We
were led to this formulation by the fact that even when procedures
were used to align waveforms on P300 and re-average, in all subjects the evoked P300 was larger in amplitude than the emitted
P300 under the same experimental conditions (Ruchkin & Sutton,
1978).[4] It seemed to us that this difference in amplitude might
be due to the fact that uncertainty was more clearly and sharply
resolved by the occurrence of a stimulus than by its absence.

Recently, we made a direct experimental attack on the question
by studying time judgment and emitted potentials at two time intervals (Ruchkin & Sutton, in press, a). We took advantage of the
well-known fact that the variability of time judgment increases the
longer the interval to be judged. We were able to show that the
decrease in P300 average amplitudes (compensated for latency) as a
function of time interval went hand-in-hand with the increase in
variability in time judgment as a function of time interval.

When we turned to the literature we found ample support for the
equivocation formulation. Adams and Benson (1973) had shown that
P300 amplitude in response to a feedback stimulus of constant intensity signalling successful performance varied as a function of
the intensity of the feedback stimulus used to signal unsuccessful
performance. An inverse version of this paradigm in which P300
amplitude in response to the feedback stimulus signalling unsuc-
cessful performance was found to vary as a function of the intensity of the feedback stimulus used to signal successful performance
was recently done in Donchin's laboratory (Johnson & Donchin, in
press). In both versions as feedback stimulus contrast for

---

[4]To the extent that latency compensation procedures that have been
utilized will err, they will tend to overestimate smaller underlying signals more than larger underlying signals. Therefore, if
any error has crept into our findings it is likely that the differences between evoked P300s and emitted P300s are even larger
than we have reported (Ruchkin & Sutton, 1978; Ruchkin & Sutton,
in press, a).

successful and unsuccessful performance decreased, equivocation increased and presumably was the reason for the decrease in P300 amplitude.

Hillyard, Squires, K.C., Bauer, and Lindsay (1971) investigated the relationship between detectability (d') of low intensity signals and P300 amplitude. They reported that P300 increased as detectability improved up to a level of about 90 per cent correct responses. The falloff of P300 with increase of detectability above 90 per cent has always been something of a paradox. However, in a recent attack Ruchkin and I have made on the problem, we have been unable to replicate the falloff of P300 at high levels of detectability (unpublished data).

Paul (Paul & Sutton, 1972), in our laboratory, using an experimentally manipulated criterion, found that P300 amplitude for hits increased as the subject's criterion became more strict. In other words, as the hits average was increasingly limited to trials about which the subject was more certain, P300 amplitude was largest. Squires, K.C., Squires, N.K., and Hillyard (1975) who also used a fixed stimulus intensity had subjects respond with a numeric confidence rating. P300 amplitude was larger for more confident ratings.

Support for the equivocation concept has been obtained in a number of other studies and with a variety of experimental paradigms (Donchin, 1968; Ford, Roth, & Kopell, 1976; Lang, Gatchel, & Simons, 1975; Mast & Watson, 1968; Ritter, Simson, & Vaughan, 1972; Simons & Lang, 1976; Squires, K.C., Hillyard, & Lindsay, 1973; Squires, K.C., & Squires, N.K., 1975; Squires, K.C. et al., 1975; Squires, N.K., Donchin, Squires, K.C., & Grossberg, 1977).

The Kutas et al. (1977) data are an elegant demonstration of the stimulus evaluation time formulation and represent a significant advance beyond the formulation, presented in Sutton, Tueting, Zubin, and John (1967), that P300 occurs at the point in time at which uncertainty is resolved. There are two points that I would like to make about the relationship between equivocation and stimulus evaluation time. First, when Ruchkin and I formulated the equivocation concept, we made no comment about P300 latency although we were aware that in some paradigms reduced amplitude is associated with increased latency (see for example, Ford et al., 1976; Squires, N.K. et al., 1977). Partly this was due to the fact that we were not impressed by the generality of this association. Partly we were not happy with our ability to measure P300 latency given the broadness of the component. Second, at the time we developed the equivocation formulation we were thinking in terms of equivocation with respect to sensory discriminability. In some of the experimental paradigms, the differences between stimuli were below 100%

discriminability in the psychophysical sense; and in the experimental paradigms where the differences between stimuli were above
100% discriminability in the psychophysical sense, the stimuli
still yield reaction time differences due to intensity differences
and/or contrast (Ford et al., 1976; Johnson & Donchin, in press;
Squires, N.K. et al., 1977; Thurmond & Alluisi, 1963). We did not
then, and we do not now, know whether the equivocation formulation
developed in relation to sensory discriminability, can be extended
to the complexity of semantic categorization of clearly discriminable words as used by Kutas et al. (1977).

Rist and Towey in our laboratory have more recently come up
with an apparent exception to the equivocation formulation which
we cannot as yet account for (unpublished data). Working with the
"oddball" paradigm, they had subjects silently counting rare clicks
(20% probability). In some blocks of trials the oddballs were 5
dB softer than the frequent clicks and relatively difficult to
discriminate; in other blocks of trials the difference was 10 dB
and relatively easy to discriminate. P300 amplitude was found to
be essentially the same for the two oddballs. However, there was
a latency shift, later for the 5 dB P300. Johnson and Donchin (in
press) recently also reported no amplitude differences across a
range of intensity differences for 50:50 probability in the counting paradigm. They did not report their latency data. What it is
about the silent counting paradigm that weakens or eliminates the
equivocation effect is unclear.

## UTILITY AND CONFIRMATION-DISCONFIRMATION

Johnston's findings are of great interest to me because they
parallel a number of experiments which we have done in recent years
in our own laboratory. We thought our laboratory was going to be
closed down by the vice squad when we had subjects gamble for as
high as 50¢ a prediction. I am impressed with Johnston's courage
in upping the ante to $2. But our findings with respect to the
effect of the size of the bet are, even without factor analysis,
unequivocally in the P300 region. In Fig. 3 are some data from an
experiment by Steinhauer and Hakerem of our laboratory. Since the
results are so consistent across subjects, I have taken the liberty
of presenting the data as grand averages across subjects. These
are waveforms when the subjects win. Note we had two conditions:
one in which the subject decided on the value of the bet, and one
as in Johnston's experiment where the computer decided on the value
of the bet. In our data, both in the subject bet condition and in
the computer bet condition, P300 is larger the greater the value
of the bet. Here we are in complete agreement with the Johnston
findings. In Fig. 4 are the grand averages for the lose trials.
Here again we found that P300 was larger the greater the amount of

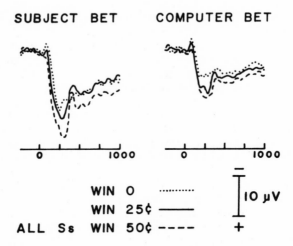

Fig. 3  Grand means across 8 subjects of vertex ERP waveforms (ear-lobe reference) for the "win" trials in the subject bet and computer bet conditions at 3 payoff levels.

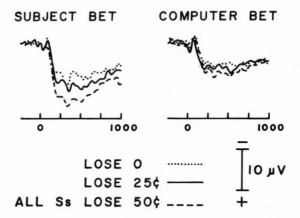

Fig. 4  Grand means across 8 subjects of vertex ERP waveforms (ear-lobe reference) for the "lose" trials in the subject bet and computer bet conditions at 3 payoff levels.

money lost under both betting conditions.  We depart here somewhat
from Johnston's findings in that his Factor 1 did not relate to
the amount of money lost; and although his Factor 2 did relate to
the amount of money involved, it did not do so for winning and
losing analyzed separately.

An examination of the factor loadings for Factor 1 shows clear
peaks of activity in the region of the N250 component and in the
region of the P300 component.  In our data, under the subject bet
condition, three components, P200, N250, and P300 were found to be
related to the amount of money bet for both the win and lose trials.
trials.[5,6]  In the computer bet condition, all three components
were found to be related to the amount of money bet when the subject wins; but in contrast to Johnston's findings, we did find
that P300 was also related to the amount of money bet when the subject loses.  While it may be that the differences in findings for
the lose trials between Johnston's and our computer bet condition
are due to procedural differences, I wonder whether it is not possible that Johnston's negative findings in this instance are due
to an overreliance on factor analysis.  If he were to return to
the original waveforms and measure specific components, it is possible that he would also find that P300 is related to the amount
of money bet in the lose trials.

The possibility that factor analysis may mask findings when un-
aided by an examination of the original waveforms is illustrated
more clearly in relation to the differences Johnston reports with
respect to confirmation-disconfirmation.  This problem of correlates of confirmation-disconfirmation has distressed our laboratory for many years.  As far back as 1965, we reported that P300
was larger for wrong guesses than for right guesses (Sutton et al.,
1965).  But this was a statistical finding.  It did not hold in
all subjects, nor indeed in all studies.  More recently, Tueting,
Hammer, Hakerem and I retackled the problem systematically with a
design which separated win-lose from confirmation-disconfirmation

---

[5]In the factor loadings of Johnston's Factor 1, there is a relatively small negative peak of activity at 150 milliseconds.  However, since I do not know how to interpret the polarity information in his factor loadings, it is difficult to tell whether this
peak of activity has any relationship to our P200 findings.

[6]Because we have used grand averages across subjects in Figs. 3
and 4 the details of specific components such as P200 and N250 are
lost in latency jitter across subjects and cannot be distinguished.
For the statistical analyses, these components were of course measured in the individual subject waveforms.

(Sutton, Tueting, Hammer, & Hakerem, in press).[7]  In the win-lose
comparison, we again found our statistical effect in the P300
region.  But in the P200-N250 region, the difference was consistent
and in the same direction in 12 out of 13 subjects.  The 13th subject was a child, who seemed to have confused the instructions.  A
sample subject is shown in Fig. 5.  Note the right hand section of
the figure which illustrates the differences between winning and
losing.  In this design, the subject could win either by making a
right prediction or by making a wrong prediction.  The way we did
this was by having a rule that two right predictions in a row, or
two wrong predictions in a row resulted in winning money.  However,
one right and one wrong, in either order, resulted in losing money.
That is why there are both win and lose waveforms superimposed
under the word "Right" and under the word "Wrong."  In both cases,
P300 is larger for the lose waveform in this subject, but this is
the finding that I have pointed out tends to be statistical in
nature.  The finding which occurs in 12 out of 13 subjects is that
the lose waveform is more negative in the P200-N250 region.

On the left hand side of the figure are shown differences between confirmation and disconfirmation where confirmation-disconfirmation has no differential implications for winning or losing --
these are the waveforms to the first members of the pair of guesses
in the structure of rules as described above.  Similarly to the
win-lose difference, there is greater negativity in the disconfirm
waveform than in the confirm waveform in the P200-N250 region.
This was also found in the overwhelming majority of subjects.

In Johnston's chapter, based on his factor analysis, he emphasizes the P300 findings with respect to confirmation-disconfirmation (which in his experiment is the same as win-lose).  However,
examination of the factor loadings for his Factor 1, as I have
noted above, shows maxima of activity in the regions of the N250
and P300 components.  In our data, the waveforms for the individual subjects show the P300 findings to be statistical in nature;
more subjects have larger P300s for the lose condition.  However,
when we examined the P200 and N250 components, which involve
smaller effects in terms of amplitude, we found that all but one
subject in the sample had more negativity for lose than for win:
P200 is less positive and N250 is more negative in the lose,
exactly as illustrated in the sample waveforms in Johnston's chapter.

Our current interpretation of the several studies that have

_____

[7]In previous studies which compared correlates of being right vs.
being wrong, the relationship between confirmation and winning on
the one hand, and disconfirmation and losing on the other, has been
an uncontrolled variable.

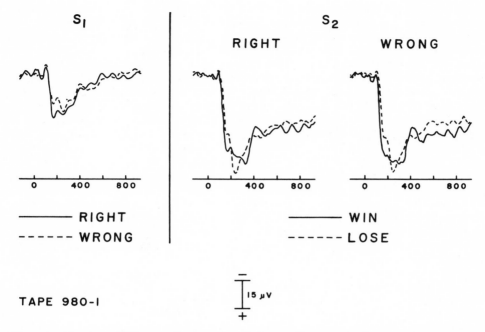

Fig. 5  Vertex ERP waveforms (earlobe reference) for one subject
for $S_1$ -- confirmation-disconfirmation and $S_2$ -- win-lose (from
Sutton et al., in press).

shown statistical findings in the P300 region in relation to correct and incorrect guesses is that they probably reflect uncontrolled differences between subjects or interaction between subjects
and the nature of the task.  Our speculation is that some subjects
focus on the incorrect trials for determining their strategy, whereas other subjects focus on correct trials.  Other subjects may fluctuate.  Different tasks may bring out these propensities to a
greater or lesser degree.  Thus any tendency which would make the
win or the lose trials more salient for different subjects (or for
different designs) would result in correspondingly larger P300 amplitudes for the more salient category.  In contrast, the finding
in the P200-N250 region while smaller in amplitude appears to be
consistent across subjects.

     Some comment should also be made about the difference between
the subject bet and the computer bet conditions.  Examination of
Figs. 3 and 4 shows that P300 was much larger for the subject bet
condition than for the computer bet condition.  Furthermore, as

noted above in the subject bet condition, findings were consistent
in relation to utility across all three components: P200, N250,
and P300 for both win and lose trials. In the computer bet condition, only P300 showed a consistent relationship to utility across
win and lose trials. Our interpretation of the difference between
the subject bet and computer bet conditions is that they differ on
a dimension of subject involvement. Despite the fact that the subject was involved in the same amount of risk -- monetary rewards
and penalties were the same -- the act of deciding the value of
the bet created a different level of commitment to the outcome.

## "MEANING" AND EVENT RELATED POTENTIALS

I would like now to comment about the concept of "meaning," a
theme which recurs in several of the chapters. Johnston arranged
his experiment so that conjunction between the subject's prediction and the identity of the subsequent stimulus had the meaning
of winning money and disjunction had the meaning of losing money.
In the experiments of Tueting, Hammer, Hakerem and myself, we
played a more complicated game. Two conjunctions in sequence, or
two disjunctions in sequence had the meaning of winning money. In
our situation therefore, the subject could win money on an incorrect prediction. In still other experimental paradigms target
stimuli are distinguished from non-target stimuli; rare events
from frequent events; high payoff events from low payoff events.
These are all meanings that are imparted to stimuli by the instructions, the experimental design, or the nature of the subject's
task.

I could go on with many more examples. What they would illustrate is that where we have most successfully nailed down event
related potential correlates of meaning, we have done so in relation to the salience aspect of meaning: we are dealing with events
which by some maneuver or other have been made important to the
subject. We are usually dealing with task relevant stimuli. Some
uncertainty has been resolved: a subject discovers that a guess
or a discrimination is correct or incorrect. Money may be won or
lost. In these situations, we are dealing in some sense with
salience, i.e., with an importance or value sense of the term
meaning.

There are quite other senses of the meaning concept barely
scratched by research with event related potentials. For example,
whether in one's own language or in a foreign language one might
be studying, one understands perfectly the meaning difference between "this is the hat of my aunt" and "this is the pen of my
uncle." But this meaning difference does not lie in their value
or importance to us, it lies in the specificity of their referents.

"Hat" is a different object from "pen," differently shaped, of different materials, serving different functions. "Aunt" is a closely related kin term to "uncle," but clearly distinguished by sex.

Some years ago, we showed that circles produced different event related potentials from squares, while large and small figures of the same shape produced event related potentials which were relatively similar (John, Herrington, & Sutton, 1967). We thought this might imply correlates of the meanings of circleness vs. squareness. But we did the experiment with relatively primitive technology. A recent sophisticated replication was more cautious in its interpretations (Purves, 1976). Brown, Marsh, and Smith (1976) have shown differences between the same words used as verbs and nouns, but here too, despite the elegance of the experiments, much cleaning up remains to be done. Chapman has shown event related potential correlates of the categories of Osgood's semantic differential. However, significantly for this discussion, his strongest findings are for the value dimension. Begleiter, Gross, and Kissin (1967) have shown differences between stimuli which have been endowed with different affective significance. On the negative side, Thatcher (1977) did not find differences between synonyms and antonyms.

It is against this background of relatively preliminary results in the area of correlates of meaning, other than its salience aspect, that the findings reported in Molfese's chapter have to be evaluated. When we examine his experimental design, we find subjects were in a two choice situation: They pressed one telegraph key for meaningless CVC syllables and another telegraph key for meaningful CVC syllables. What is equivocal in the structure of the design is that the differences that emerge need not be correlates of linguistic meaningfulness as opposed to meaninglessness. Rather, it is just as plausible an interpretation of the design that linguistic meaningfulness is the property which one set of stimuli shared which made them more important or salient. Given the fact that it is so well established that we can get evoked potential correlates of the importance or value dimension, it seems more likely that we are observing correlates of importance vs. unimportance.

The problem of establishing correlates of conceptual or referential meaning goes beyond the problem of experimental design, and the success or failure of the effort may ultimately depend on the state of our analysis of meaning systems such as language. The issue of the correlates of "hat" vs. "pen" is a misleading example, or at the very least a long way away from the capabilities of our present tools. The efforts to obtain event related potential correlates of large categories of analysis are much more to the point.

But what should these large categories be?  That a category, or a duality, can be abstracted from the use of language, does not mean that the brain is physiologically organized that way.  Perhaps the success in finding correlates for nouns vs. verbs and the failure to find differences between antonyms and synonyms, has something to do with the noun/verb distinction being a grammatical property of language, which the antonym/synonym distinction is not -- perhaps this is telling us something about the way the brain processes linguistic meaning.  Where does one go from here?  Does one go on various fishing expeditions?  Plants vs. animals?  Solids vs. liquids?  Living vs. non-living objects?  Interrogative vs. declarative forms?  Perhaps, some of that is in order.  I suspect that examination of the literature of the various aphasic disorders may give some clues for reasonable next steps; and perhaps the attempts in linguistic theory to develop the universal properties of language may be significant.  I also think bootstrap or iterative operations are called for, i.e., the utilization of positive findings to reorder our psychological constructs to lead to new event related potential experiments.


## ACKNOWLEDGMENTS

I am indebted to Dr. Daniel Ruchkin for substantive advice with respect to a number of issues dealt with in this chapter.  I am extremely grateful to Dr. Muriel Hammer for a critical review of the manuscript.  Ms. Marion Hartung rendered invaluable editorial assistance.


## REFERENCES

Adams, J.C., & Benson, D.A.  Task-contingent enhancement of the auditory evoked response.  Electroencephalography and Clinical Neurophysiology, 1973, 35, 249-257.

Begleiter, H., Gross, M.M., & Kissin, B.  Evoked cortical responses to affective visual stimuli.  Psychophysiology, 1967, 3, 336-344.

Brown, W.S., Marsh, J.T., & Smith, J.C.  Evoked potential waveform differences produced by the perception of different meanings of an ambiguous phrase.  Electroencephalography and Clinical Neurophysiology, 1976, 41, 113-123.

Donchin, E.  Average evoked potentials and uncertainty resolution.  Psychonomic Science, 1968, 12, 103.

Donchin, E., Kubovy, M., Kutas, M., Johnson, R., Jr., & Herning, R.I.  Graded changes in evoked response (P300) amplitude as a function of cognitive activity.  Perception & Psychophysics, 1973, 14, 319-324.

Ford, J.M., Roth, W.T., & Kopell, B.S.  Auditory evoked potentials to unpredictable shifts in pitch.  Psychophysiology, 1976, 13, 32-39.

Friedman, D., Hakerem, G., Sutton, S., & Fleiss, J.L.  Effect of stimulus uncertainty on the pupillary dilation response and the vertex evoked potential.  Electroencephalography and Clinical Neurophysiology, 1973, 34, 475-484.

Hillyard, S.A., Squires, K.C., Bauer, J.W., & Lindsay, P.H.  Evoked potential correlates of auditory signal detection.  Science, 1971, 172, 1357-1360.

John, E.R., Herrington, R., & Sutton, S.  Effects of visual form on the evoked response.  Science, 1967, 155, 1439-1441.

Johnson, R., Jr., & Donchin, E.  On how P300 amplitude varies with the utility of the eliciting stimuli.  Electroencephalography and Clinical Neurophysiology, in press.

Kutas, M., McCarthy, G., & Donchin, E.  Augmenting mental chronometry: the P300 as a measure of stimulus evaluation time.  Science, 1977, 197, 792-795.

Lang, P.J., Gatchel, R.J., & Simons, R.F.  Electrocortical and cardiac rate correlates of psychophysical judgment.  Psychophysiology, 1975, 12, 649-655.

Mast, T.E., & Watson, C.S.  Attention and auditory evoked responses to low detectability signals.  Perception & Psychophysics, 1968, 4, 237-240.

Mowrer, O.H.  Preparatory set (expectancy) -- Further evidence of its 'central' locus.  Journal of Experimental Psychology, 1941, 28, 116-133.

Mowrer, O.H., Rayman, N.N., & Bliss, E.L.  Preparatory set (expectancy) -- An experimental demonstration of its 'central' locus.  Journal of Experimental Psychology, 1940, 26, 357-372.

Paul, D.D., & Sutton, S.  Evoked potential correlates of response criterion in auditory signal detection.  Science, 1972, 177, 362-364.

Purves, S.J.S.  The effect of the geometric form and meaning of the stimulus on the configuration of the visual evoked response.  Unpublished doctoral dissertation, The University of British Columbia, 1976.

Ritter, W., Simson, R., & Vaughan, H.G.  Association cortex potentials and reaction time in auditory discrimination.  Electroencephalography and Clinical Neurophysiology, 1972, 33, 547-555.

Ruchkin, D.S., & Sutton, S.  Emitted P300 potentials and temporal uncertainty.  Electroencephalography and Clinical Neurophysiology, in press. (a)

Ruchkin, D.S., & Sutton, S.  Equivocation and P300 amplitude.  In D. Otto (Ed.), Multidisciplinary perspectives in event-related brain potential research.  Washington, D.C.: U.S. Government Printing Office, in press. (b)

Ruchkin, D.S., & Sutton, S.  Latency characteristics and trial-by-
    trial variations of emitted cerebral potentials.  In J.E.
    Desmedt (Ed.), Progress in clinical neurophysiology.  (Vol.
    6).  Cognitive components in cerebral event-related potentials
    and selective attention.  Basel: S. Karger, 1978.
Simons, R.F., & Lang, P.J.  Psychophysical judgment: electro-
    cortical and heart rate correlates of accuracy and uncertainty.
    Biological Psychology, 1976, 4, 51-64.
Squires, K.C., Hillyard, S.A., & Lindsay, P.H.  Cortical potentials
    evoked by confirming and disconfirming feedback following an
    auditory discrimination.  Perception & Psychophysics, 1973,
    13, 25-31.
Squires, K.C., & Squires, N.K.  Vertex evoked potentials in a
    rating-scale detection task: relation to signal probability.
    Behavioral Biology, 1975, 13, 21-34.
Squires, K.C., Squires, N.K., & Hillyard, S.A.  Decision-related
    cortical potentials during an auditory signal detection task
    with cued observation intervals.  Journal of Experimental Psy-
    chology: Human Perception and Performance, 1975, 1, 268-279.
Squires, N.K., Donchin, E., Squires, K.C., & Grossberg, S.  Bi-
    sensory stimulation: inferring decision-related processes from
    the P300 component.  Journal of Experimental Psychology: Human
    Perception and Performance, 1977, 3, 299-315.
Sutton, S., Braren, M., Zubin, J., & John, E.R.  Evoked potential
    correlates of stimulus uncertainty.  Science, 1965, 150, 1187-
    1188.
Sutton, S., Tueting, P., Hammer, M., & Hakerem, G.  Evoked poten-
    tials and feedback.  In D. Otto (Ed.), Multidisciplinary per-
    spectives in event-related brain potential research.  Washing-
    ton, D.C.: U.S. Government Printing Office, in press.
Sutton, S., Tueting, P., Zubin, J., & John, E.R.  Information de-
    livery and the sensory evoked potential.  Science, 1967, 155,
    1436-1439.
Thatcher, R.W.  Evoked potential correlates of hemispheric laterali-
    zation during semantic information processing.  In S. Harnad,
    R. Doty, L. Goldstein, J. Jaynes, G. Krauthamer (Eds.), Later-
    alization in the nervous system.  New York: Academic Press,
    1977.
Thurmond, J.B., & Alluisi, E.A.  Choice time as a function of stimu-
    stimulus dissimilarity and discriminability.  Canadian Journal
    of Psychology, 1963, 17, 326-337.
Tueting, P., & Levit, R.A.  Long-term changes of event-related po-
    tentials in normals, depressives and schizophrenics.  In J.E.
    Desmedt (Ed.), Progress in clinical neurophysiology.  (Vol. 6).
    Cognitive components in cerebral event-related potentials and
    selective attention.  Basel: S. Karger, 1978.
Tueting, P., Sutton, S., & Zubin, J.  Quantitative evoked potential
    correlates of the probability of events.  Psychophysiology,
    1970, 7, 385-394.

# VISUAL EVOKED POTENTIALS AND AFFECTIVE RATINGS OF SEMANTIC STIMULI

H. Begleiter, B. Porjesz, and R. Garozzo

State University of New York
Downstate Medical Center
Brooklyn, New York

In the last decade it has become quite evident that .event-related brain potentials not only reflect changes in the physical parameters of a stimulus but are also quite sensitive to psychological variables. The relationship between event-related brain potentials and concomitant ongoing cognitive processing has been the subject of numerous investigations which have been thoroughly reviewed (Regan, 1972; Beck, 1975; Callaway, 1975; Thatcher and John, 1977).

A number of investigators have studied the question of whether the processing of specific informational content of a stimulus is reflected in the morphological characteristics of the evoked brain potential. Lifshitz (1966) used groups of photographs intended to induce positive, neutral or negative affective states. Potentials evoked by the three classes of stimuli were found to be different in some subjects. Begleiter, Gross and Kissin (1967) studied the influence of affective meaning on visual evoked potentials, by means of a classical conditioning procedure. Previously meaning-less figures (CS) were conditioned to elicit a positive, negative or neutral affective response (CR). Waveforms of the evoked potentials were found to differ significantly across the three effective conditions. These results have been replicated by Gliddon, Busk and Galbraith (1971). Using the same conditioning procedures previously used in our laboratory, Lenhardt (1973) reported results quite consistent with ours. In another approach, Shevrin (Shevrin and Fritzler (1968; Shevrin, Smith, and Fritzler, 1971) reported that stimuli presented subliminally with the use of a tachistoscope, resulted in significantly different evoked potentials.

In 1967, John, Herrington and Sutton reported that different words equated for the area covered by the printed letters elicited different evoked potential waveforms. Differences in evoked potentials, concomitant with differences in semantic meaning were also reported by Begleiter and Platz (1969). Changes in evoked potentials related to semantic stimuli have also been reported by a number of investigators (Buchsbaum and Fedio, 1969; Morrell and Salamy, 1971; Matsumiya, Tagliasco, Lombroso and Goodglass, 1972; Wood, Goff and Day, 1971; Neville, 1974; Ratliff and Greenberg, 1972; Thatcher, 1976; Friedman, Simson, Ritter and Rapin, 1975a; 1975b; Chapman, Bragdon, Chapman and McGrary, 1977).

In all of the aforementioned studies, the observed relationship between stimulus meaning and evoked potentials was not independent of changes in the physical structure of the stimuli. In order to establish robust relationships between stimulus content and neuroelectric events, it is critical to control for the effects of the physical structure of the stimuli (Schwartz, 1976). In recent years, some investigators have made use of a paradigm in which evoked potentials are recorded to identical stimuli under different conditions. This design makes it possible to vary the meaning of the stimulus by embedding it in different contexts, by using the same stimulus to deliver different kinds of information or by presenting the same stimulus under different psychological sets.

Jenness (1972) reported that identical stimuli conveying different informational contents result in significantly different evoked brain potentials. Brown, Marsh and Smith (1973; 1976) found that evoked potentials to the word "fire" differed when the word appeared in the phrases "sit by the fire" and "ready, aim, fire." When the word appeared in the initial position in the phrases "fire is hot" or "fire the gun" the evoked potentials to the word fire were not significantly different. The findings indicate that context-produced differences in the meaning of a word produced significant differences in evoked potential waveform. A related experiment was conducted by Teyler, Roemer, Harrison and Thompson (1973). The authors instructed the subjects to think about one or the other of two meanings of ambiguous words during the presentation of click stimuli. The results of this experiment indicated that thinking about the noun and verb meanings of the ambiguous words produced differential waveforms to the click stimuli.

The technique for classification of evoked potentials according to the subjective interpretation of the stimulus has been utilized in experiments using other than semantic stimuli. Spunda, Radil-Weiss, and Radilova (1975) used a necker cube as a pattern stimulus. They reported different evoked potentials to the same stimulus depending on the subjective perception of the stimulus. A recent study by Johnston and Chesney (1974) illustrates the

use of context-sensitive symbols as an elegant approach for investigating the representation of meaning in the brain.  Evoked potentials to the same symbol were recorded in two different contexts.
In one, the symbol was embedded in the temporal context of numbers,
in the other it appeared in the temporal context of letters.  Their
findings indicate that the frontal evoked potentials reflect the
change of meaning of a symbolic stimulus when it appears in different temporal contexts.  More recently, Begleiter and Porjesz (1975)
studied evoked potentials to physically identical stimuli in trials
resulting in different behavioral decisions.  The authors report
that when a subject is presented with a stimulus of medium intensity and decides that it is "bright," the evoked potential to that
stimulus is quite different from the evoked potential elicited by
an identical stimulus that he decides is "dim."  Significantly different evoked potentials to the same physical stimulus were obtained
in trials that resulted in different behavioral decisions.

Taken together these studies strongly support the notion that
when the physical characteristics of the stimulus are held constant,
it is quite possible to obtain differences in evoked potential which
are attributable to the context of the stimulus and to its subjective informational content.

We now report a study in which evoked potentials to the same
semantic stimuli were recorded under two different task conditions.
In one condition the subjects are attending to the structural content of the words by identifying certain letters.  In the second
condition, the subjects are attending to the connotative content
of the words, and the individual letters are less important.


METHODS

Ten, right-handed males with a mean age of 23 volunteered to
participate in the experiment.  Gold electrodes (Grass instrument)
were attached with collodion at F3, F4, C3, C4 P3 and P4 in accordance with the 10-20 electrode system of the International Federation (Jasper, 1958).  All recordings were referential to linked
ears with differential ear resistance maintained below 500 ohms and
electrode resistance kept below 4000 ohms; an electrode placed on
the nasion served as subject ground.  The frequency bandpass of the
recording system (Grass polygraph, Model 78B) was set between 0.1
to 100 Hz.  Eye movements were continuously monitored with EOG
averages using the same gain frequency response.

In order to cull a sizeable number of appropriate words for
this experiment, we asked 245 medical students to rate 439 five-
letter words on a seven point semantic differential scale going
from pleasant to unpleasant.  From the ratings, we chose the 62
most positive words,  the 62 most neutral words and the 62

most negative words, thus obtaining a total of 186 words which
were used as visual stimuli in our study.

A computer-controlled CRT display system (Tektronix #635) presented the words individually to a dark-adapted subject seated in
a darkened, sound-treated chamber (IAC enclosure). All words were
randomly presented foveally, as briefly flashed stimuli subtending
a visual angle 11.8° with a duration of 20 ms. The interstimulus
interval (ISI) was randomized between 3.5 to 6 seconds. During
that interval a fixation target was present in the form of a dimly
illuminated dot on the CRT. Stimulus presentation and data collection were achieved on line with the use of a PDP 11-40 computer.
Individual evoked potentials were digitized for 50 msec. prior to
stimulus presentation and for 450 msec. post-stimulus presentation.

Each subject participated in two experimental runs. In the
Letter Identification run (LI) the subject was told to actively
attend to a series of words (N=186); each time a word was presented
he was asked to press one of five buttons to indicate the position
of the last vowel in that word. In the middle of the run the position of the five buttons was switched. In the Affective Rating run
(AR) each subject was requested to press one of the buttons to
indicate his personal rating of the affective loading imparted by
each word. Button 1 indicated a positive loading, Button 2 slightly
positive, Button 3 neutral, Button 4 slightly negative and Button 5
indicated a negative loading. For half of the Ss this order was
reversed. All subjects were asked to use both hands to press the
buttons and were not instructed to press the buttons as quickly as
possible. In the middle of each run, the amplifiers and A/D converters used to record from each hemisphere were reversed in order
to correct for amplifier or A/D converter bias.

At the end of the experiment, all individual evoked potentials
were retrieved and averaged in accordance with the various behavioral response conditions, as follows:
Composite 1: Evoked potentials in the LI run were averaged for each
response condition (button press to indicate the position of the
last vowel). There were five possible button-pressing responses.
Composite 2: Evoked potentials in the AR run were also averaged for
each response condition (button press indicating affective loading)
separately, yielding 5 averaged evoked potentials.
Composite 3: Evoked potentials to all stimuli in LI run were also
averaged in accordance with their respective responses in the AR
run. Condition 3 enabled us to compare the evoked potential to a
word when the subject was rating its affective loading, to the
evoked potential to the very same word when the subject responded
by indicating the position of the last vowel.

In this paper we will only report our findings recorded at P3
and P4. Evoked potential recordings are illustrated in Figure 1
and are reported here in terms of peak-to-peak amplitudes and

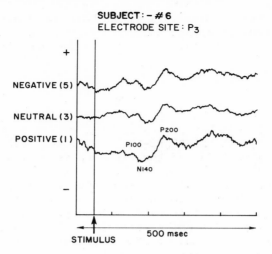

FIGURE 1

Visual evoked potentials obtained from left parietal of a subject.
The three traces represent the averaged evoked potentials in composite 2 when the subject was pressing one of five buttons to indicate his affective ratings of semantic stimuli.  The top trace
represents the average evoked potentials to stimuli rated negative,
the middle trace is evoked by stimuli rated neutral and the bottom
trace is obtained to stimuli rated positive.

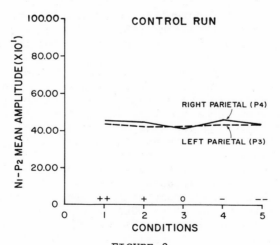

FIGURE 2

N1-P2 amplitude of evoked potentials recorded at left and right
parietal electrodes.  The evoked potentials were obtained in the
LI run when the subject was pressing a button to indicate the
position of the last vowel.  (composite 1)

latencies.  Preliminary statistical analyses were accomplished with
the use of analyses of variance for 2 factors with repeated measurements, performed on all individual amplitudes and latencies (Winer,
1962).


                                  RESULTS

     We performed a number of analyses of variance on the peak-to-
peak amplitudes (P1-N1, N1-P2, P2-N2, N2-P3) and latencies (P1, N1,
P2, N2, P3) for electrodes at the right parietal (P4) and left parietal (P3) electrodes.  The means of the five averaged evoked potentials obtained in Composite 1 (searching for the position of the
last vowel) were subjected to an alalysis of variance.  The F ratios
for all amplitudes and latencies of evoked potentials obtained at
both electrode sites were not significant.  The identical statistical analyses was performed on the five averaged evoked potentials
derived in Composite 3.  These are evoked potentials to identical
semantic stimuli in the LI run averaged in accordance with their
respective affect rating in the AR run.  F ratios for all amplitudes
and latencies at both parietal leads were not significant (Figure 2).

     An analysis of variance was also performed to compare the five
averaged evoked potentials obtained in Composite 2.  These are
evoked potentials to semantic stimuli presented in the affective
rating run (AR).  The only statistically significant differences
(P<.01) were obtained for the N1-P2 amplitude (140-200 msec) at the
right (P4) and left parietal (P3).  Individual comparisons of all
possible pairs of evoked potential means (N1-P2 component) obtained
during the affective rating runs (AR) are summarized in Table 1 for
the right parietal and summarized in Table 2 for the left parietal.

     Finally, we compared the five averaged evoked potentials ob-
tained in the AR run, when the subject was rating the affective
loading of each word, to the averaged evoked potential to the identical words but when the subject performed the letter identification
task (Composite 3).  The analysis of variance yielded F ratios which
indicated that there were no significant difference for latencies
of evoked potential components obtained at both P3 and P4.  The only
statistically significant differences were obtained for the N1-P2
amplitude (140-200 msec.) at both P3 and P4.  The analysis of variance performed on the N1-P2 component recorded at P3 yielded an F
ratio of 21.46 significant at p<.0001 level (Figure 3).  The analysis of variance performed on the N1-P2 component recorded at P4
yielded an F ratio of 4.36 significant at p<.01 level (Figure 4).
Because we found significant differences in evoked potentials obtained to the identical words under the two different task conditions
we proceeded to perform t tests for correlated means.  The results
are summarized in Table 3.

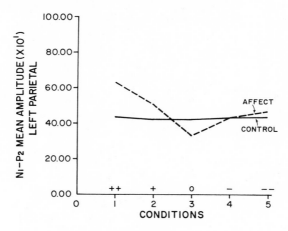

FIGURE 3
N1-P2 amplitude of averaged evoked potentials recorded at left
parietal (P3). The solid line represents the five averaged evoked
potentials obtained in the control condition (composite 3). The
broken line represents the averaged evoked potentials obtained in
the AR run when the subjects pressed one of five buttons to indicate the affective rating of each semantic stimulus.

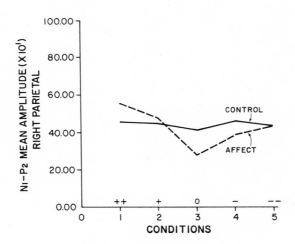

FIGURE 4
N1-P2 amplitude of averaged evoked potentials recorded at right
parietal (P4). The solid line represents the five averaged evoked
potentials obtained in the control condition (composite 3). The
broken line represents the averaged evoked potentials obtained in
the AR run when the subjects pressed one of five buttons to indicate the affective rating of each semantic stimulus.

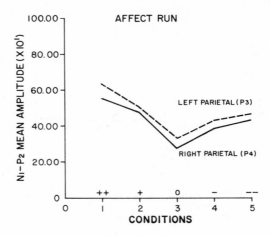

FIGURE 5

N1-P2 amplitude from left and right parietal recordings obtained
in the AR run.


TABLE 1

|  | Positive Affect Rating | Slightly Positive Affect Rating | Neutral Rating | Slightly Negative Affect Rating | Negative Affect Rating |
|---|---|---|---|---|---|
| Positive Affect Rating |  | N.S. | 4.35 p<.01 | N.S. | 2.45 p<.05 |
| Slightly Positive Affect Rating |  |  | 3.13 p<.01 | N.S. | N.S. |
| Neutral Rating |  |  |  | 2.56 p<.05 | 3.21 p<.01 |
| Slightly Negative Affect Rating |  |  |  |  | N.S. |
| Negative Affect Rating |  |  |  |  |  |

Individual t-test comparisons of N1-P2 amplitude means for all five
averaged evoked potentials obtained during the Affect Rating run at
the right parietal electrode (P4).

TABLE 2

|  | Positive Affect Rating | Shortly Positive Affect Rating | Neutral Rating | Slightly Negative Affect Rating | Negative Affect Rating |
|---|---|---|---|---|---|
| Positive Affect Rating |  | 5.39 p<.001 | 9.71 p<.001 | 8.94 p<.001 | 4.00 0<.001 |
| Slightly Positive Affect Rating |  |  | 6.83 p<.001 | 2.48 p<.05 | 1.85 p<.05 |
| Neutral Rating |  |  |  | 4.76 p<.01 | 4.56 p<.01 |
| Slightly Negative Affect Rating |  |  |  |  | N.S. |
| Negative Affect Rating |  |  |  |  |  |

Individual t-test comparisons of N1-P2 amplitude means for all five averaged evoked potentials obtained during the Affect Rating run at the left parietal electrode (P3).


In order to assess possible hemispheric differences we compared all amplitudes and latencies across tasks between right and left parietal recordings. While none of the statistical tests reached significance, it should be noted (Figure 5) that the N1-P2 component was suggestive of a possible hemispheric difference.

TABLE 3

| | Right Parietal (P4) | | Left Parietal (P3) | |
|---|---|---|---|---|
| | t-test | p value | t-test | p value |
| Positive Affect Rating<br><br>Composite 3 | 1.87 | < .05 | 6.89 | < .001 |
| Slightly Positive<br>Affect Rating<br><br>Composite 3 | | N.S. | 3.01 | < .01 |
| Neutral Rating<br><br>Composite 3 | 2.75 | .05 | 3.33 | .01 |
| Slightly Negative<br>Affect Rating<br>vs<br>Composite 3 | | N.S. | | N.S. |
| Negative Affect Rating<br>vs<br>Composite 3 | | N.S. | 1.83 | < .05 |

Individual t-test comparisons for N1-P2 amplitude of averaged evoked potentials obtained in Condition 2 (Affect Rating) versus Condition 3 (composite of identical words obtained while performing Letter Identification) for electrodes P3 and P4.

## DISCUSSION

Our results indicate that tasks requiring different kinds of information processing may involve different neurophysiological transactions which are reflected in scalp-recorded evoked potentials. In the present study, the physical structure of the stimuli was identical across runs. In one run, the subjects performed an analytical task by extracting specific structural features from the semantic stimuli. In the second run they performed a more global or wholistic task by rating the connotative meaning of the words. Our findings suggest that certain aspects of the evoked potential waveform may reflect neural activity correlated with the subjective connotative meaning imparted by the stimulus that are not attributable to changes in the physical characteristics of stimulus. When the subject is engaged in a task requiring active and sustained attention to specific alphabetical features, which may also impede his active processing of connotative meaning, the scalp-recorded potentials appear to be similar across the five groups of words (Composite 3). However, when the subject is requested to respond to each word by rating his feelings about the word, the evoked potentials to the various groups of words ranging from positive to negative are quite different from one another. At both the left and right parietal, the comparison of evoked potentials to the same words obtained between Composite 2 and Composite 3 yielded significant results for only the N1-P2 component. These differences were statistically significant for all but one condition, namely the slightly unpleasant condition.

It is quite possible that the 5 point affective rating scale which we arbitrarily imposed on the subject does not in any way represent a scale with equal incremental steps. Consequently the difference between the slightly negative and negative conditions may be quite negligible and may be less than is necessary to be reflected in the N1-P2 component of the evoked potential. This possibility is suggested by the individual statistical comparisons between all possible pairs of evoked potential means within the affect rating run. Comparisons of all evoked potential pairs were significant except for the comparison of the slightly unpleasant condition with the unpleasant condition.

The results obtained at the right hemisphere electrode site are not as striking as those obtained at the left and suggest that the left hemisphere may be more involved, and/or more responsive to connotative meaning elicited by semantic stimuli. It should be noted that the amplitude of the N1-P2 component is somewhat greater over the left hemisphere than on the right. However, in our study these results are only suggestive and are not statistically significant. Our findings do suggest the use of caution in the interpretation of the asymmetric role of the cortical hemispheres in dealing

with semantic information.  The lack of hemispheric asymmetry in
the processing of linguistic material has been reported by a number
of investigators (Shelburne, 1972, 1973, Galambos et al, 1975, and
Friedman et al., 1975a; 1975b).

In general our findings are in keeping with earlier reports
from our laboratory (Begleiter and Platz, 1969; Begleiter, Gross,
and Kissin, 1967) in which we suggested that the processing of specific connotative content of a stimulus is encoded in the waveform
of the human evoked potential.  Our present results and those of
other investigators suggest that internal experiences of feelings
or mental imagery about semantic stimuli may indeed be reflected
in the electrical activity of the human brain.  We do not suggest
that this neural representation of feelings is determined by the
specific affective state which a word explicitly names or describes,
so that the evoked potential obtained to the word LOVE does not
represent an electrical sign of the specific feeling of love but may
possibly represent the general connotative properties of the word
which might possibly vary from individual to individual.

In the last decade numerous investigations have demonstrated
that event-related brain potentials are quite sensitive in encoding
the content of the eliciting stimulus.  Our present findings and
those of other investigators strongly suggest that the connotative
meaning may well be reflected in the neuroelectric activity elicited
by semantic stimuli.

ACKNOWLEDGMENTS

This work was supported by NIAAA grant# AA-02686.

REFERENCES

Beck, E.C.  Electrophysiology and behavior.  In Annual Review of
Psychology.  Rosensweig, M.R. and Porter, L.W. (Eds.).  Annual Review Inc., Palo Alto, 1975, 26:233-262.

Begleiter, H. and Platz, H.  Cortical evoked potentials to semantic
stimuli.  Psychophysiol.  1969, 6:91-100.

Begleiter, H. and Porjesz, B.  Evoked potentials as indicators of
decision-making.  Science, 1975, 187:754-755.

Begleiter, H., Gross, M.M., and Kissin, B.  Evoked cortical responses
to affective visual stimuli.  Psychophysiol.  1967, 3:336-344.

Brown, W.S., Marsh, J.T., and Smith, J.C.   Contextual meaning effects on speech-evoked potentials.  Behav. Biol.  1973, 9:755-761.

Brown, W.S. and Marsh, J.T., and Smith, J.C.   Evoked potential waveform differences produced by the perception of different meanings of an ambiguous phrase.  Electroenceph. clin. Neurophysiol. 1976, 41:113-123.

Buchsbaum, M. and Fedio, P.   Visual information and evoked responses from the left and right hemispheres.  Electroenceph. clin. Neurophysiol.  1969, 26:266-272.

Callaway, E.  Brain Electrical Potentials and Individual Psychological Differences.  Grune and Stratton, New York, 1975.

Chapman, R.M., Bragdon, H.R., Chapman, J.A., and McCrary, J.W.  Semantic meaning of words and average evoked potentials.  In Progress in Clinical Neurophysiology.  Desmedt, J.E. (Ed.) vol.3, S. Karger, Basal (Switzerland), 1977, pp.36-47.

Friedman, D., Simson, R., Ritter, W. and Rapin, I.   Cortical evoked potentials elicited by real speech words and human sounds.  Electroenceph. clin. Neurophysiol.  1975a, 38:13-19.

Friedman, D., Simson, R., Ritter, W., and Rapin, I.   The late positive component (P300) and information processing in sentences. Electroenceph. clin. Neurophysiol.  1975b, 38:255-262.

Galambos, R., Benson, P., Smith, T.S., Shulman-Galambos, C. and Osier, H.   On the hemispheric differences in evoked potentials to speech stimuli.  Electroenceph. clin. Neurophysiol.  1975, 39:279-283.

Gliddon, J.B., Busk, J., and Galbraith, G.C.   Visual evoked responses to emotional stimuli in the mentally retarded.  Psychophysiol. 1971, 8:576-580.

Jasper, H.H.   The ten twenty electrode system.  Electroenceph. clin. Neurophysiol.  1958, 10:371-375.

Jenness, D.   Stimulus role and gross differences in the cortical evoked response.  Physiol. and Behav.  1972, 9:14-146.

John, E.R., Herrington, R.N., and Sutton, S.   Effects of visual form on the evoked response.  Science.  1967, 155:1439-1442.

Johnston, V.S. and Chesney, G.L.   Electrophysiological correlates of meaning.  Science.  1974, 186:944-946.

Lenhardt, M.L.   Effects of frequency modulation on auditory averaged evoked response.  Audiology.  1971, 10: 18-22.

Lifshitz, K.  The averaged evoked cortical responses to complex visual stimuli. Psychophysiol.  1966, 3:55-68.

Matsumiya, Y., Tagiliasco, V., Lombroso, C.T., and Goodglass, H. Auditory evoked response:  meaningfulness of stimuli and interhemispheric asymmetry. Science.  1972, 175:790-792.

Morrell, L.K. and Salamy, J.G.  Hemispheric asymmetry of electrocortical response to speech stimuli.  Science.  1971, 174:164-166.

Neville, H.  Electrographic correlates of lateral asymmetry in the processing of verbal and nonverbal auditory stimuli.  J. Psychol. Res.  1974, 3:151-163.

Ratliff, S.S. and Greenberg, H.J.  The averaged encephalic response to linguistic and nonlinguistic auditory stimuli.  J. Audit. Res. 1972, 12:14-25.

Regan, D.  Evoked Potentials in Psychology, Sensory Physiology and Clinical Medicine.  Chapman and Hall, London, 1972.

Schwartz, M.  Averaged evoked responses and the encoding of perception.  Psychophysiol.  1976, 13:546-553.

Shelburne, S.A.  Visual evoked responses to word and nonsense syllable stimuli.  Electroenceph. clin. Neurophysiol.  1972, 32:17-25.

Shelburne, S.A.  Visual evoked responses to language stimuli in normal children.  Electroenceph. clin. Neurophysiol. 1973, 34: 135-143.

Shevrin, H. and Fritzler, D.E.  Visual evoked response correlates of unconscious mental processes.  Science.  1968, 161:295-298.

Shevrin, H., Smith, W.H. and Fritzler, D.E.  Average evoked response and verbal correlates of unconscious mental processes.  Psychophysiol. 1971, 8:149-162.

Spunda, J., Radil-Weiss, T. and Radilova, J.  A technique for on-line classification of evoked potentials into two groups according to subjective interpretation of the stimulus.  Electroenceph. clin. Neurophysiol.  1975, 39:411-413.

Teyler, T.J., Roemer, R.A., Harrison, T.F., and Thompson, R.F. Human scalp-recorded evoked-potential correlates of linguistic stimuli.  Bull. Psychom. Soc.  1973, 1:333-334.

Thatcher, R.W. and April, R.S.  Evoked potential correlates of
semantic information processing in normals and aphasics.  In R.
Riebert (Ed.).  The Neuropsychology of Language:  Essays in Honor
of Eric Lenneberg.  Plenum Press, New York, 1976.


Thatcher, R.W. and John, E.R.  Functional Neuroscience Vol. I
Foundations of Cognitive Processes.  Lawrence Erlbaum Assoc.,
New Jersey, 1977.

Winer, B.J.  Statistical Principles in Experimental Design.  New
York: McGraw-Hill, 1962.

Wood, C.C., Goff, W.R., and Day, R.S.  Auditory evoked potentials
during speech perception.  Science.  1971, 173:1248-1251.

# FUNCTIONAL LANDSCAPES OF THE BRAIN: AN ELECTROTOPOGRAPHIC PERSPECTIVE

Robert W. Thatcher and Eileen B. Maisel

Brain Research Laboratories and Department of
Psychiatry, New York University School of Medicine,
550 First Avenue, New York, New York 10016

The title "Functional Landscapes of the Brain" was borrowed
from a particularly elegant study of regional cerebral blood
flow changes during cognitive performance by Ingvar and Risberg
(1967). Ingvar and colleagues (Risberg and Ingvar, 1973; Ingvar
and Schwartz, 1974; Ingvar et al,1975a) used radioactive xenon
to monitor the metabolic regulation of cerebral blood flow (rCBF)
which was regionally specific and accompanied problem solving and
abstract thinking (Ingvar and Risberg, 1967; Risberg and Ingvar,
1973), voluntary hand movements (Ingvar et al,1975a), speech and
reading (Ingvar and Schwartz, 1974), and electrical cutaneous stimulation (Ingvar et al, 1975b). This work represents the first
comprehensive quantitative topographic analysis of regionally
specific physiological changes accompanying higher mental activity.

However, a major drawback of blood flow methods is that temporal resolution is on the order of seconds. In contrast, the
method of evoked potential (EP) analysis offers the possibility of
studying topographic correlates of mental activity on the order of
milliseconds. The advantage of finer time resolution lies in the
fact that those vital processes intermediate between the presentation of information and the final motor output can be brought
under closer scrutiny. As discussed elsewhere (Thatcher, 1976),
this is one of the major advantages of electrophysiological tests
in contrast to psychometric tests. That is, only electrophysiological measures allow for the dissection of the millisecond transformations of sensory information to higher levels of cascading
cognitive processing which occur before motor output and are fundamental to correct and adaptive performance.

In the present paper, preliminary attempts to develop an

143

"Electrotopographic Task Analysis" (ETA) will be presented. This approach involves applying multivariate statistics to evoked potentials obtained during the performance of cognitive tasks. The full spectrum of multivariate techniques have not, as yet, been applied. This must await further study. However, the novel use of the varimax factor analysis will be emphasized as a method to dissect early (0 to≈ 250 msec) and late (≤250 to 700 msec) evoked potential components which are specific to various aspects of cognitive performance and show regional specificity.

## THE NEUROCOGNITIVE TEST BATTERY

The present chapter addresses itself to the application of evoked potentials in active task challenges. The work presented in this chapter dates back to 1973 where the "Background Information Probe" (BIP) paradigm was first presented at a conference on "Behavior and Brain Electrical Activity" (Thatcher and John, 1975).

BIP is a general procedure designed to control for background excitability states that precede and follow information delivery (Thatcher, 1977a). The procedure, which is illustrated in Figure 1, involves the presentation of a variable number of random dot displays (controls), then an information stimulus (the standard,

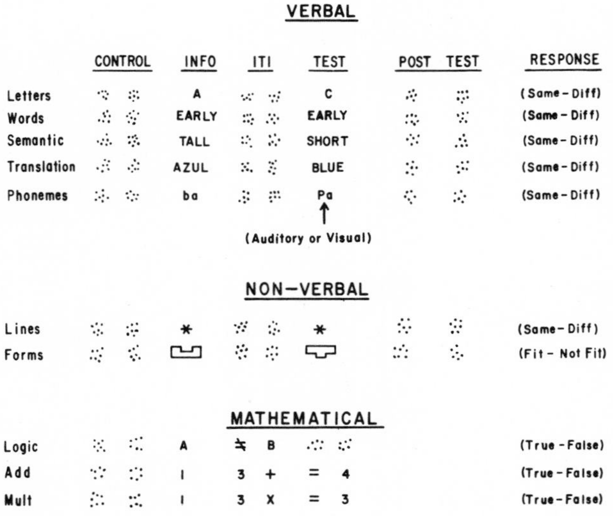

**VERBAL**

|  | CONTROL | INFO | ITI | TEST | POST TEST | RESPONSE |
|---|---|---|---|---|---|---|
| Letters |  | A |  | C |  | ( Same – Diff ) |
| Words |  | EARLY |  | EARLY |  | (Same – Dif f) |
| Semantic |  | TALL |  | SHORT |  | (Same – Diff) |
| Translation |  | AZUL |  | BLUE |  | (Same – Diff) |
| Phonemes |  | ba |  | Pa ↑ |  | (Same – Diff) |

(Auditory or Visual)

**NON–VERBAL**

| Lines |  | * |  | * |  | (Same – Diff) |
|---|---|---|---|---|---|---|
| Forms |  | ⊔ |  | ⊽ |  | (Fit – Not Fit) |

**MATHEMATICAL**

| Logic |  | A | ⋚ B |  | (True – False) |
|---|---|---|---|---|---|
| Add |  | 1 | 3 + = 4 |  | (True – False) |
| Mult |  | 1 | 3 X = 3 |  | (True – False) |

Fig. 1.   Examples of items in the Neurocognitive Test Battery

e.g. a letter or word) followed by a second series of random dot displays (intertest interval or ITIs) followed by a second infor- mation stimulus (test stimulus) that matches or mismatches the standard. In some of the tasks a third series of random dot dis- plays are presented following the test stimulus in order to further investigate excitability changes as well as to delay responses so as to avoid contamination by movement artifact. All of the displays within a task are equal in duration (20 msec), intensity, and in retinal area subtended (foveal). The interstimulus inter- vals are typically 1 second but can be varied. Intertrial inter- vals are usually 4 seconds during which subjects differentially respond to match (same), mismatch (different) and, in some tasks, an uncertain, no operation or neutral condition. A more detailed description of the procedure is presented elsewhere (Thatcher, 1976; 1977a).

It should be emphasized that this is only a prototype test battery. To date, subjects have been run on the letter and word matching tasks, the synonym and antonym task, the Spanish-to- English and English-to-Spanish task, the logic and mathematical tasks, and the form matching tasks. The complete battery has not, as yet, been standardized on a population of normals. Given the difficulty in obtaining government funding this test battery may never be applied in its entirety. It is presented here to illus- trate and describe an hypothesized approach to neurocognitive assessment, namely, an evoked potential active task challenge that contains procedural invariants as controls that, theoretically, facilitate diagnostic and prognostic assessment. It can be seen in Figure 1 that all of the various tasks share the general cognitive challenge of delayed matching to sample. That is, a general demand on a subject's attention, the maintenance of the memory of the standard display and a subsequent comparison (some- times at a concrete level and sometimes at more abstract levels) is required in all tasks. The aim of the test battery is to provide a series of tasks which are short in duration and thus not overly fatiguing and which challenge different aspects of cognitive func- tion involving ascending or descending levels of complexity. Each of the tasks require a subject's continual attention since the subjects cannot predict exactly when the information display will occur. Examination of AEP variance to the random dot control stim- uli may help in assessing attention fluctuations. Attention can also be assessed by separately averaging all the EPs elicited on correct trials in comparison to incorrect trials (this assumes that the subject's attention is needed for greater than chance correct performance).

The procedural invariants are an integral part of the test battery and are designed to maximize the following comparisons: 1) Within-Subject-Within-Task Differences; 2) Within-Subject-

Between-Task Differences;  3) Between-Subject-Within-Task Differences;  4) Between-Subject-Between-Task Differences.  The first
set of comparisons are between the AEPs elicited by succeeding
random dot displays that precede information.  This represents
the control differences which yield information about within subject variance.  As will be shown later (see fig. 2), stable and
reproducable control AEPs facilitate the interpretation of the
varimax factor analysis.  Other Within-Subject-Within-Task differences are between AEPs elicited by identical random dot displays
that precede and follow the standard stimulus (during the rehear-
sal period, see Thatcher, 1976; 1977a; 1977b), between AEPs elicited
by the standard stimulus and physically identical test stimuli, and
between AEPs elicited by test stimuli that match the standard stimulus in comparison to identical test stimuli that mismatch.  These
and other comparisons in the delayed letter matching task are
shown in Table I.

     The Within-Subject-Between-Task analyses involve differences
within a subject for control, standard, ITI and test conditions
across tasks.  These comparisons can provide important information
about changes in AEP component latencies and anatomical topography
which occur as a function of the nature of the task (Thatcher, 1976).

     The Between-Subject-Within-Task analyses involve first compu-
ting the Within-Subject-Within-Task differences and then comparing
any individual subject with any other subject or any individual
with the group mean (of the same age or a different age).  Z transforms can be used, for instance, to compare the changes between
control and the standard stimulus or between the standard and test
stimuli, etc., for an individual with respect to the group mean.
In this way, differences in "cognitive style" may be revealed as
groups or clusters within the normal population (sometimes with
membership = 1) as well as statistically significant deviance from
normal in one or more scalp locations which may be related to a
disability.  Of course, large Ns and careful assessment of variance
is necessary to adjust statistical thresholds so as to minimize
false positives and false negatives.

     The Between-Subject-Between-Task comparison is similar to the
previous analysis but involves computing a difference across tasks
for an individual with respect to any other individual or group.
This analysis may eventually help in providing relevant neurophysiological information about a subject's strengths and weaknesses
in cognitive function.  Again, large Ns and replications of the
discriminate functions are needed to establish the full diagnostic
effectiveness of this approach.

     It is believed that the meaningfulness of these various com-
parisons are maximized by the procedural details of the paradigm

Table I: AEP COMPARISONS THAT DISTINGUISH "CONTENT" vs "OPERATION" [a]

| CONTROL ANALYSES | OPERATION IS CONSTANT WHILE INFORMATION VARIES | INFORMATION IS CONSTANT WHILE OPERATION VARIES |
|---|---|---|
| Control$_1$ AEP vs Control$_2$ | "A" Standard AEP vs "B" Standard | "A" Match AEP vs "A" Mismatch |
| Control$_1$ AEP vs ITI$_{1-n}$ | "B" Standard AEP vs "C" Standard | "B" Match AEP vs "B" Mismatch |
| Control$_1$ AEP vs Standard (A,B,C) | "C" Standard AEP vs "A" Standard | "C" Match AEP vs "C" Mismatch |
| Control$_1$ AEP vs Match (A,B,C) | "A" Test AEPs vs "B" Test AEPs | "A" Standard AEP vs "A" Test |
| Control$_1$ AEP vs Mismatch (A,B,C) | "B" Test AEPs vs "C" Test AEPs | "B" Standard AEP vs "B" Test |
| | "C" Test AEPs vs "A" Test AEPs | "C" Standard AEP vs "C" Test |

itself, that is, the use of psychophysically controlled stimuli, unpredictable stimulus contents and the invariance of the operat- ions of delayed matching invoked in different cognitive tasks. Also, the fact that the procedure requires attention, is interes- ting to subjects, and minimally fatiquing, helps reduce variance which, in turn, enhances meaningful comparisons.

Another important factor, unique to these procedures, is that stimuli are not presented repeatedly or redundantly. For instance, in the synonym-antonym task (Thatcher, 1977b), 48 different words are presented in a session and subjects are run on only two sess- ions. In the logic task the letters A, B, C and D are presented but in continually different logical contexts (Thatcher and Maisel, unpublished). Thus, habituation of the content of specific stim- uli and redundancy in general is minimized.

Finally, the technique of embedding information within a series of meaningless stimuli should be discussed. The study of background excitability changes using non-contingent probes pre- sented in the same or a different modality is a widely used tech- nique in human and, particularly, animal research (Gershuni et al, 1960; Kitai et al, 1965; Morrell and Morrell, 1965; Khachaturian and Gluck, 1969; Ciganek, 1969; John et al, 1973a; Hudspeth and Jones, 1975). A number of studies (Gastau et al, 1957; John and Killam, 1960; Khachaturian and Gluck, 1969; Khachaturian et al, 1974) and, most recently, a particularly elegant study by Hudspeth and Jones (1975) report systematic changes in the coher- ence of anatomically distributed electrode sites during condition- ing. These changes were complex, often involving regionally specific increases or decreases in coherence. As hypothesized more fully elsewhere (Thatcher, 1976; Thatcher and John, 1977) background neural excitability states represent the initial state from which trajectories of information flow originate. For this reason, it is believed that attempts to quantitize or measure EP waveforms to non-contingent probes is a necessary and vital adjunct to the understanding of the brain's response to information.

## APPLICATION OF VARIMAX FACTOR ANALYSIS

The historical development of the field of human electrophysi- ology illustrates the frequent controversies that occur as a new science or scientific technique emerges. The application of ortho- normal systems of equations (such as exponential, fourier, walsh analysis, etc.) and multivariate statistics to the analysis of EP data is one example of where controversy still exists. The metho- dological details and advantages of the application of these methods to EP data analysis, however, is beyond the scope of the present chapter. Several excellent reviews of this subject are available (Glaser and Ruchkin, 1976; John et al, 1977). Suffice it to say, that different procedures are suitable for different purposes and often involve different assumptions about the natural structure of the data.  At this early stage of development it is our strategy to be open to any and all methods of analysis and not to purposely exclude any one or, conversely, to use only one method. However, in comparison to peak-to-peak or baseline-to-peak EP component analysis, there are several distinct advantages to the use of multivariate statistics.  One, is that peak-to-peak or baseline-to-peak component analysis implicitly emphasize the independence of the EP components.  In contrast, multivariate statistics (such as factor analysis and discriminant analysis) emphasize the covariance of the sequence of time points that comprise the EP.  The multivariate approach assumes ignorance of the independence or dependence of the various EP components and asks, simply, which set of covarying time points are distinguishable from other sets of covarying time points.  Another advantage of the use of multivariate statistics is that such methods provide for the analysis of large numbers of EPs in a maximally simplistic and parsimonious manner, a feature useful in large population studies.

One method used extensively by the present authors is the varimax rotation of the principal-component axes of the factor analysis (Kaiser, 1958; Harmon , 1967).  The varimax rotation has the advantage of facilitating the physiological interpretation of the factors since an AEP tends to have a high coefficient for only one factor, and each factor has zero, or near zero, coefficients for at least some of the AEPs.  This minimax constraint tends to produce a type of cluster analysis in which a set of AEPs, with shared waveform characteristics, load maximally on one factor and contribute minimally to any other factor (see John et al, 1973 b Thatcher and John, 1975; Thatcher 1976; 1977a; 1977b).

The computer program that we use[1] provides the option of performing the factor analysis on a set of amplitude normalized AEPs. The normalization process, which involves setting the total variance of each AEP equal to unity,[2] constrains the factor analysis such that differential loadings on orthogonal factors occur <u>as a function of AEP waveshape, independent of amplitude</u>.  Averaged EPs which differ only in amplitude may suggest a quantitative difference in function but not a qualitative difference.  That is, increased amplitude represents either an increase in the number of generators (e.g. glial cells and/or neurons) or greater synchrony with equal population size (Thatcher and John, 1977).  AEP waveform changes, on the other hand, reflect alterations in the spatio-temporal distribution of active generators which indicate a qualitative, and not simply, a quantitative difference in function.

An example of the results of varimax factor analysis of amplitude normalized AEPs from the delayed letter matching paradigm is shown in Figure 2. The top row of waves are AEPs from the various conditions of the letter-matching experiment (controls, standard, ITIs and test). The 4 waves in the column on the left are the orthogonal factors, which in this case accounted for 93% of the variance of all the AEPs. The first factor is called a control factor because it loads primarily on AEPs elicited by the random dot controls (the factor loadings on the AEPs are represented by scaling the amplitude of the factors by their weighting coeffic- ients, see Thatcher and John, 1975 for details). The second factor is called a post-information factor because it loads un- differentially on all information bearing stimuli (Info, Diff. and Same). The third factor is called an information factor since it differentially loads on the first letter and the matching test test stimulus but not on the mismatching test stimulus. And

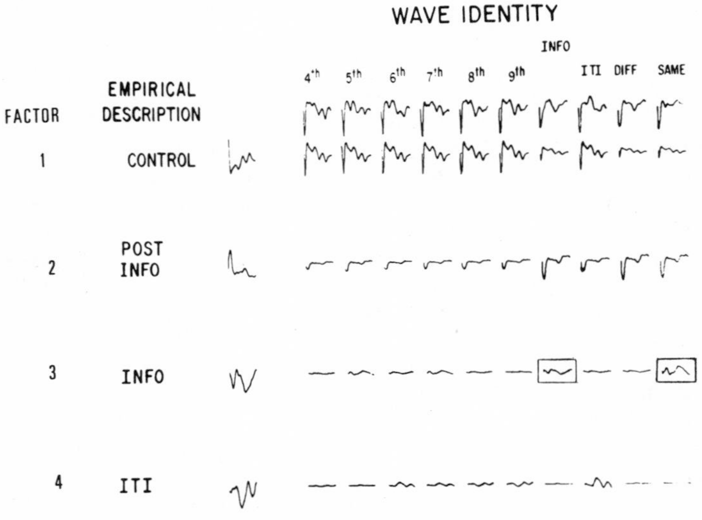

WAVE IDENTITY

Fig. 2. The top are AEPs (N = 52 for all AEPs except same and different AEPs where N = 26) starting with the fourth control dis- play and extending to the test. The four factors (accounting for 93% of the variance) are in the first column of waves on the left. The empirical description of factors was determined by the relat- ive contribution of a factor to a specific variable of the experi- ment. Note that the information factor (factor 3) loads heaviest on the AEP produced by the information display and on the AEP elic- ited by the test stimulus that "matches" (same) the standard dis- play but not on the AEP elicited by the "mismatch" (diff) stimulus. Factors are inverted because they are negatively correlated (from Thatcher and John, 1975).

finally, the fourth factor is called an ITI factor since it loads
on the first ITI.    Thus, orthogonally different factors loaded
on AEPs which were determined by the critical variables of the
experiment.[3]

The results of the varimax factor analysis in Figure 2 represents a "within derivation" analysis.    That is, all of the AEPs
were from one derivation $(O_1)$ but were elicited by different stimulus conditions.    Another method of analysis involves a "between
derivation" factor analysis.    That is, AEPs obtained simultaneously
from all derivations but for only one stimulus condition at a time.
The latter analysis is important since it provides topographic
information.    An example of such an analysis is shown in Figure 3.
This analysis was performed on AEPs elicited in the logic task.

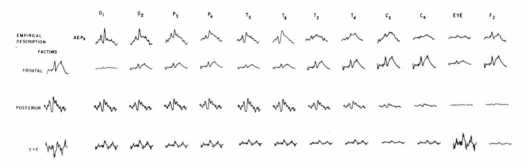

Fig. 3   Top row are AEPs (N=24; analysis epoch = 786 msec)
from 12 different derivations elicited by random dot stimuli in
the logic task.    The three factors (column on left) account for
96% of the variance.    Factor loadings are represented by amplitude
scaling of the factor waveshapes.    The first factor is called a
"frontal factor" since it loads most heavily on frontal derivations
$(T_3, T_4, C_3, C_4, F_z)$; the second factor is called a "posterior factor"
since it loads most heavily on posterior derivations $(O_1, O_2, P_3, P_4,$
$T_5, T_6)$; the third factor is called an "eye factor" since it loads
most heavily on the eye lead.

The three factors in the column on the left account for 96% of the variance. It can be seen that factor one loads slightly on $P_3$ and $P_4$ but heavily on anterior derivations, particularly, $T_3$, $T_4$, and $C_3$, $C_4$. In contrast, factor 2 loads heavily on the posterior derivations, $0_1$, $0_2$, $P_3$, $P_4$, $T_5$ and $T_6$. Factor 3 is a unique factor loading primarily on the eye lead. In general the eye lead loads on an orthogonally different factor than do the scalp leads (Thatcher, 1977b). Differential factor loadings between match and mismatch AEPs and control and standard and ITI AEPs occur maximally in posterior derivations and are absent or attenuated in anterior derivations (see Figures 6 and 7). These consistent findings show that the various phenomena observed in these studies are not due to eye-movements. Another consistent finding revealed by the between derivation factor analysis (such as in figure 3 and table 2) is an anterior-posterior split or differential factor loadings in the anterior-posterior plane. That is, posterior derivations usually load on one factor while anterior derivations load on an orthogonally different factor (Thatcher, 1976). It has been shown that the anterior-posterior split can be altered, systematically, as a function of the various conditions of the BIP procedure (Thatcher, 1977a; 1977b).

Table 2 shows an example of changes in the anterior-posterior dimension, as well as between homologous derivations in the letter matching paradigm. The anterior-posterior split between factors 1 and 2 at $T_3$ is seen in the control condition. Note also that in the control condition there is an absence of interhemispheric asymmetries. That is, homologous electrode pairs load on the same factor. However, as seen in Table 2, a markedly different organization appears when information is presented to the subject. That is, interhemispheric asymmetries appear in which AEPs from the left and right hemisphere load on orthogonally different factors. Also, the anterior-posterior split disappears and is replaced by a uniform left side loading. That is, $P_3$, $T_5$, $T_3$ and $F_7$ all load on the same factor. This analysis suggests a functional organization. That is, there is a change in the topographic organization of AEP waveforms as a function of the presentation of information and this change involves an increased commonality of waveform across widely distributed, but lateralized, scalp regions. It is important to note that the interhemispheric asymmetries in table 2, which occur to the presentation of information, represent asymmetries in AEP waveform independent of amplitude. Thus, with this analysis the functional topography can be studied in terms of either amplitude changes or changes in AEP morphology.

## LOGIC OF NEGATION AND EQUIVALENCE

There are many different logical systems. For example, there is the classical Aristotelian logic, single valued logical systems

TABLE 2

BETWEEN-CONDITION VARIMAX FACTOR ANALYSIS[a]

| Derivations | $O_1$ | $O_2$ | $P_3$ | $P_4$ | $T_5$ | $T_6$ | $T_3$ | $T_4$ | $F_7$ | $F_8$ | EYE | $F_z$ |
|---|---|---|---|---|---|---|---|---|---|---|---|---|
| Control Factors | | | | | | | | | | | | |
| 1 | 0.89 | 0.88 | 0.65 | 0.85 | 0.67 | 0.46 | 0.06 | 0.40 | 0.06 | 0.06 | 0.00 | 0.06 |
| 2 | 0.06 | 0.04 | 0.15 | 0.07 | 0.11 | 0.05 | 0.63 | 0.44 | 0.91 | 0.83 | 0.34 | 0.67 |
| 3 | 0.00 | 0.00 | 0.00 | 0.00 | 0.06 | 0.03 | 0.29 | 0.02 | 0.00 | 0.02 | 0.00 | 0.10 |
| 4 | 0.00 | 0.00 | 0.01 | 0.00 | 0.02 | 0.06 | 0.01 | 0.00 | 0.00 | 0.01 | 0.65 | 0.01 |
| First Letter Factors | | | | | | | | | | | | |
| 1 | 0.90 | 0.96 | 0.42 | 0.57 | 0.22 | 0.17 | 0.02 | 0.08 | 0.01 | 0.01 | 0.00 | 0.11 |
| 2 | 0.04 | 0.00 | 0.35 | 0.10 | 0.54 | 0.18 | 0.95 | 0.35 | 0.90 | 0.04 | 0.00 | 0.28 |
| 3 | 0.01 | 0.02 | 0.00 | 0.07 | 0.06 | 0.10 | 0.00 | 0.42 | 0.04 | 0.95 | 0.08 | 0.17 |
| 4 | 0.00 | 0.00 | 0.15 | 0.16 | 0.07 | 0.52 | 0.00 | 0.06 | 0.00 | 0.00 | 0.14 | 0.32 |
| 5 | 0.00 | 0.00 | 0.00 | 0.01 | 0.00 | 0.00 | 0.00 | 0.00 | 0.00 | 0.00 | 0.77 | 0.00 |

[a] Varimax factor analysis on amplitude-normalized AEPs from 12 derivations for two different experimental conditions in subject D.D. Each row represents the loading of AEPs from different anatomical derivations on a single factor. Each column represents the factor structure for a given derivation. Results show that AEPs from anterior derivations ($T_3$ thru $F_z$) load on different factors than do AEPs from the posterior derivations ($O_1$ thru $T_6$)

(Lewis and Langford, 1932), doubled valued or probalistic systems
(Reichenbach, 1949) and Whitehead and Russell's (1925) axiomatic
system. All of these systems rely on the concepts of "sameness"
and "difference" including Whitehead and Russell who proved that
the foundations of axiomatic mathematics is based on logic. George
Boole (1951) developed an algebra based entirely on binary classifications which involve the concepts of "sameness" and "difference".
These concepts are unique for having played an important role in
the history of psychology, mathematics and physics. Recently,
G. Spencer Brown (1973) developed a logical notation which formal-
ized in an elegant manner, the concepts of "sameness" and "difference". For instance, twenty-eight pages of complex notation from
the "Principia Mathematica" (p. 98-126) was reduced to a single
symbolic statement by the formal application of the concept of
difference.

Recognition of the fundamental position of the concepts of
sameness and difference led to the development of the test battery
in Figure 1. That is, the general operation of representational
matching is held constant while the content and complexity of tasks
varies across items. Given the importance of logic in the development of cognition, a specific logic task was devised. The paradigm, which is represented in Table 3 (for letters A and B only),
involves presenting a variable number of random dot control displays followed by a letter (A, B, C or D),followed by an operation sign ( = or ≠ or a no operation ♩ ), followed by a second
letter (A, B, C or D). The number of illuminated dots is the
same for all displays. The displays are 20 msec in duration and

Table 3. True, False, and No Operation (NOP) Statements

| Function | First Letter | Operation | Second Letter |
|----------|--------------|-----------|---------------|
| True | A | = | A |
| True | B | = | B |
| True | B | ≠ | A |
| True | A | ≠ | B |
| False | B | = | A |
| False | A | = | B |
| False | A | ≠ | A |
| False | B | ≠ | B |
| NOP | A | ♩ | A |
| NOP | B | ♩ | B |
| NOP | A | ♩ | B |
| NOP | B | ♩ | A |

are presented at a repetition frequency of .66/sec.   The subjects
are instructed to move a lever to the left if the syllogistic
statement is true (e.g. A = A; A ≠ B, etc.), to the right if it
is false (e.g., A ≠ A, A = B, etc.) and both left and right in
the no operation condition (e.g., A ◪ B, A ◪ A, etc.).   All conditions are counterbalanced, there are 48 trials per session and
each subject is run on at least two sessions.   In this experiment
concordance or disconcordance between letters occurs equally probably.   Thus, the letter or perceptual aspect of the match-mismatch
procedure is the same as in test item one (see figure 1).   The
difference in this experiment is that the operator determines
whether the second letter matches a logic truth function or not.
If matching of internal representational systems contributes to
late EP positivity, then one might expect that matching of sensory
representations with logic representations would also contribute
to late positivity.   The no operation condition (NOP) should provide valuable information about logic operations since letter AEPs
in this condition can be contrasted with the logic conditions.
The subjects were not asked to match letters, although the letters
were presented successively as in the delayed letter matching
experiment.   Seven subjects (5 males, 2 females ranging in age
from 23 to 35) have been run thus far.   Figure 4 shows AEPs from
one subject to second letters in the three conditions (truth,
falsity, no operation).   It can be seen that the EPs elicited by
second letters in the truth condition exhibit greater late positivity than EPs elicited by the same letters in the false and no
operation conditions ( 't' tests are shown at the bottom of the
figure ).

     An example of AEPs from the various conditions is shown in
Figure 5.   At the bottom of the figure are AEPs elicited by the
random dot controls which can be compared to the AEP elicited by
the first letter.   The latency and shape of the late components of
the AEPs elicited by the operator signs (=,≠ & ◪ ) are different
depending on the operation, while second letter AEPs are different
depending on the logical condition.

     Topographic analyses using the varimax factor analysis reveal
different factor structures from different derivations depending
on the different aspects of the task.   A 3-dimensional representation of these findings is shown in Figures 6 and 7.   The vertical
axis represents the factor coefficients beginning at .25.   The
factors are on the left and the various experimental conditions
are on the right.   These analyses are from the grand averages computed by summing AEPs from all seven subjects.    In the occipital
derivations (Fig. 6) factor 1, with a pronounced early component,
accounts for the variance due to the control AEPs. Factor 2, with
a pronounced late component, accounts for the variance due to the
letters and operator symbols.   Very little variance is accounted

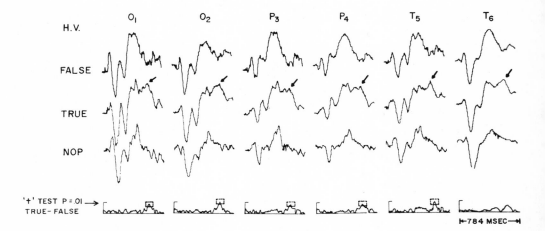

Fig. 4.   AEPs (N = 24) from 1 subject elicited by the second letter of a logic statement (truth e.g., A = A; false e.g., B = A; and no operation A ≠ A).   t-tests between true and false conditions are shown at bottom.   Arrows point to enhanced late positivity. (Horizontal line represents p = 0.01, two-tailed).

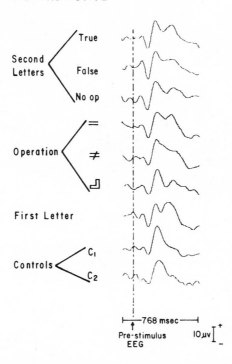

Fig. 5.   Example of AEPs from 1 subject ($T_5$) elicited by the various stimuli in the logic task.

for by factor 3, thus most of the variance due to the various conditions of the experiment is accounted for by two factors.  Since the two factors differentiate the response to random dots versus letters and operators, the occipital regions ($O_1$ and $O_2$) are given the functional description of differentiating and formating information input.  A somewhat different picture is seen in the parietal and posterior temporal derivations ($P_3$, $P_4$ and $T_5$, $T_6$).  In these derivations the factor analysis differentiates between first letters (factor 2) and second letters (factor 3) as well as between the controls (factor 1) and first and second letters.  Accordingly, the parietal and posterior temporal derivations are given the functional description of mediating, primarily, secondary operations since there is a differential loading on orthogonal factors between first letters and second letters and a somewhat different factor structure for operators versus second letters.  This type of structure was not observed in the occipital derivations.  Note that factor 1, which describes the control space, exhibits an early component, factor 2 a late component and factor 3 a complex early-late complex.

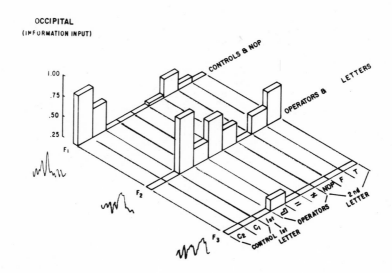

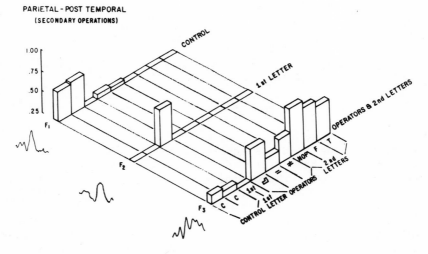

Fig. 6.   3-dimensional display of factor analysis of grand
mean AEPs (7 subjects) from two different topographic regions.
The conditions of the experiment are represented on the right, the
factor waveshapes are on the left and the factor loadings are represented by the height of the bars (beginning at .25).   Note that
factor differentiation between first and second letters occurs
only in the parietal-posterior temporal derivations.   See text
for functional descriptions.

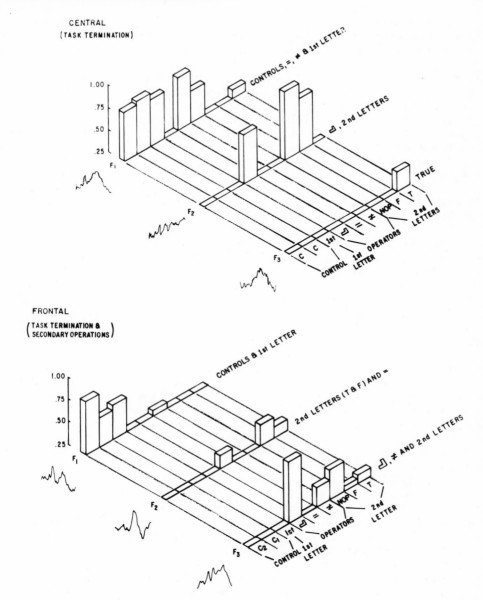

Fig. 7. 3-dimensional display of factor analysis of grand mean AEPs (7 subjects) from two different topographic regions. Explanation of the axes is same as in fig. 6. Note that, in contrast to the analyses in fig. 6, there is no factor differentiation between the random dot controls and first letters in these anterior derivations (i.e., central = $T_3, T_4, C_3, C_4$ and frontal = $F_z$). See text for functional descriptions.

A distinctly different factor structure is seen in anterior derivations (Figure 7). For example, in the central derivations (this same basic factor structure was present in $T_3$, $T_4$, $C_3$ and $C_4$) there is no differentiation (see factor 1) between controls and first letters and the "equals" and "not equals" operators. On the other hand, factor 2 shows heavy loadings for the no operation operator and second letters (NOP and false). In this task the no operation symbol which follows the first letter ( ✔ ) "closes" or terminates the task in the sense that the subjects know immediately what their response must be. Similarly, the presentation of the second letters "closes" the task and also determines the subject's response. Thus, the no operator symbol and the second letters have in common task closure or termination. Accordingly, the central derivations (including $T_3$ and $T_4$) are given the functional description of mediating task termination or closure.

The frontal ($F_z$, Figure 7) derivation exhibited a functional structure that was a combination of both the central and the parietal - posterior temporal regions. That is, there was no distinction between first letters and controls. Also, differential loadings occurred to the no operation symbol and the NOP second letter (and somewhat to the $\neq$). However, some differentiation occurred within the second letters (see factor 2) and between the second letters and the operators.

Thus, in summary, the factor analysis reveals differential AEP loadings according to the critical variables of the task which differ in the anterior-posterior plane. All of the AEPs within an analysis were amplitude normalized and no consistent evidence of interhemispheric asymmetries was observed. These results suggest the feasability of an "Electrotopographic Task Analysis" That is, different regions of the scalp exhibit AEP waveforms that change, differentially, as a function of task demands. The analysis suggests that the occipital regions are involved in information reception, the parietal and posterior temporal regions in secondary and abstract operations, the central regions in task termination and the frontal regions are complexly involved in both central and parietal functions. However, this is not to be interpreted as evidence for strict localization of function since shared functional structures are seen spanning the entire anterior-posterior plane. Also, the data are preliminary in that these particular phenomena were observed in this one experiment and need to be replicated in this and variations of this task. It should be noted, however, that orthogonal factor loadings between controls and words in the synonym-antonym task occur primarily in left side derivations ($P_3$ and $T_5$) and not in the right (see Table 4). Also, a complex anterior-posterior shift in shared factors from left side derivations has been noted in both the delayed letter matching experiment (see Table 2 and Thatcher, 1977a) and the synonym-antonym task (Thatcher, 1977b). This suggests that the exact topography is some-

what unique to each task.  More work is needed before definitive
statements about function can be made.

## DELAYED SEMANTIC MATCHING

Another example of the application of BIP is in the delayed
semantic task involving synonym, antonym and neutral word pairs.
In this task delayed word pairs such as "large"- "little" (antonym),
"small"-"little" (synonym), or "down"-"little" (neutral) are presented.  There are 36 different first words and 12 different second words in a session of 36 trials.  Thus, the same 12 second
words are presented in three different semantic contexts with
the three semantic conditions counterbalanced across trials
(Thatcher, 1976; 1977b).  This task requires remembering the first
word and then comparing the meaning of the second word.

Figure 8 shows an example of AEPs elicited by first words,
random dot controls and second words.  In this experiment only
synonyms and antonyms were presented.  The AEP response to the
first words (top row) was confined largely to occipital and parietal derivations.  A similar anatomical distribution was elicited

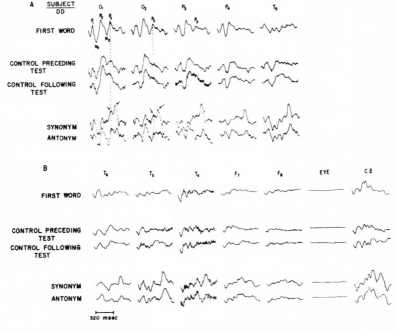

Fig. 8.  AEPs from delayed semantic matching task (from Thatcher, 1976).

by control stimuli, although the latter elicited a significantly
attenuated $N_3$-$P_3$ complex in comparison to first and second words.
The bottom two rows show AEPs to the synonyms and antonyms.  A
very prominent late positive response (P-400) occurred in widespread regions (even $F_7$ and $F_8$) at 440 msec for the synonyms and
460 msec for the antonyms.  Interhemispheric asymmetries were
dynamic, occurring only to the second and not to the first words.
The asymmetries were maximal in $T_5$ vs $T_6$ involving both the early
and late components.  An anterior-posterior gradient of asymmetry
with maximal temporal involvement was noted in a second semantic
experiment that required a Spanish to English and English to
Spanish language translation (Thatcher, 1976, 1977c).  Figure
9 shows an example of AEP waveform asymmetries in $T_5$ vs $T_6$ derivations elicited during the language translation task.  Note that
the component asymmetries occur primarily to second words and not
to the controls or the first words.  This indicates that interhemispheric waveform asymmetries are maximized when higher level
language processes are challenged.  Unlike other tasks (e.g., logic,

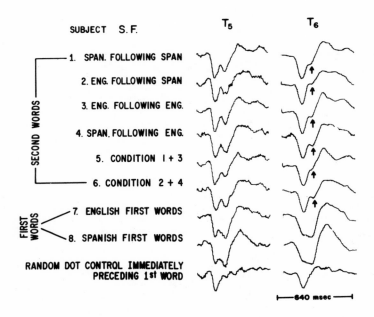

Fig. 9.  AEPs from Spanish-to-English and English-to-Spanish
translation task (from Thatcher, 1977c).

form matching, mathematics, etc.), the semantic tasks, such as those involving language translations or synonym-antonym comparisons, result in pronounced interhemispheric waveform asymmetries which occur independent of AEP amplitude (Thatcher, 1977b).

Another example of a functional topography revealed by the normalized factor analysis is seen in Table 4. The rows represent the various conditions of the synonym-antonym-neutral task while the columns represent the orthogonal factors that describe the AEPs elicited by the task conditions. This factor analysis was performed on the grand averages from all eight subjects performing in the task. It can be seen in Table 4 that in the $P_3$ and $T_5$ derivations AEPs elicited by the random dot controls and the AEPs elicited by words load on orthogonally different factors (factors 1 and 2) where as, in $P_4$ and $T_6$ or the right side derivations, very little factor differentiation between controls and words is observed. This data provides another example of a functional interhemispheric asymmetry in which the signal-to-noise ratio, represented by the brain's responses to randomness versus words, is greater from the left hemisphere than from the right.


## DISCUSSION

A topographical perspective of brain function is desirable for both basic research purposes and clinical applications. Many attempts toward the development of EEG and EP topographic analyses have been made (see Regan, 1972; and John, 1977 for reviews of this literature). For example, Livanov (1962) and Gavrilova (1970) showed increased coherence of frontal-occipital EEG during mental activation (such as problem solving). Callaway (1975) and Callaway and Harris (1974) demonstrated left hemisphere increases in coherence (using the information theory coupling coefficient) during verbal tasks and right hemisphere increases during spatial tasks. Also, many workers have shown AEP and EEG interhemispheric asymmetries during verbal and spatial tasks (see Donchin et al, 1977 and Thatcher, 1977b for reviews). However, no global and comprehensive electrophysiological analysis has demonstrated reliable and regionally specific changes in brain physiology as a function of the qualitative aspects of a task. As discussed in the introduction, electrophysiology is lagging in that qualtitative physiological profiles have been provided by Ingvar and colleagues in their studies of regional blood flow changes.

Theoretically, electrophysiological analyses offer the advantage of very fine time resolution (on the order of milliseconds). This is important since the series transformations from patterns of energy falling on receptors, to spatial temporal electrophysiological activity (ionic flows), to intermediate molecular activity

TABLE 4.  EVOKED POTENTIAL FACTOR LOADINGS FOR LEFT AND RIGHT HEMISPHERE DERIVATIONS FROM THE DELAYED SEMANTIC MATCHING TASK

| | Left Parietal | | | Right Parietal | | |
|---|---|---|---|---|---|---|
| | Factors | | | Factors | | |
| | 1 | 2 | 3 | 1 | 2 | 3 |
| Control - | 0.69 | 0.11 | 0.06 | 0.80 | 0.00 | 0.00 |
| Control - | 0.92 | 0.03 | 0.01 | 0.83 | 0.06 | 0.00 |
| 1st Word - | 0.25 | 0.62 | 0.10 | 0.97 | 0.00 | 0.00 |
| ITI-1 - | 0.89 | 0.04 | 0.01 | 0.65 | 0.01 | 0.06 |
| ITI-2 - | 0.02 | 0.00 | 0.98 | 0.00 | 0.00 | 0.99 |
| ITI-3 - | 0.61 | 0.24 | 0.00 | 0.60 | 0.37 | 0.03 |
| Neu. - | 0.40 | 0.31 | 0.25 | 0.91 | 0.03 | 0.00 |
| Ant. - | 0.21 | 0.47 | 0.30 | 0.97 | 0.00 | 0.01 |
| Syn. - | 0.25 | 0.44 | 0.29 | 0.98 | 0.00 | 0.00 |

| | Left Posterior Temporal | | | Right Posterior Temporal | | |
|---|---|---|---|---|---|---|
| | Factors | | | Factors | | |
| | 1 | 2 | 3 | 1 | 2 | 3 |
| Control - | 0.80 | 0.08 | 0.00 | 0.50 | 0.32 | 0.18 |
| Control - | 0.89 | 0.06 | 0.00 | 0.42 | 0.41 | 0.07 |
| 1st Word - | 0.23 | 0.73 | 0.03 | 0.86 | 0.03 | 0.02 |
| ITI-1 - | 0.80 | 0.11 | 0.01 | 0.66 | 0.24 | 0.04 |
| ITI-2 - | 0.04 | 0.00 | 0.95 | 0.00 | 0.98 | 0.01 |
| ITI-3 - | 0.81 | 0.11 | 0.00 | 0.27 | 0.61 | 0.08 |
| Neu. - | 0.31 | 0.54 | 0.12 | 0.96 | 0.01 | 0.01 |
| Ant. - | 0.21 | 0.69 | 0.10 | 0.95 | 0.01 | 0.03 |
| Syn. - | 0.25 | 0.65 | 0.08 | 0.95 | 0.02 | 0.03 |

Neu. = neutral second word; Ant. = antonym second word; Syn. = synonym second word.  Underlines represent maximum factor loadings for a given condition on a single factor.

(biogenic amines, enkephalin, cyclic AMP, etc.), to macromolecular representations (proteins, aminoacids, etc.) can theoretically be monitored and quantified by a combination of topographic analyses. The brain's responses to drugs, recovery of function following trauma and the evaluation of remediation may someday rely on such measures.

The present chapter emphasizes the application of the varimax factor analysis in the development of an electrophysiological task analysis. The central idea of this approach is two-fold: One, in the between derivation analysis, the idea is to find AEP waveforms that are shared by a subset of topographic regions during a particular cognitive function but are not shared during other cognitive functions; and,two, in the within derivation analysis, the idea is to find AEP waveform differences within a given region that occur to different aspects of a task (also, between tasks or between groups). The varimax analysis maximally finds a subset of waves that reflect commonality or shared processes. An underlying supposition of this approach is that temporal patterns which occur nearly contiguously in different brain regions reflect a common function. Conversely, dissimilar temporal patterns represent a difference in function.

Given the goal of finding commonalities and differences in waveforms, it should be noted that factor analysis posseses a number of weaknesses that do not make this method ideal (see Cooley and Lohnes, 1971). Multidimensional scaling, cluster analysis, minimal spanning trees, and discriminate analysis offer greater promise, if used appropriately, to reveal replicable and invariant processes in time and space related to particular aspects of cognitive function.

In summary, the attempt at an electrophysiological task analysis presented here is still only preliminary. The data obtained to date, however, shows that the use of an active task with non-contingent probes and built in invariances reveals regionally specific electrophysiological profiles related to different aspects of cognitive function. Furthermore, these profiles reflect shared wave processes within subsets of anatomical derivations.

## FOOTNOTES

[1]

The factor analysis program was written by Dr. Paul Easton for the PDP-12 computer

[2]

The amplitude normalization process involves first computing the epoch mean voltage $\overline{X} = 1/N \sum x_i$, where $x_i$ equals the voltage values in each sample bin. Then a DC level is computed $(\overline{X} - x_i)$ and normalized $\overline{Y}^2 = \dfrac{(\overline{X} - x_i)^2}{(\overline{X}^2 - \overline{x}_i^2)} Y2$. Unity variance is set for all the AEPs by scaling each voltage value so that $\overline{Y}^2 = 1$.

[3]

The replicability of the factor analyses can be judged by a) 43 out of 43 subjects run in the various tasks to date show differential loadings on control AEPs versus information AEPs; b) 38 out of 43 subjects show a unique ITI factor; c) 7 out of 9 subjects run in the delayed letter matching task showed higher loadings between match and standard AEPs than between mismatch and standard AEPs; and, d) 39 out of 43 subjects showed an anterior-posterior factor structure with one factor loading heavily on anterior derivations ($T_3$ thru $F_z$) and another factor loading heavily on posterior derivations ($O_1$ thru $T_{5\&6}$).

## REFERENCES

Boole, G.  1951.  An Investigation of the Laws of Thought. New York, Dover Publications, Inc. (Originally published in 1854.)

Brown, G. S. 1973. Laws of Form. New York, Bantam Books.

Callaway, E. and Harris, P. R. 1974.  Coupling between cortical potentials from different areas.  Science, 183:873-874.

Callaway, E. 1975.  Brain potentials and predictors of performance.  In N. Burch and H. Altshuler (eds.), Behavior and Brain Electrical Activity, p. 473.  New York, Plenum Press, Inc.

Gavrilova, N. A. 1970.  Spatial syncrhronization of cortical potentials in patients with disturbances of association.  In V. S. Rusinov (ed.), Electrophysiology of the Central Nervous System, p. 129. New York, Plenum Press, Inc.

Ciganek, L. 1969.  Visually evoked potential correlates of attention and distraction in man.  Psychiat. Clin., 2:95-108.

Cooley, W. and Lohnes, P. 1971. Multivariate Data Analysis. New York, John Wiley and Sons, Inc.

Donchin, E., Kutas, M., and McCarthy, G. 1977. Electrocortical indices of hemispheric utilization. In S. Harnar, R. Doty, L Goldstein, J. Jaynes, and G. Krauthamer (eds.), Lateralization in the Nervous System, p. 339. New York, Academic Press.

Gastaut, H., Jus, A., Jus., C., Morrell, F., Storm Van Leeuwen, W., Dongier, S., Naquet, R., Regis, H., Roger, A., Bekkering, D., Kamp, A., and Werre, J. 1957. Etude topographique des reactions electroencephalographiques conditionness chez l'homme. Electroenceph. Clin. Neurophysiol., 9:1-14.

Gershuni, G. V., Kozhevnikov, V., Maruseva, A. M., Avakyan, R., Radionova, E., Altman, J., and Soroko, V. 1960. Modifications in electrical responses of the auditory system in different states of the higher nervous activity. Electroenceph. Clin. Neurophysiol. 13:115-124.

Glaser, E. M., and Ruchkin, D. S., 1976. Principles of Neurobiological Signal Analysis. New York, Academic Press.

Harmon, H. H., 1967. Modern Factor Analysis. Chicago, Univ. of Chicago Press.

Hudspeth, W. J. and Jones, G. 1975. Stability of neural interference patterns. In P. Greguss (ed.), Holography in Medicine: Proceedings of the International Symposium on Holography in Biomedical Sciences. London: IPC Science and Technology Press.

Ingvar, D. H., and Risberg, J. 1967. Increase of regional cerebral blood flow during mental effort in normals and in patients with focal brain disorders. Exp. Brain Res., 3:195-211

Ingvar, D. H. and Schwartz, M. S. 1974. Blood flow patterns induced in the dominant hemisphere by speech and reading. Brain, 97:274-288.

Ingvar, D. H., Risberg, J., and Schwartz, M. S. 1975a. Evidence of subnormal function of association cortex in presenile dementia. Neurol., 25:964-974.

Ingvar, D. H., Rosen, I., and Elmsvist, D. 1975b. Effects of sensory stimulation upon regional cerebral blood flow. (abstr) VII Int. CBF Symposium, Aviemore, Holland, June.

John, E. R. 1977. Functional Neuroscience, Vol. II, Clinical Applications of Neurometrics. E. R. John and R. W. Thatcher (eds.) New Jersey, L. Erlbaum Assoc, Inc.

John, E. R. and Killam, K. F. 1960.  Electrophysiological correlates of differential approach-avoidance conditioning in the cat. J. Nerv. Ment. Dis., 131:183-196.

John, E. R., Bartlett, F., Shimokochi, M., and Kleinman, D. 1973a. Neural readout from memory.  J. Neurophysiol., 36:893-924.

John, E. R., Walker, P., Cawood, D., Rush, M., and Gehrman, J. 1973b. Factor analysis of evoked potentials.  Electroenceph. Clin. Neurophysiol., 34:33-43.

John, E. R., Ruchkin, D. S. and Vidal, J. J.  1977 (in press) Measurement of event-related potentials. In Proc. NIMH Conf. on Event-Related Potentials in Man, Arlinghouse, MD.

Kaiser, H. F. 1958. The varimax criterion for analytic rotation in factor analysis.  Psychometrika, 23:187-192.

Khachaturian, Z. S. and Gluck, H. 1969. The effects of arousal on the amplitude of evoked potentials.  Brain Res. 14:589-606.

Khachaturian, Z. S., Chisholm, R. and Kerr, J. 1973.  The effects of arousal on evoked potentials to relevant and irrelevant stimuli.  Psychophysiol., 10:194.

Kitai, S. T., Cohen, B., and Morin, F. 1965.  Changes in the amplitude of photically evoked potentials by a conditioned stimulus. Electroenceph. Clin. Neurophysiol., 19:344-349.

Lewis, C. I. and Langford, C. H. 1932.  Symbolic Logic.  New York, The Century Company.

Livanov, M. N. 1962. Spatial analysis of the bioelectric activity of the brain.  In Information processing in the nervous system, Proceedings of the 22nd International Congress of Physiological Science. p. 899. Leiden.

Morrell, F., and Morrell, L. 1965.  Computer aided analyses of brain electrical activity.  In L. D. Proctor and W. R. Adey (eds.), The Analysis of Central Nervous System and Cardiovascular Data Using Computer Methods. p. 441. Washington, D. C.: NASA, U. S. Government Printing House.

Regan, D. 1972.  Evoked Potentials in Psychology, Sensory Physiology and Clinical Medicine.  London, Chapman Hall, Ltd.

Reichenbach, H. 1949.  The Theory of Probability; An Inquiry into the Logical and Mathematical Foundations of the Calculus of Probability.  Berkeley, Univ. of Calif. Press.

Risberg, J. and Ingvar, D. H. 1973.  Patterns of activation in the grey matter of the dominant hemisphere during memorization and reasoning.  Brain. 96:737-756.

Thatcher, R. W. 1976.  Electrophysiological correlates of animal and human memory.  In R. D. Terry and S. Gershon (eds.), Neurobiology of Aging. New York, Raven Press.

Thatcher, R. W. 1977a.  Evoked potential correlates of delayed letter matching.  Behav. Biol., 19:1-23.

Thatcher, R. W. 1977b.  Evoked potential correlates of hemispheric lateralization during semantic information processing.  In S. Harnar, R. Doty, L. Goldstein, J. Jaynes, and G. Krauthamer (eds.),  Lateralization in the Nervous System, p. 429. New York, Academic Press.

Thatcher, R. W. 1977c.  Electrophysiological techniques in clinical neurology.  In The Proceedings of the 17th Annual San Diego Biomedical Symposium.  New York, Academic Press (in press).

Thatcher, R. W. and John, E. R. 1975.  Information and mathematical quantification of brain state.  In N. Burch and H. Altshuler (eds.), Behavior and Brain Electrical Activity, p. 303. New York, Plenum Press, Inc.

Thatcher, R. W. and John, E. R.  Functional Neuroscience, Vol. I: Foundations of Cognitive Processes. New Jersey, L. Erlbaum Assoc, Inc. 1977.

Whitehead, A. N., and Russell, B. 1925.  Principia Mathematica, second edition, Vol. I.  Cambridge (England), The University Press.

# CONNOTATIVE MEANING AND AVERAGED EVOKED POTENTIALS

Robert M. Chapman

Psychology Department and Center for Visual Science

University of Rochester

Rochester, N.Y. 14627

## ABSTRACT

The effects of two kinds of experimental manipulation of semantic meaning were studied in Evoked Potentials (EPs), brain responses recorded from scalp monitors. Both kinds of semantic manipulation were based on Osgood's rating analyses which described three primary dimensions of connotative meaning: Evaluation, Potency, and Activity (E, P, and A). One kind of experimental variable was the semantic class of the stimulus word (E+, E-, P+, P-, A+, A-). The other kind of experimental variable was the semantic dimension of the rating scale (E, P, A) which the subject used to make semantic judgments about the stimulus words. These variables were experimentally combined in that for each trial the subject used a designated semantic scale to judge a specified stimulus word while brain activity was recorded. Using multivariate procedures, both stimulus word class and scale dimension effects on the EPs were found. Individual subject analyses demonstrated the generality of the results by showing successful discrimination of word classes and scale dimensions for each of the ten subjects analyzed separately.

------------

Supported in part by NIH Research Grant 5 R01 EY01593 and the Advanced Research Projects Agency (Contract N00014-77-C-0037). The author thanks John W. McCrary and John A. Chapman for their collaboration in this research and Janice K. Martin for her assistance.

# INTRODUCTION

Although a relatively young field, the study of language and evoked potentials is gaining momentum and sophistication (for review: Chapman, 1976; Chapman, in press, a). The work in this field is particularly difficult since linguistic problems as well as problems inherent in EP research need to be considered. A central problem involves distinguishing language effects per se from other effects, such as lower order sensory and motor effects, as well as higher order effects such as general states and cognitive processes. One strategy is to systematically relate EP effects to intra-linguistic variation within the conceptual framework provided by one of the well-delineated subfields in linguistics.

In order to investigate brain responses related to semantic meaning, we extended the technique of averaging the EEG to averaging EPs across a number of words belonging to the same semantic class (Chapman, 1974b; Chapman, Bragdon, Chapman, and McCrary, 1977). With the aid of a quantified theory of connotative semantic meaning, we found brain activity from the human scalp which is related to semantic meaning. In order to control commonly confounding variables, the subject's task was held constant, the presentation sequences were randomized, and the semantic classes were represented by a relatively large number of different words in two lists. With regard to the specificity of the linguistic effects, six different semantic classes were distinguished.

We specified and controlled internal semantic meaning using the conceptions and materials provided by Osgood's analyses of semantic meaning (Miron and Osgood, 1966; Osgood ,1971; Osgood, May, and Miron, 1975). Those analyses indicate that the connotative meaning of a word may be represented by its position in a space spanned by three semantic dimensions: Evaluation, Potency, and Activity (E, P, and A). We selected words (Heise, 1971) which are relatively "pure" in the sense that they score high or low on one of the dimensions and are relatively neutral on the other two. Thus, we used six semantic meaning classes (E+, E-, P+, P-, A+, A-) representing the positive and negative extremes of the Evaluation, Potency, and Activity dimensions.

The degree of specificity of language effects found in EPs depends on the dimensionality of the EP measures themselves (Chapman, in press, b). It is helpful to use EP measures which can focus on linguistic parts of EPs. Two possible techniques are: (1) to use the difference between EPs with and without the particular linguistic processing; and (2) to use multivariate statistical analyses which take into account all of the time points within the EPs as well as their relationships. Thus, the dimensionality of the interpretations of linguistic specificity is limited by the dimensionality of the EP measures and the dimensionality of the experimental design.

In this paper new data relating EP effects to the semantic dimension of the subjects' task (semantic differential) are given after briefly reviewing Osgood's analysis of connotative meaning and our previous results relating EP effects to connotative classes of stimulus words.

## Osgood's Analysis of Connotative Meaning

The work of Osgood and his associates is an exemplar of the psychophysics of semantic meaning (e.g. Osgood, 1952; Osgood, 1971). Their work has led to the idea that connotative meaning space can be reasonably spanned by three dimensions. Thus, any connotative semantic meaning may be specified by three numbers which represent the amount of three components "in" the stimulus (usually a word).

Their analysis used semantic differential measures of meaning. The basic measure in the semantic differential technique is obtained by collecting from the subject a match between a stimulus word and a 7-point scale, defined by a pair of polar terms (e.g., good-bad). These matches were made between a large number of words and a large number of polar terms (adjective pairs). A multivariate analysis applied to these data showed a large portion of the total variance in judgments of verbal meaning could be accounted for in terms of three underlying orthogonal factors which have been called Evaluative, Potency, and Activity (E,P,A). Some of the semantic differential scales dominantly loaded on the E, P, and A semantic dimensions are schematically depicted in Figure 1.

These semantic differential techniques have been applied to 23 different language/culture groups around the world. Although the words were different and translated words may occupy different positions in the three-dimensional connotative meaning space, the analyses repeatedly derived the same E, P, and A dimensions for spanning those meaning spaces. These cross-cultural analyses as a whole suggest that human beings share a common framework within which they allocate concepts in terms of their semantic meanings. This communality overrides gross differences in both language and culture.

This quantitative system does not deal with denotative meaning per se which would appear to have many more dimensions. Rather it deals with connotative (affective) aspects of semantic meaning. In color measurement, trichromatic specification says little about

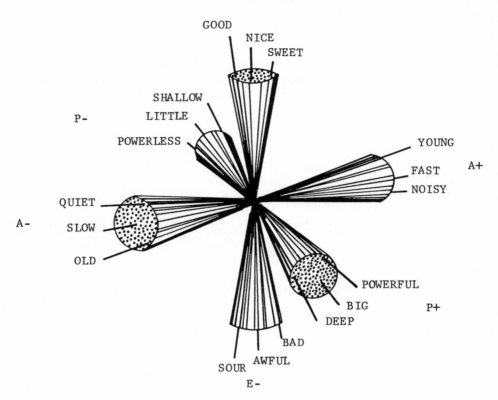

Figure 1.  The Evaluation (E), Potency (P), and Activity (A)
structure of connotative meaning.  Some of the
semantic differential scales dominantly loaded
on E, P, and A.  Based on Osgood (1964).

spatial patterns although the same visual stimuli involve both
spatial and color aspects.  Similarly, tri-connotative
specification of semantic meaning says little about denotative
meaning.

There is available, then, Osgood's well-defined,
objectively-measured, widely-tested, fundamental analysis of
semantic meaning.  It enables one to work within a domain which is
explicitly delimited, which has dimensions that are quantified,
and which readily lends itself to objective replication.

## Evoked Potentials and Connotative Meaning

When a stimulus word is presented, it evokes a number of neural processes, some of which are concerned with meaning. The detection of semantic meaning in EPs permits a more direct examination of language and its neurophysiological processes, and this opens new areas of research and application. Our data are encouraging in that significant effects related to Osgood's semantic dimensions have been shown (Chapman, 1974b; Chapman, Bragdon, Chapman, and McCrary, 1977; Chapman, McCrary, Chapman, and Bragdon, in press). Other work has also indicated effects (Begleiter, Gross and Kissin, 1967; Begleiter, Gross, Projesz and Kissin, 1969; Begleiter and Platz, 1969).

For our research we selected words on the basis of Osgood's Evaluative, Potency and Activity dimensions of connotative meaning (Heise, 1971). Six semantic meaning classes (E+, E-, P+, P-, A+, A-) representing the positive and negative extremes of each of the three dimensions were used. Twenty words from each of the six semantic classes were randomly assigned to a list. Two such lists were constructed with different words, except for the P- category where the same words were used. The words belonging to these semantic meaning classes were visually presented and the average EPs for these classes were analyzed. The physical parameters of the stimuli (various spatial characteristics) vary from one word to the next but the physical parameters tend toward the same average for the various groups of words (Chapman, McCrary, Chapman, and Bragdon, in press). Using two lists provided an additional control. While the background EEG is averaged to obtain EPs, the physical characteristics of the words are averaged to control for their effects and the meanings of the words are averaged to provide a common core of connotative meaning. The words within each list were given in different random orders from run to run, so that the subjects could not anticipate either a semantic class or a particular word. Thus, differences in the EPs to these semantic categories can be associated with post-stimulus processing of semantic information, with the comparison of responses to the two lists helping establish the reliability and generality of the effects. Because the brain responses to be compared were derived from semantic categories which are randomly interspersed, it is difficult to attribute the obtained differences to anything other than semantic processing or effects arising from semantic processing.

In our initial research on semantic meaning (Chapman, 1974b; Chapman, Bragdon, Chapman, and McCrary, 1977) we used a scoring template approach to compare EPs to word classes from opposite ends of Osgood's dimensions. For the scoring template for the Evaluative dimension, the average EP (from CPZ) for E- words was subtracted from that of E+ words, averaged over three

subjects on two word lists.  This scoring template was then used
to measure each EP by computing the Pearson product-moment
correlation coefficient using the 102 corresponding time points of
the scoring template and the EP.  This yielded a single measure
for each EP reflecting its similarity to the scoring template.
Using this measure significant differences were found between EPs
for E+ and E- word classes.  (The EP template measures were
z-transformed [arc-tanh] before applying t-tests for correlated
measures).  The t values for all 12 subjects were in the predicted
direction, i.e., positive.  For the three subjects involved in the
development of the scoring template, 81% of their EPs were
correctly classified into E+ or E- word classes on the basis of
the relative magnitudes of their correlations with the E template.
A somewhat smaller, but significant, success rate was obtained for
the nine subjects in the independent cross-validation group.  P
(Potency) and A (Activity) templates derived in the same way had
somewhat lower success rates in discriminating P+ from P- and A+
from A- word classes, respectively.  The relative strengths of the
EP effects found for the E, P, and A dimensions might be expected
from Osgood's analysis.  Evaluation has been found to be the most
pervasive aspect of connotative meaning, followed by the Potency
and then the Activity dimensions.  The use of a scoring template
to measure EPs for semantic effects was an exploratory technique.

Encouraged by these template results we have continued our
research on semantic meaning and EPs with the aid of multivariate
statistical techniques (Chapman, 1976; Chapman, McCrary, Chapman
and Bragdon, in press; Chapman, in press, a, b).  One of the
problems was coping with the large individual differences in EP
waveforms.  These overall waveform differences, while not the
semantic effects of interest, were relatively stable
characteristics of each individual subject.  This problem was
solved by standardizing the EPs for each subject separately
(transforming to z-scores at each time point) before proceeding
with the analysis.  A varimaxed principal components analysis was
computed on the standardized EPs from a group of 10 subjects in
order to obtain component scores.  These EP component scores were
used in a multiple discriminant analysis to develop classification
functions for the six semantic word classes.  The success rates in
classifying EPs to the semantic classes were significantly better
than chance.  Classification functions were developed separately
for the EP data from each list of words and the results
cross-validated by several procedures:  (i) jackknifed
(one-left-out procedure), (ii) other word list, and (iii) new
subject.

When the EPs were classified to word classes from opposite
ends of each semantic dimension separately (E+ vs. E-, P+ vs. P-,
A+ vs. A-), the average apparent success rate was 97% and the
jackknifed cross-validation success rate was 90% (chance was 50%).

When the same classification functions were applied to the EP data
obtained from the other word list, the overall sucess rate was
73%.

Multidimensional analyses considered the EP data for all three
semantic dimensions at once, in which case six semantic classes
were discriminated from each other (E+, E-, P+, P-, A+, A-).  The
classification rates were significantly better than chance.
Overall, the jackknifed success rates (where each EP is left out
of the development set and then classified) were 42% for List 1
and 43% for List 2 data, some 2.5 time better than chance (16.7%).
The other-list cross-validations averaged 40%.  Thus combinations
of components of these EPs were powerful detectors of semantic
differences.

It is to be noted that all of the above success rates were
obtained across subjects.  That is, the same classification
functions were used for all ten subjects.  This is evidence that
not only can EP effects be found that relate to connotative
semantic meaning but these EP effects tend to be the same in
different individuals.

A further test of the generalizability of the findings was
made by applying the classification functions to a new subject,
one not used in developing the analysis.  After standardizing his
EPs and using component scoring and discriminant functions
developed from the separate group of 10 subjects, 42% of the new
subject's EPs were correctly classified into the six semantic
classes, essentially the same rate as the jackknifed accuracy of
the group of 10 subjects and significantly better than chance
(16.7%).

SEMANTIC-DIFFERENTIAL SCALES AND SEMANTIC WORD CLASSES

In the results summarized above, the subject's task was simply
to repeat each word aloud after it was flashed.  It was of
interest, for several reasons, to change to a semantic-
differential judgment task, one in which the subject makes
a judgment about each word on a designated bipolar adjective
scale.  This was the task that Osgood used to develop his semantic
data and quantitative information about the loadings of various
scales on Osgood's dimensions is available.  This made it possible
to select judgment scales that strongly represented each of the E,
P, and A semantic dimensions.

In our previous research internalized representation of
semantic meaning was manipulated by carefully selecting stimulus
words.  Another aspect of internalized representation may relate
to an individual's semantic expectancies.  When the same word is

presented on different occasions, a subject may be seeking
different kinds of semantic information.  That is, a subject may
have various kinds of semantic expectancies and, consequently, the
semantic information in the words may be processed along various
semantic dimensions.  For example, an individual might be
primarily concerned with potency (powerful-powerless) when a
stimulus word "official" occurs or he might be primarily concerned
with evaluation (good-bad).  Do the Evoked Potentials related to
the word "official" vary for these different semantic
expectancies?  Do these different semantic expectancies have their
own EP effects?

     In order to study questions of this sort, we manipulated the
semantic expectancy by assigning various semantic differential
scales to the subjects at different times (Table I).  The
subject's task was the semantic differential task, as used by
Osgood in developing his semantic analysis.

     A further reason to change the subject's task from repeating
the word to giving a numerical judgment (+3 to -3) was as an
additional control for speech effects.  The same vocalizations
were made to all word classes, as well as for all scale
dimensions.

     Thus, this research studied two kinds of experimental
manipulation of semantic meaning:  word class of the stimulus word
(E+, E-, P+, P-, A+, A-), and scale dimension (E, P, A) which the
subject used to make semantic differential judgments about the
stimulus words (Fig. 2).  Five bipolar scales that were heavily
loaded on (correlated with) each of Osgood's semantic dimensions
(E, P, and A; see Table I) were selected (Osgood, 1964).  Each of
these 15 scales was used with each stimulus word.  Thus, the
effects of two kinds of experimental manipulation of semantic
meaning were studied: (1) the semantic class of the stimulus word,
and (2) the dimension of the semantic scale (E, P, A) which the
subject used to make semantic-differential judgments about the
stimulus words.  These variables were experimentally combined in
that for each trial the subject used a designated semantic scale
to judge a specified stimulus word.  Separate analyses identified
word class and scale dimension effects in the EPs at better than
chance levels.

## Synopsis of Procedure

     During each experimental run, 120 words were flashed in random
order while the subject's EEG was recorded.  For each run, there
were 20 words representing each of six classes of semantic meaning
lying at the positive and negative extremes of each of the Osgood
dimensions:  Evaluation, Potency, and Activity.  The subject was

Table I

Loadings of Semantic Differential Scales on
Evaluation (E), Potency (P), and Activity (A) *

| SCALE | | E | P | A |
|---|---|---|---|---|
| **E Dominantly** | | | | |
| E1 | nice-awful | .96 | -.02 | -.09 |
| E2 | sweet-sour | .94 | .02 | -.04 |
| E3 | good-bad | .93 | .03 | -.05 |
| E4 | heavenly-unheavenly | .93 | .00 | -.21 |
| E5 | mild-harsh | .92 | -.20 | -.06 |
| **P Dominantly** | | | | |
| P1 | big-little | -.05 | .81 | -.24 |
| P2 | powerful-powerless | .16 | .75 | .18 |
| P3 | deep-shallow | -.11 | .69 | -.32 |
| P4 | strong-weak | .04 | .68 | .13 |
| P5 | long-short | .02 | .64 | -.23 |
| **A Dominantly** | | | | |
| A1 | fast-slow | -.14 | .22 | .64 |
| A2 | young-old | .39 | -.42 | .56 |
| A3 | noisy-quiet | -.39 | .25 | .56 |
| A4 | alive-dead | .52 | .13 | .55 |
| A5 | known-unknown | .16 | .10 | .48 |

------------
* American English semantic differential loadings reported in
Osgood, 1964.  Loadings shown are for the first listed adjective
of each pair.  "Good", "Powerful", and "Fast" are represented
by the positive poles of E, P, and A.

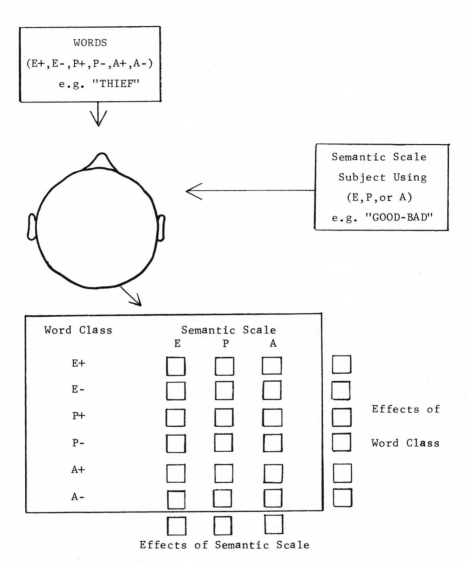

Figure 2.  Experimental Design
Two kinds of experimental manipulation of semantic meaning.

assigned a particular semantic scale for use during the run in judging each word as it was presented. The EEGs for the 20 stimulus words representing each semantic class were averaged for the run to obtain the evoked potentials (EPs) used in subsequent analyses. A total of 30 such runs was required to complete the collection of 180 such averaged EPs for each individual across all experimental conditions:

(1) Six semantic classes of stimulus words,
(2) Two different lists of words (to control for specific stimulus characteristics or properties other than connotative meaning),
(3) Three semantic task dimensions, each represented by five different scales (to control for specific scale properties other than dominant semantic dimension).

## METHOD

The research steps are summarized in the Flow Chart of Experiment (Table II).

The six semantic categories were represented by the same word lists used previously (Chapman, 1974b; Chapman, Bragdon, Chapman, and McCrary, 1977; Chapman, McCrary, Chapman, and Bragdon, in press). The words within each list were given in different random orders from run to run, so that the subjects could not anticipate the semantic class of the stimulus words during the experiment.

Five scales that are heavily loaded on each of Osgood's three semantic dimensions (Evaluation, Potency, and Activity) were selected (Osgood, 1964). Each of these 15 semantic scales (Table I) was used with each stimulus word. This required 15 runs with List 1 and 15 runs with List 2, making a total of 30 runs for each subject. The scales were given in different random orders for each subject.

Before each run the subject was assigned a semantic scale, e.g. "nice-awful," which he was to use on all 120 words in that run. The subject was asked to rate each stimulus word on the designated semantic scale using values from +3 to -3. The instructions to the subject when the scale was "nice-awful" were: If the meaning of the word to you is more nice than awful, then give a + rating, with a 1, 2, or 3 to express various degrees of niceness. On the other hand, if the meaning of the word to you is more awful than nice, give a - rating using 1, 2, or 3 to indicate the degree of awfulness. If the word is perfectly neutral on that scale, give a "zero." For each scale, regardless of whether it was "nice-awful," "big-little," "fast-slow," or some other scale,

Table II

FLOW CHART OF EXPERIMENT

--------
2 LISTS OF WORDS SELECTED
FOR 6 SEMANTIC CLASSES:
   E+,E-,P+,P-,A+,A-
   BASED ON OSGOOD'S
3-DIMENSIONAL ANALYSIS

--------
5 SEMANTIC DIFFERENTIAL
SCALES SELECTED FOR EACH OF
3 DIMENSIONS: E, P, A
BASED ON OSGOOD'S ANALYSES

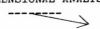          

--------
WORDS FLASHED ON CRT
EEG RECORDED
SUBJECT GIVES SEMANTIC DIFFERENTIAL

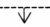

--------
EVOKED POTENTIALS (N=20) COLLECTED
FOR EACH SEMANTIC WORD CLASS
WITH EACH SEMANTIC SCALE

--------
VARIMAXED PRINCIPAL COMPONENTS ANALYSIS
ON EPs OF 102 TIME POINTS,
COMPONENT SCORES COMPUTED FOR EACH EP.

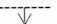

--------
DISCRIMINANT ANALYSES USING
COMPONENT SCORES TO CLASSIFY
EPs INTO:

--------
SEMANTIC
WORD
CLASSES (6)
--------

--------
SEMANTIC
SCALE
DIMENSIONS (3)
--------

numerical values from +3 to -3 were used.  After each word was
flashed the subject gave his semantic differential rating aloud.

A computer-generated display system presented each word as a
briefly flashed stimulus on a CRT (Fig. 3).  The subject sat in a
dark, sound-damped chamber.  The average word subtended a visual
angle of 1.5 degrees with a duration of 17 msec.  Each letter was
formed by lighting appropriate positions in a 5 by 7 matrix.  A
fixation target was presented (0.5 sec. duration) one second
before each word.  After each word was flashed the subject gave
his semantic differential rating (+3 to -3) toward the end of the
2.5 sec. interval between each word and the fixation stimulus for

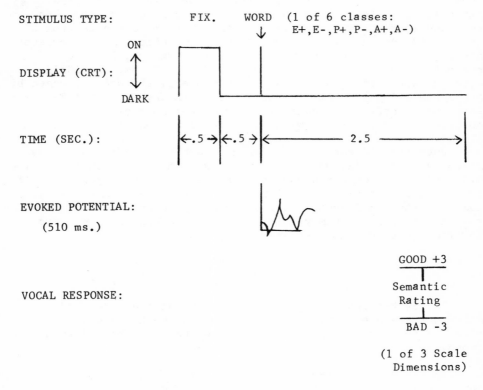

Figure 3
Diagram of Single Trial.

the next trial. This task assured that each stimulus word was perceived and provided access to a behavioral measure. The brain activity following these word stimuli was averaged separately for each of the semantic meaning classes in conjunction with each semantic scale. The sequence for each word presentation (a trial) within each run was as follows:

(1) Fixation target on for 0.5 sec.
(2) Blackout for 0.5 sec.
(3) Stimulus word flashed (approximately 17 msec.)
(4) Blackout for 2.5 sec., during which time the subject gave a number representing his semantic judgment of the word on a designated scale.

An experimental run consisted of 120 words presented in this fashion.

During experimental runs, the subject's EEG was picked up from standard Grass electrodes (silver cup shape) which were attached by bentonite CaCl paste. The data reported here were recorded from a scalp location one-third of the distance from CZ to PZ (CPZ recorded monopolar to linked earlobes). The frequency bandpass of the recording system (Grass polygraph, FM tape recorder, operational amplifiers) was 0.1 to 70 Hz. Beginning with the word stimulus and lasting 510 msec., EPs were averaged by a program using 102 time points (5 msec. interval). Each EP was based on 20 different words of the same semantic class. Eye movements were monitored with EOG (electrooculogram).

Data from 10 subjects are presented here. Each subject was given 30 runs of 120 words (20 words in each of 6 semantic meaning classes) spread over a number of sessions. For each subject half of the runs used List 1 (each run with one of 15 semantic scales) and the other half used List 2 (each run with one of the 15 semantic scales) randomly interspersed. The EPs used in these analyses were averages across 20 words (N=20).

RESULTS

The Evoked Potentials for the six semantic classes had different average waveforms. For Figure 4 the EP data were standardized separately for each of the ten subjects and then averaged.

Individual analyses have been done for each of the ten subjects. The generality of the results is demonstrated by sucessful discriminations of word classes and scale dimensions for each subject. The various steps in the data analyses are summarized in Table II. The first step was to obtain measurements

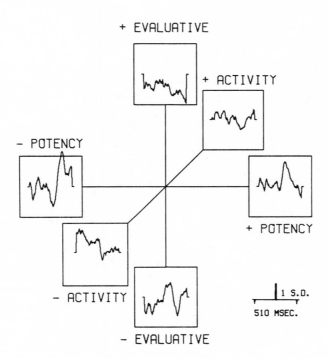

Figure 4. Average Evoked Potentials (EPs) for six semantic classes
after standardization. The semantic word classes are based on
Osgood's Evaluation, Potency, and Activity dimensions which define
a three-dimensional connotative meaning space, represented schematically here. The EPs cover 510 msec (102 time points X 5 msec)
along the horizontal, beginning at the time the words were flashed.
The vertical axes for the EPs are in standard units (z scores).
For the Standardized Potentials each subject's data at each time
point were transformed to z scores (means=0 and standard deviation=
1). Averages include data for two word lists and ten subjects.
Monopolar recordings (bandpass: 0.1 to 70 Hz) from a scalp location
1/3 of the distance from Cz to Pz. Positive is up.

of components of the brain potentials by use of a varimaxed
principal components analysis.  The next step was to assess the
extent to which these components contained semantic information
related to (1) the semantic categories of the word stimuli and (2)
the semantic dimensions represented by the task scale.
Discriminant analyses were used to develop classification
functions relating the component measures to these types of
semantic groups.

The principal components analysis closely followed the
procedures used previously (Chapman, 1974a; Chapman, McCrary,
Bragdon, and Chapman, in press).  Two general steps are involved:
(1) determing the EP components, and (2) measuring how much of
each component is in each EP.  These steps were done by a
varimaxed principal components analysis computed by BMDP4M Factor
Analysis Program (Dixon, 1975).  The EP data entered into the
analysis were the EP amplitude measurements obtained at the 102
successive time points for each of the EPs.  The BMDP4M Program
transformed the data matrix to a correlation matrix.  The
product-moment correlation coefficients computed for each pair of
time points comprised the 102 x 102 matrix to which principal
component analysis was applied.  Unities were retained in the
diagonal.  The number of components to be retained was set at the
number of eigenvalues equal to or greater than unity.  The
retained components were rotated using the normalized varimax
criterion (Kaiser, 1958).  Scores were computed for each of the
original EPs on each of the varimaxed principal components.  These
component scores (factor scores) measure the contributions of the
components to the individual EPs.  These component scores were
compared for the various semantic classes of words.

Having reduced the dimensionality of the EP from 102 measures
to a much smaller number of principal components, the next step
was evaluating the extent to which these components contained
semantic information and, more specifically, the utility of that
information in discriminating and predicting semantic class of
EPs.  This evaluation was accomplished by multiple discriminant
analyses.  The aim of the discriminant analyses was to predict the
semantic class membership of the EPs on the basis of the EP
measures (component scores).  The discriminant analyses were done
by the BMDP7M Stepwise Discriminant Analysis Program (Dixon,
1975).  This program was applied to the component scores derived
from the principal components analyses.  A set of linear
classification functions was computed by choosing the independent
variables in a stepwise manner.  Using these functions, the
probabilities of each EP belonging to each semantic class were
computed.

Two separate multiple discriminant analyses, one for each word
list, were performed on each subject's EP data to determine the

ability of the EP component measures to discriminate simultaneously among all six of the semantic classes of stimulus words.  The success rates of classifying EPs into the appropriate semantic classes were averaged for the two word lists and are presented in Table III.

The overall success rate (pooling lists and subjects) in classifying EPs involved in the computation of the discriminant analyses and classification functions was 43.5 percent.  The success was well beyond the chance level of 16.7 percent.  These results were cross-validated by two procedures:  (1) jackknifed cross-validation and (2) other-list cross-validation.  The jackknifed procedure assesses the classification success when EPs are left out of the development set one at a time and the discriminant functions so developed are used to classify the EPs as they are left out.  This technique is used to estimate the success which would be expected in classifying other, additional EPs obtained using the development list.  An overall success rate of 31.0 percent was obtained with this procedure.  In the other-list cross-validation, the classification rules developed for EPs obtained with one word list are used to classify EPs collected with the other list of word stimuli.  This provides a further check on generalizability of the discriminant functions and tests their likely success rate in classifying other, additional EPs obtained using a different set of words.  As shown in Table III, the overall accuracy in classifying such other-list EPs was 26.8 percent for these ten subjects.

Since all six semantic classes of stimuli were represented simultaneously in these analyses, the success rate expected by chance was 16.7 percent.  The success rates were all well beyond this chance level (chi-squares in Table III).

In addition to semantic class of the stimulus words, the semantic dimension of the subjects' task was investigated.  The average EP data for E, P, and A semantic differential tasks are shown in Figure 5 as Standardized Potentials.  An additional discriminant analysis was performed for each of the ten subjects to evaluate the extent to which the EP component measures also contain information about the semantic nature of the subject's task (Table III, 3 Scale Dimensions).  The specific aim of the analysis was to determine whether functions of these EP components could be developed to differentiate among EPs according to the semantic dimension of the scale being used by the subject to make judgments about the stimuli being presented.  The overall success rate of these functions in correctly classifying the EPs used in their development was 47.4 percent.  This rate of success was better than the chance rate of 33.3 percent.  The jackknifed cross-validation, using the one-left-out procedure described

Table III

Percentages of EPs Correctly Classified

6 Semantic Groups of Words
3 Semantic Dimensions of Scales
2 Word Lists

| Subject | 6 Semantic Groups Multi-Dimensional Analysis | | | 3 Scale Dimensions | |
| | Develop-ment | Cross-Validation Jack-knifed | Other List | Develop-ment | Jackknifed Cross-Validation |
| --- | --- | --- | --- | --- | --- |
| A | 46.1 | 31.6 | 30.6 | 54.4 | 50.6 |
| B | 36.1 | 28.9 | 23.3 | 47.8 | 41.7 |
| C | 57.2 | 38.4 | 30.0 | 47.2 | 47.2 |
| D | 38.4 | 28.4 | 23.9 | 45.0 | 38.9 |
| E | 35.6 | 24.4 | 28.9 | 43.3 | 40.6 |
| F | 39.4 | 31.7 | 13.8 | 47.2 | 44.4 |
| G | 40.6 | 32.2 | 27.2 | 46.1 | 42.2 |
| H | 43.3 | 30.6 | 25.6 | 45.0 | 42.8 |
| I | 48.9 | 30.0 | 31.7 | 48.9 | 46.1 |
| J | 49.4 | 33.4 | 32.8 | 48.9 | 44.4 |
| OVERALL | 43.5 | 31.0 | 26.8 | 47.4 | 43.9 |
| CHANCE EXPECTATION | 16.7 | 16.7 | 16.7 | 33.3 | 33.3 |
| CHI-SQUARE df = 1 | 931.2 | 263.2 | 131.8 | 159.4 | 89.8 |

Each individual percentage based on 180 EPs.

All values of Chi-square corrected for discontinuity.

Chi-square (df=1, p=.001) = 10.8

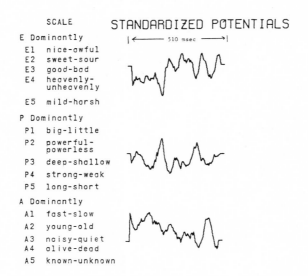

Figure 5. Standardized Evoked Potentials (from CPZ) for semantic differential task scales which are dominantly loaded on Evaluation (E), Potency (P), and Activity (A) semantic dimensions. Data averaged across stimulus word classes, two word lists, and ten subjects. See Figure 4 legend for information about Standardized Potentials. The vertical scale is indicated by the peak-to-peak amplitude of 0.26 z-score units for the response to E scales.

previously, resulted in the correct identification of the semantic
dimension of the task scale of 43.9 percent of the EPs.  This is
an indication of the likely success to be obtained in classifying
other, additional EPs obtained with the subjects while using these
semantic differential scales.  The chi-square statistics indicate
that these rates of correct classifications are well beyond chance
expectations.

The individual analyses (Table III) indicate that EP data
from each of the subjects could be used individually to
discriminate successfully among semantic word groups (stimuli) and
among semantic scale dimensions (tasks).  The success rates varied
little among the ten subjects and lend further concrete support to
the ubiquitous nature of semantic effects in EPs.  These
individual analyses corroborate that the successful
classifications found in group analyses are not due to a few
exceptional subjects.

The identifications of stimulus word classes and task
semantic dimensions were not all equally successful.  Generally,
the A+ class of words (words connoting high activity) is a less
distinct word class than the others, and the Activity scale
dimension is less distinct than the Evaluation and Potency scale
dimensions.  This may be due to the tertiary role that the A
dimension plays in semantic-differential judgments.  Osgood and
others have generally found that the E and P dimensions are more
distinct and account for considerably more variance in semantic
differential judgments than the A dimension.  Table I shows that
the A scales have lower loadings on their dominant dimension and
higher loadings on their non-dominant dimensions than do the E or
P scales.  In a similar vein, the average values for the word
classes on their respective dominant dimensions (Heise, 1971) were
only +1.0 and -0.8 for the A+ and A- word classes, whereas they
were +2.0 and -1.3 for the E+ and E- classes and +1.9 and -0.6 for
the P+ and P- classes.  These semantic quantifications derived
from behavioral measurements are consonant with our classification
rates derived from brain response measures.

Are different EP components involved in the two kinds of
semantic processes studied:  (i) semantic dimension of judgement
scale and (ii) connotative meaning of stimulus words?  Or are
these similar phenomena in terms of their EP effects?  Three
discriminant analyses were available for each subject: one
discriminating among the three task scale dimensions and two (one
for each word list) differentiating among the six semantic classes
of word stimuli.  The first EP component to enter each of these
discriminations was noted for each subject and frequency counts
were made of how often the EP component entered (1) was the same
for the two stimulus word class discriminations and (2) was the
same for the task scale dimension discrimination and either or

both of the word class discriminations (Fig. 6).  In 40% of the
pairs of stimulus word discriminations, the first EP components
were identical.  However, the first component entering the
discrimination of task scale dimensions matched those entering
either of the stimulus word discriminations only once out of 20
possible matches.  The difference is statistically reliable
(Fisher's exact probability=.03).  The first two EP components
entering each discriminant analysis were also compared.  They were
identical on 50% of the possible occasions for the two word lists
(discriminating semantic word classes).  The first two scale
components matched those in either of the word list analyses 15%
of the possible times (6 out of 40).  These differences in

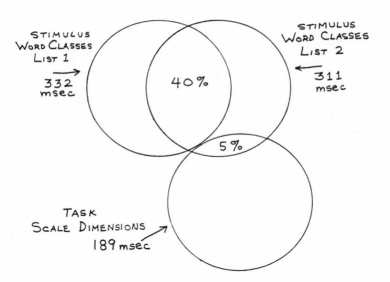

Figure 6.  Overlap among first EP components
to enter each of three kinds of discriminant
analyses and mean latencies of maximum loadings
of first EP components to enter.

frequencies of matches are statistically reliable (corrected chi-square=7.43, df=1, p<.01).  Thus, EP components contributing most to distinguishing among stimulus word classes are seldom those which contribute most to distinguishing task scale dimensions.

In a different approach to the same question, the EP latencies which correlated maximally (maximum loading) with the first EP component entering each of the discriminations were tabulated.  The mean latencies for the separate word list analyses, 332 msec. and 311 msec., did not differ significantly (t=.62, df=9).  The mean of such latencies for the first components entered in discriminating task scale dimensions was 189 msec., which differed reliably from the mean latency for the stimulus word class discriminations (t=3.15, df=9, p<.02).  Thus, the EP time points which correlate maximally with the components most important to distinguishing task scale dimensions are significantly earlier than the time points most important to discriminating stimulus word classes (Fig. 6).

## DISCUSSION

These findings suggest that internal representations of meaning can be assessed by analyzing electrical brain responses. Can these findings be attributed to variables other than connotative meaning?  Since the semantic classes were presented randomly, the obtained differences cannot be attributed to any pre-stimulus variables, e.g., expectancy, arousal, attention, etc. Since the subject's task (perceive word and form a semantic rating on a designated scale) was constant, the obtained differences do not relate to general post-stimulus variables, e.g., differential information processing, response preparation, uncertainty resolution, etc.  It is not likely that the EP differences are related to different muscle activity since (i) the numerical ratings were spoken after the 510 msec. EP interval and (ii) the same numerical responses were given to various semantic classes. Analyses of the EOG data show that eye movements do not explain the EP effects.  Since many different words were the stimuli for each semantic class and the EP results generalized across two such lists of words, it does not seem likely that the results are due to the physical differences in the visual stimuli.  The same aspect of the experimental design guards against interpretations based on surface linguistic features.  Finally, distinguishing six semantic classes indicates a degree of specificity which generally taxes interpretations in terms of variables other than connotative meaning.

Previous research investigated EP effects associated with the same six semantic classes of words when the subjects' task was merely to repeat each word after it was flashed (Chapman, 1974; 1976; in press, a; Chapman, Bragdon, Chapman and McCrary, 1977; Chapman, McCrary, Chapman and Bragdon, in press).  In the present experiment the subject's task was to give semantic differential ratings of each word on semantic scales predominantly loaded on one of three semantic dimensions.  Does the increased task complexity prevent discriminating the word class by brain response measures?  Does the use of different scales, loaded on different semantic dimensions, interfere with identifying the word class of stimulus words?  Do the various semantic expectancies engendered by prior assignment of semantic scales interfere with identifying the stimulus word classes?

The present results indicate that semantic effects of stimulus words continue to be detectible in EPs when the subject is engaged in a semantic task considerably more complex than only repeating the stimulus words.  The added complexity of the experimental conditions clearly does not obscure the semantic word effects.

In addition, the results provide evidence that EP effects may also be used to discriminate among semantic expectancies, sets or contexts (E, P and A scale tasks) regardless of the semantic location of the stimulus words (E+, E-, P+, P-, A+, A-).  Semantic judgements were elicited from the subjects using 15 scales selected to represent the E, P, and A dimensions.  The subjects' internal semantic events were manipulated by the subjects' task which is set prior to delivering the stimulus word.  In this sense, the task provides a semantic context or expectancy within which the stimulus word is to be evaluated.  We are not using semantic expectancy here to mean the subjects' expectancy of a particular stimulus word or word class (which were randomized), but rather to mean the subjects' previously established context (delineated by dominant dimension of semantic scale) which the subject expects to apply to flashed stimulus words.  The task scale dimension variable was manipulated in this experimental design independently of the stimulus word class.  It was not previously known whether the task scale dimensions would have distinctive effects in EPs and, if so, whether these effects would interact with those associated with stimulus word class. The present results indicate that the semantic context established by various scales does have its own EP effects, which do not appear to interact with detection of stimulus word class.

In a manner which parallels our conclusions about identifying stimulus word class, there is some generality to identifying task scale dimension.  A number of semantic differential scales were used to represent each semantic dimension (five adjective pairs for each) in order to establish general relationships to EPs, not tied to particular exemplars of the semantic scales.  This parallels the use of many exemplars of stimulus word class in establishing the generality of those EP effects.

The scale dimensions could be identified by separate analyses of each individual's data (Table III). The success of these analyses supports the universality of the EP effects across individuals.

Analyses of the EP components involved in the discriminations indicate that the components reflecting the greatest differences among task scale dimensions are different from the EP components which discriminate maximally among semantic classes of stimulus words. The maximal representation of effects in the EPs occurs significantly earlier for the task scales than for the stimulus words. These findings support the conclusion that these are different kinds of semantic effects. Moreover, the earlier maximal representation in the EPs of the task scales fits the interpretation of a semantic expectancy established by the semantic differential scale assigned to the subject before the stimulus words are flashed. These data lead to the hypothesis that, following the presentation of each stimulus word, a process relating to the semantic differential scale used to judge the word occurs before the connotative meaning of the stimulus word is fully developed.

In general, the research provides evidence that two kinds of semantic variables can be independently and simultaneously identified in EPs: (1) the semantic class of stimulus words and (2) the semantic dimension of semantic-differential scales being used to judge stimulus words. These findings have important implications for applications as well as a basic understanding of the processes. In this experiment, two kinds of semantic effects were registered in the EP and could be used to assess different semantic aspects: (1) the processing of the semantic meaning in stimulus words, regardless of the semantic expectancies of the subject, and (2) the semantic expectancies of the subject, regardless of the semantic content of stimulus words.

## REFERENCES

Begleiter, H., Gross, M.M. and Kissin, B.  Evoked cortical responses to affective visual stimuli.  Psychophysiology, 1967, 3, 336-344.

Begleiter, H., Gross, M.M., Porjesz, B. and Kissin, B.  The effects of awareness on cortical evoked potentials to conditional affective stimuli.  Psychophysiology, 1969, 5, 517-529.

Begleiter, H. and Platz, H.  Cortical evoked potentials to semantic stimuli.  Psychophysiology, 1969, 6, 91-100.

Callaway, E.  Brain Electrical Potentials and Individual Psychological Differences.  New York: Grune and Stratton, 1975.

Chapman, R.M.  Latent components of average evoked brain responses
  functionally related to information processing.  In International Symposium on Cerebral Evoked Potentials in Man,
  pre-circulated abstracts.  Brussels: Presses Universitaires de
  Bruxelles, 1974a, 38-42.

Chapman, R.M.  Semantic meaning of words and average evoked
  potentials.  In International Symposium on Cerebral Evoked
  Potentials in Man, pre-circulated abstracts.  Brussels: Presses
  Universitaires de Bruxelles, 1974b, 43-45.

Chapman, R.M. (Chair.)  ERPs and Language.  Transcript of panel at
  Fourth International Congress on Event Related Slow Potentials of
  the Brain (EPIC IV), David A. Otto, Program Chairman, 4-10 April,
  1976, Hendersonville, N.C.

Chapman, R.M.  Language and evoked potentials.  In D.A. Otto (Ed.),
  Multidisciplinary Perspectives in Event-Related Brain Potential
  Research.  U.S. Government Printing Office, Washington, D.C.,
  in press (a).

Chapman, R.M.  Method of EP analysis in linguistic research.  In
  D.A. Otto (Ed.), Multidisciplinary Perspectives in Event-Related
  Brain Potential Research.  U.S. Government Printing Office,
  Washington, D.C., in press (b).

Chapman, R.M., Bragdon, H.R., Chapman, J.A. and McCrary, J.W.
  Semantic meaning of words and average evoked potentials.  In J.E.
  Desmedt (Ed.), Progress in Clinical Neurophysiology.  Vol. 3:
  Language and Hemispheric Specialization in Man: Cerebral
  Event-Related Potentials.  Basel: Karger, 1977, 36-47.

Chapman, R.M., McCrary, J.W., Bragdon, H.R., & Chapman, J.A.  Latent
  components of event-related potentials functionally related to
  information processing.  In J.E. Desmedt (Ed.), Progress in
  Clinical Neurophysiology.  Vol. 6: Cognitive Components in
  Cerebral Event-Related Potentials and Selective Attention.  Basel:
  Karger, in press.

Chapman, R.M., McCrary, J.W., Chapman, J.A., & Bragdon, H.R.  Brain
  responses related to semantic meaning.  Brain and Language,
  in press.

Dixon, W.J. (Ed.)  BMDP Biomedical Computer Programs.  Berkeley:
  Univ. of California Press, 1975.
  Programs developed at Health Sciences Computing Facility, UCLA;
  sponsored by NIH Special Research Resources Grant RR-3.

Heise, D.R.  Evaluation, potency, and activity scores for 1551 words: a merging of three published lists.  Chapel Hill, N. C., Univ. of N. Carolina, December 1971.

Kaiser, H.F.  The varimax criterion for analytic rotation in factor analysis.  Psychometrika, 1958, 23, 187-200.

Miron, M.S. & Osgood, C.E.  Language behavior: The multivariate structure of qualification.  In R. B. Cattell (Ed.) Handbook of Multivariate Experimental Psychology.  Chicago: Rand-McNally & Co., 1966, 790-819.

Osgood, C.E.  The nature and measurement of meaning.  Psychological Bulletin, 1952, 49, 197-237.

Osgood, C.E.  Semantic differential technique in the comparative study of cultures.  Amer. Anthro., 1964, 66, 171-200.

Osgood, C.E.  Exploration in semantic space: A personal diary.  Journal of Social Issues, 1971, 27, 5-64.

Osgood, C.E., May, W.H., and Miron, M.S.  Cross-Cultural Universals of Affective Meaning.  Urbana, Ill.: University of Illinois Press, 1975.

Rummel, R.J.  Applied Factor Analysis.  Evanston: Northwestern Univ. Press, 1970.

# COGNITION AND THE BRAIN

Walter Ritter

Lehman College, CUNY and Albert Einstein College of
Medicine
Bronx, New York

The aim of this paper is to put the search for brain correlates of stimulus meaning, the general topic of the first section
of this book, into the broad perspective of cognition and the
brain. I shall begin by making a brief statement of some of the
major points of view to be developed, along with a rough outline
of the paper.

The reason why science is an empirical discipline is because
the knowledge it acquires about the world is related, directly
or indirectly, to experience. A physicist, for example, may
develop complex formulations as to the structure of the atom, but
the ultimate test of whether his theories are related to reality
rests upon some predictable effect upon experience. In more general terms, the reason why people believe that something is real,
or is a part of reality, is because it is related to their own
experience in one way or another, or because they believe the
assertions of other people who report that they have had the relevant experiences.

For the brain scientist concerned with cognition, the first
thing of importance the brain does is to make experience possible.
The reason for that is because experience is the basis for all
cognition (or knowledge) of the world, whether personal or scientific. The first portion of this paper, then, deals with some
ideas fundamental to cognitive psychology as it relates to epistemology. A basic question of cognition concerns what it is that
we have experience of. To say that we have experience of the world,
though obviously relevant, is too simple a description of the ac-

*This work was supported by Grant HD 10804 from NICHD.

tual state of affairs. Our experience of the world depends on
a series of transformations which ultimately transform events in
the environment and the brain, which only have physical attributes,
into biophysical events in the brain which have the psychological
attributes of conscious experience. It is these psychological
attributes which form the basis of experience of and knowledge
about the world. Throughout this paper I have adopted the convention of psychophysics which distinguishes between physical and
psychological attributes of stimulation. The physical attributes
of stimulation are those that are measurable with instruments,
such as the amplitude and frequency of sound waves. The psychological attributes of stimulation are those which are experienced
by the subject, such as loudness and pitch.

Our knowledge of the world does not consist of isolated, un-
connected pieces of experience. Instead, we develop an integrated
conception of reality which depends upon but goes well beyond individual experiences. Since the psychological attributes of experience are qualitatively different than the physical attributes
of the environment, and since people experience the world in
somewhat different ways, I shall refer to personal reality as the
integrated conception of reality developed by each individual
based on his conscious experience of the world. The second thing
of importance which the brain does related to cognition, then, is
the construction of personal reality, since it is the fundamental
medium for complex knowledge of the world.

From these considerations, it should be clear that conscious
experience plays an essential role in cognition. Since our knowledge of the world, whether personal or scientific, affects the
manner in which we interact with the environment, then conscious
experience is part of the complex, causal network of events which
occur in the nervous system. Thus, a major argument of this paper
is that in order to comprehend cognition and the brain, it is
necessary to understand how brain activity affects, and in turn
is modified by, conscious experience. The position that consciousness is an epiphenomenon of brain activity is rejected because it
removes from cognition the essential role which experience plays
in the development of personal and scientific conceptions of reality and the effects they have on behavior.

The first half of the paper, therefore, deals with stimulus
meaning within the context of cognitive psychology and the development of personal reality. Language meaning is dealt with as the
most extensive and effective manner of encoding and communicating
conscious experience. The second half of the paper focuses on ways
in which the biophysical transformations of the brain could be related to the interaction between conscious and non-conscious brain
activities and discusses strategies for relating brain processes
to cognition.

## COGNITIVE PSYCHOLOGY

The most significant way in which psychology and brain research meet and influence one another today is through the concepts
of information processing developed in cognitive psychology.  The
basic idea of cognitive psychology is that our knowledge of and
interaction with the world is accomplished through a variety of
transformations associated with information processing.  In his
classic book, Cognitive Psychology, Neisser suggested that "the
term 'cognition' refers to all the processes by which the input is
transformed, reduced, elaborated, stored, recovered and used"
(1967, p.4).  It is helpful, in this regard, to recall the lovely
passage which appears on the first page of Neisser's book:

> Physically, this page is an array of small mounds
> of ink, lying in certain positions on the more highly
> reflective surface of the paper.  It is this physical
> page which Koffka and others would have called the
> "distal stimulus," and from which the reader is hope-
> fully acquiring some information.  But the sensory in-
> put is not the page itself;  it is a pattern of light
> rays, originating in the sun or in some artificial
> source, that are reflected from the page and happen
> to reach the eye.  Suitably focused by the lens and
> other ocular apparatus, the rays fall on the sensi-
> tive retina, where they can initiate the neural pro-
> cesses that eventually lead to seeing the so-called
> "proximal stimuli." ... the proximal stimuli bear
> little resemblance to either the real object that
> gave rise to them or to the object of experience that
> the perceiver will construct as a result (1967, p.3).

The three fundamental phenomena referred to in this quote, namely
the "real object," the "pattern of light rays which strike the
eye" and the "object of experience," are qualitatively different
from one another, that is, reflect transformations in kind.  We
are not normally aware of the transformations which occur between
objects in the world and our awareness of them.  The world is
always experienced directly, with no sense, for example, that
between a table and the perception of it are streaming photons and
numerous electrical impulses traveling along the optic nerve.  The
fact of these transformations, however, can be appreciated upon
reflection on certain experiences.  One of the most striking occurs
when we become so absorbed in reading a novel that, instead of
perceiving the page and its words, we see people and places, and
enter the world of the novel.  Upon reflection, it is apparent
that in this situation the difference between the distal object
(the "small mounds of ink" on the page) and the object of experience is even greater than usual:  there have been additional transformations from the registration and comprehension of the words on

the page to the images, emotions and meanings of the plot.  What
we take note of is that we have no awareness of seeing the page or
the words on it.  But it is apparent that the words must have been
registered and comprehended in us in order for the people and places
of the novel to appear before us.  It is inescapable that processes
inside us must occur, outside of our awareness and, all the evidence
suggests, inside our brain.  But there is the far more reaching
realization that what happens when reading a novel is representative
of all experience.  There are always intermediaries between the
object and the experience of it, which we have no awareness of,
such as the photons.

A conception crucial to the notion of the transformations involved in information processing is that conscious experience of
the world is a construction, to use Neisser's term.  Since the real
object and the object of experience are not identical, due to the
number of transformations that occur between them (or, more exactly,
that there is in principle no way of establishing their identity,
and that all the evidence suggests that the probability of their
being identical is very low), then the object of experience includes
features not contained in the real object, and vice versa.  The
simplest reason why perception is a construction is because it
adds features to stimuli which they do not have (more complex constructions are discussed later).  The added features are experienced
as being attributes of the stimulus, and this is called naive realism.  The constructionist view rejects naive realism and is thereby
consistent with a host of considerations from epistemology and
the natural sciences (Russell, 1948).  For brain scientists the rejection of naive realism is perhaps most succinctly captured in the
basic idea of psychophysics that psychological and physical attributes of stimulation (for example, color and wavelength of light,
respectively) are distinct and not to be confused with one another.
Thus, when a person tastes a piece of chocolate, he experiences
it as having sweetness (i.e., that it is the chocolate that is
sweet).  But what psychophysics tells us is that the chocolate is
composed of certain chemicals, and that chemicals do not have sweetness.  Rather, when these chemicals are placed on the tongue, a
series of transformations take place in the nervous system which
eventually lead to the experience of sweetness.  One of the few
contemporary theorists to cautiously suggest that naive realism
might actually be true is Gibson.  The interested reader can find
a summary and critique of Gibson's views, as well as obtain relevant references, in an article by Henle (1974).  In any case, the
view that I shall develop is based on the more commonly held assumption that naive realism is false.

If naive realism is false, meaning that the object of experience is qualitatively different than the real object in the environment, then on what basis can the constructions of perception

constitute the grounds for personal and scientific knowledge of
the world?  This question has been dealt with extensively by
Russell (1948) with regard to science;  my emphasis shall be on
personal knowledge.


## The Physical Environment

Many correlations have been established between the physical
and psychological attributes of stimulation.  The energy sources
for perceptions in the various sensory modalities have been generally determined (light waves for vision, sound waves for sound,
etc.).  Also, variation of specific energy sources are related to
variations in perception within sensory modalities.  These correlations are sufficiently universal among humans that particular
colors have been related to particular wavelengths of light,
certain tastes to certain chemicals, and so on.  The extent and
reliability of these correlations is such as to suggest that they
depend upon inherited characteristics of our nervous systems.
Variations in stimulation from the environment, therefore, produce
correlated variations in perception (for those energies in the
environment to which our receptors respond).  Patterns of inter-
sensory input are integrated in perception (as when we see someone's lips moving and hear what is said).  Objects in the environment which have certain configurations of physical features, therefore, can produce perceptions which integrate the correlated psychological attributes in such a way as to permit recognition of
that object, so long as there are structural correspondences
between the physical nature of the object, the physical stimulation which it generates or reflects, and the perception which
occurs in the brain.  Since variations in physical attributes of
stimulation from the environment correlate with variations in the
experienced psychological attributes, the latter can be used as a
basis for useful knowledge of the environment.  For example, a
certain potentially dangerous animal (such as a bull) may be experienced as making particular sounds and having a distinguishing
pattern of coloring.  Whether or not the animal makes sound or has
color does not matter.  The animal may actually emit sound waves
and reflect light waves of particular frequencies, as psychophysics indicates, nevertheless if a person acts in terms of the
experienced psychological attributes of sounds and colors this
will increase his chances of survival.  Furthermore, if the person
warns his children about animals who make certain sounds and have
certain colors, their chances of survival will also increase.

The covariation between physical and psychological attributes
of stimulation also constitutes the empirical basis of science.
Newton, who rejected naive realism, showed that light from the sun
is composed of a variety of different light waves on the grounds

of the perception of the spectrum of colors produced by the inter-
position of a prism between the source of light and the perceiver.

The meaning or usefulness of the information obtained from
physical stimulation, however, is not contained in the stimulation
itself.  Gibson (1966), for example, draws the distinction between the information contained in the pattern of stimulus energies associated with perception of the location, size, movement,
and so on, of an object, and the "affordances" which that object
may have for the perceiver.  If food smells repulsive, for example, that suggests the food may be decaying and dangerous to eat.
But another creature, say some kind of scavenger, may find the
same food smells perfectly delicious.  The meaning of the information which stimulation conveys, then, can vary across species
(assuming that other species have conscious perceptions, which it
seems to me terribly anthropocentric to deny given the similarities in nervous systems, the gradual pace with which changes
occur in evolution, and numerous encounters with my pet dog over
which foods she prefers to eat).

The meaning of stimulus information also varies across and
within persons, depending on their age, experience, general state,
and intentions.  For persons armed with weapons, an identical
stimulus array associated with the bull mentioned before might
convey the presence of a source of food rather than danger.  Thus,
the sound waves and light waves associated with the animal do not
of themselves contain meaning, but rather are a potential source
of useful knowledge about the world.  The same holds true for
science:  the meaning drawn from empirical investigations is not
contained in the physical stimulation associated with the observations which support or disconfirm hypotheses.

The degree of sophistication which people have developed
around the relationship between objects and the psychological
attributes of perception is such that they can learn to discriminate between change in perception due to variations in the object
and variations in themselves.  Ordinarily, when food tastes strange,
this serves as a warning that it may be dangerous to eat (i.e.,
that a change in the taste of food is correlated with a change in
the condition of the food).  However, people have learned that
changes in the taste of food may be due to changes in themselves
rather than in the food, such as when they have a cold or other
sicknesses.  We have also learned that the same food can vary in
taste as a function of emotional states, such as those associated
with being depressed, in convivial company and surroundings,
and so on.  The kind of sophisticated discriminations just described require the kind of integrated knowledge derived from a
variety of experiences which was postulated in the introduction
to be necessary for the complex construction of personal reality.

## The Human Environment

So far we have been discussing how the constructions of perception are a source of knowledge about the physical environment.
However, the bulk of our knowledge is about people, about complex
domains of experience created by humans, and about ourselves and
the manner in which we relate to the human environment.

Knowledge about the people in our environment depends upon
physical stimulation.  The only way we can know that they are
there in the first place is similar to how we know about other
objects in the environment.  But although we have perceptions
related to the physical characteristics of other persons, most of
our knowledge about them is associated with their personal realities.  We are interested in and almost constantly interacting
with how our family, friends and colleagues think and feel about
what is happening in their lives, how they feel about us, etc.
In addition to this extensive involvement with the personal realities of the people in our lives, we have knowledge about vast
domains created by the human brain.  These include art, music,
literature, the various sciences, philosophy, mathematics, law,
games (such as chess), and many others.  Most of the time spent
in school, from the first grade on, beginning with learning how
to read and write, and eventually learning to perform complex
skills (such as playing musical instruments or manipulating
laboratory devices), students acquire knowledge which has been
created by and can only be obtained from other humans.  Whereas
physical objects and stimulation are necessary for each of these
domains (the learning of philosophy, law and mathematics today
requires the use of books, and the rest are obviously dependent
on objects as well as stimulation), they are not what these areas
of human endeavor are about.

In the section on the physical environment, it was pointed
out that stimulus meaning is not contained in the physical characteristics of stimulation.  That fact is perhaps even more
striking when considering the physical stimulation upon which
knowledge of and interaction with the human environment, only
partially described above, depends.  In order to understand how
the brain is responsible for acquiring this kind of knowledge,
it is necessary to conceptualize the brain as being involved in
a domain of reality which is transmitted by but not to be found
in physical stimulation.

Consider, for example, a group of people attending a sym-
phonic concert.  The experiences of the various people will vary
depending on their interests, backgrounds, current state, etc.
Some of the things they experience will pertain to the sights
of the hall and the members of the orchestra, the sounds and

beauty of the music, and the total atmosphere of the concert hall. Whatever experience each person has phenomenologically, the colors, sounds, beauty and atmosphere will appear to them to be occurring outside of themselves (that is, in terms of naive realism). But everything just mentioned occurs solely within the conscious experiences produced by the nervous systems of the people in the hall. The philosopher, Berkeley, once asked whether there would be sound if a tree fell in the forest and no one was there. The answer, of course, is that sound waves (physical attributes of stimulation) would occur but not sounds (psychological attributes of stimulation require the presence of an organism with a nervous system that can produce conscious experience). What about the concert hall? What is present when no one is there? There would be the various forms of mass and energy which physics deals with, but no psychological attributes, such as the colors and architectural character, its special atmosphere, etc. I would like to ask the reader to pause a moment and think about what is present in his laboratory when no people (or animals) are there.

But suppose we turn Berkeley's question around and ask what is present in a concert hall while a concert is being performed. The hall, as a physical entity, still has no color or atmosphere and, in fact, is in total silence. But there is another domain of reality, shared by the musicians and the audience, which is also present. It includes the sounds and colors and atmosphere we think of as being associated with a concert, but it exists only in the human environment. The human reality of the concert, in other words, is a construction of the brain. It is both created by and experienced in the brain.

The realization that the above description is true is astonishing. It is equally astonishing to realize that our nervous system is responsible for constructing the reality of the human environment. The point of these considerations for brain scientists is that their task is to attempt to understand how the brain constructs the human reality we live in.

The concept of construction in no way implies that there is nothing outside of us, nor that people at a concert are wrong in believing that events outside of themselves can cause certain experiences. The music obviously had to be written and the orchestra had to play it in order for the audience to hear and appreciate it. Nor does the concept of construction entail believing that the experienced reality bears no relationship with the physical world.

Let us trace some of the events in the physical world and in the brain that are involved with music. A composer begins by having conscious experiences of patterns of sound which strike him as being interesting or moving or beautiful. A series of transformations occur by which he can generate sound waves (for example, by moving his fingers across a piano keyboard) which allow him to hear and then modify the music originally conceived. He eventually imagines how the music would sound if orchestrated in certain ways and then transforms these experiences into "mounds of ink" on sheets of music. At the concert hall, the musicians direct their eyes to the score and through another sequence of transformations the sound waves generated by an orchestra fill the hall. These sound waves activate the nervous systems of the members of the audience and are transformed into the experience of music. Through all of these transformations, there had to be structural correspondences which allowed the musical experience originally inside the composer's mind to produce analogous experiences inside the listener. The total sequence of transformations included physical and psychological events, in tandem. The only places where the sound of the music occurred (vs. the sound waves) was in the minds of the composer, the musicians and the audience. Music, in short, occurs only in conscious experience and is principally dependent on brain processes for its existence.

For a brain scientist to understand how the brain is involved in the production, experience, and appreciation of music, he must know of the existence of the human environment within which music exists, for it can not be found in the physical environment, or any other place for that matter. It is true that a scientist might otherwise determine that certain patterns of sound waves occur under particular circumstances, and also that human beings direct their attention to those sound waves, sometimes for rather long periods of time, even though the stimulus meaning always eludes him. But whatever hypotheses he generates as to the biological or psychological reasons for directing attention to those sound waves, he will always miss the point of what people are listening to and, therefore, why they are listening. Moreover, if the scientist did not know what people are listening to, it seems rather unlikely that he could comprehend the brain events which are involved in producing the experience of music, or even surmise that they exist. Whether or not the reader agrees with the last assertion, it should be clear that the ultimate goal of the scientific investigation of cognition and the brain should be to comprehend how the brain produces knowledge of the physical and of the human environment, since it is in terms of those environments, as just described, that we live.

## Epiphenomenalism

The contention that the constructions of perception provide useful knowledge of the physical and human environment, upon which

people act, entails the corollary that conscious experience has
causal efficacy because it is an essential part of cognition.
There has been a curious belief prominent during the present
century that consciousness is an epiphenomenon.  This belief is
most directly associated with the Behaviorist movement, which first
argued that consciousness could not be studied scientifically,
and then conveniently decided that such a state of affairs was of
no importance because consciousness has no causal effects on behavior anyway.  If the epiphenomenalist position were true, then
a scientist conceivably might understand why people sit in concert
halls in such a way that sound waves from an orchestra strike
their auditory receptors, without his knowing what music is, because the experience of music would play no role in why people are
there.

The main epiphenomenalist argument is that the nervous system
is built such that it generates in parallel the behavioral response
and the conscious experience, and that the former occurs independently of the latter.  Physical stimulation activates various
purely physical events in the nervous system which eventuate in
muscular contractions which constitute the behavior.  These activities are considered to be within the domain of physics and
chemistry and consequently to be entirely determined by the laws
of physics and chemistry.  Epiphenomenalists would presumably
agree that stimulus meaning is not contained in the physical
characteristics of stimulation, and therefore is something added
by the brain.  But since meaning is not a concept contained in
the laws of physics and chemistry, it can be dispensed with along
with the other psychological attributes of conscious experience
which are added to sensory input.  A major question for the
epiphenomenalist position is how well it can account for behavior
without reference to consciousness.

In those instances where survival is at stake, it seems
clear that individuals respond to stimulation in terms of the
quality and significance of the psychological attributes into
which the physical attributes are transformed.  James (1890)
pointed out that there is generally a substantial relationship
between foods which taste good and are nutritious, on the one
hand, and foods which taste repulsive and are harmful, on the
other hand.  This relationship fits well, he argued, with basic
conceptions of evolution:  mammals that like the taste of harmful
foods and dislike the taste of nutritious foods tend to be eliminated, and vice versa.  If conscious experience of taste bore no
causal relationship to eating behavior, then there should be no
relationship between the taste of food and its nutritious and
harmful effects.  Indeed, there should be no significant difference between the number of nutritious foods we eat which are
delicious and which are repulsive, assuming that adaptation to

the eating of appropriate nutritious foods occurred independently
of the conscious experience of taste.  There are a host of other
correlations that also are inexplicable for the epiphenomenalist
position, such as that orgasm is experienced as intensely satisfying, that stimulation which signifies danger sounds frighten-
ing, etc.

Since everyone recognizes that behavior appears to be pur-
posive, the epiphenomenalists have argued that the apparent pur-
posiveness of behavior is entirely derived from biological adaptation.  For example, the reason why food is eaten is not because
we are hungry or the way it looks and tastes, but because of
biological needs which influence brain activity in such a way as
to produce eating behavior directly, with the experience of hunger
a byproduct.  Similar arguments are made about other biological
drives, in each case the accompanying conscious experiences being
unnecessary.  But why orgasms are satisfying (versus, for example,
intolerably draining) is not dealt with.

Whereas the epiphenomenalist position scarcely accounts for
the correlations between conscious experience and adaptive behavior, the weakness of the argument is even more apparent when
faced with behaviors which are not related to survival.  Consider
the transformations of light waves into the experience of the
colors of naive realism.  When people buy furniture, rugs, cur-
tains, wall hangings, etc., and arrange them in certain patterns
in order to be pleasing and to create different kinds of atmo-
spheres in their kitchens, living rooms and bedrooms, it seems
obvious that they are doing so because of the experienced color
combinations.  Surely the color patterns so generated play no
role in biological survival.  It might be argued that the general
well being of an individual is affected by the color and atmosphere he experiences in his home, but that would be to concede
the causal efficacy of conscious experience.

But the major failing of epiphenomenalism is its inability
to reconcile itself with the nature of human cognition.  The
manner in which we have knowledge of the world is through conscious experience.  Everything that is known about the physical
environment is either based upon direct experience or, where that
is not possible (as, for example, with electromagnetic waves with
frequencies which do not activate our visual system), inferred
indirectly from other experiences.  Our knowledge of the human
environment is also mediated by conscious experience, but in this
case the very object of knowledge is often the conscious experiences of other persons.  In the study of the history of
philosophy, the object of knowledge is the conscious ideas of
certain men.  Music, as depicted earlier, exists solely as conscious experiences of people.  The object of study for music

students is not the intensity and frequency of sound waves, or the capacity, by itself, to generate particular sound waves. The object of study is the sound of music and the range of experience it can express. To grasp the historical development of music is not to know about the sequence of various sound wave patterns created by composers over time, but rather to grasp the kinds of conscious experiences produced by music of different periods and how one led to another. In these various endeavors, the commerce of the brain is with the conscious experiences of others. What is learned affects the attitudes and activities with which students later conduct their professional careers, whether they teach courses in philosophy, compose and play music, and so on. Conscious experience, therefore, is both the source of knowledge about the physical and human environment as well as the basis for behavior affected by that knowledge, which means that it has a significant role in the causal events of brain activity.

Much of what has just been said applies to the enterprise of science. Students begin by learning the ideas and methods of science, all of which were consciously devised and evaluated and must be passed on into the conscious experience of subsequent generations in order to continue. But above all, science requires conscious experience as its empirical base. One wonders how the epiphenomenalist position could ever be empirically verified, since whatever observations are required would of necessity be conscious experiences. But if conscious experience is not causal, then such observations could have no effect on subsequent brain activity and ensuing thought. Epiphenomenalogists will have to devise a new theory of knowledge which is not based on experience.

In this regard, I often have the impression that scientists forget what is fact and what is theory. The frequency of light waves, for example, has been associated with the experience of color. Some scientists seem to think that light waves constitute the real world and the conscious experiences of color associated with them some kind of unreliable, shadow events. But it is the light waves which are hypothetical (no one has ever seen them). Color is a fact. Scientific theories are held with varying degrees of confidence, and an essential tenet of science is that theories can in principle never be entirely proven. Such is not the case with conscious experience. That we experience color is not an idea to be held with varying degrees of confidence: it is a fact of human existence. Indeed, all conscious experiences are facts and represent the only things we can be certain of. Even hallucinations, though non-veridical experiences of the environment, are facts. The circumstance that conscious experiences are facts, and not fuzzy ideas in the minds of soft-minded scientists, is why observation is the cornerstone of science. That conscious experiences of the world can be non-veridical

(as in hallucinations, illusions, or the naive realism inherent
in perception which experiences psychological attributes of stimulation as being properties of the physical environment) does not
lessen their importance in science, as there is no other recourse
than to conscious experience to obtain facts for an empirical
discipline.  It does mean that scientists must incorporate in
their thinking and methods the realization that conscious experience can be non-veridical.  In other words, scientists must
give thought to and develop considerable sophistication about the
nature of conscious experience because it is their sole link to
the world around them.  If it were not possible to investigate
the nature of conscious experience, as the Behaviorists have
asserted, then scientists could not develop the sophistication
necessary to ply their trade.

     For brain scientists, then, the fact that the nervous system
produces conscious experience is essential to the study of cognition because it is the basis for all knowledge of the world.  But
it is necessary to go yet another step further and grapple with
the fact that the brain not only has the capacity to produce experience, but also that human brains can communicate their conscious experiences from one to another.  We can tell each other
about our thoughts and feelings;  poets and composers can often
generate in us experiences substantially similar to their own;
we can even compare our experiences to determine how similar they
are.  For example, it was remarked earlier that when reading a
novel, we sometimes become so involved in the meaning of the book
that we are not conscious of the words and sentences on its pages.
I have used this illustration while teaching on many occasions,
and students have generally agreed that at one time or another
they have had similar experiences.  It seems fair to infer that
the reader concurs.  What this means is that I can describe a
conscious experience of mine to you, that you can comprehend
what is said, compare it to your own experience and make a judgment as to the similarities in our experiences.  You could, if
desired, communicate back to me the degree of similarity of your
experience to mine.  It is difficult to understand how communication of conscious experience could occur if conscious experience
had no effect on brain activity.  To maintain the epiphenomenalist
view, it would be necessary to believe that neural activity in
my brain could produce conscious byproducts which have no affect
on subsequent neural activity;  that my neurons nevertheless
could fire in such a way as to produce physical events (such as
writing or speaking) which produce neural events in your brain
which yield understanding of the contents of my conscious experience;  then your neurons (having, of course, no feedback from
or knowledge of the conscious events they generate as byproducts
of their activity) would fire in such a way as to give you a
sense of how well your conscious experience compares to mine;

and, to complete the story, your neurons then fire in such a way
as to produce physical events (writing or speaking) which cause my
neurons to fire such that I find out whether your experience is
comparable to mine.  Not being in any way apprised of what has
transpired between us, my neurons then fire and generate in me
certain conclusions and further thoughts, depending on what your
reply was, as well as the impression of a coherence in my thoughts
and in our conversation about conscious experiences.  Surely a
rather implausible state of affairs.

Language

The most extensive way in which people communicate conscious
experiences to one another is through language.  The everyday
reality which each of us constructs is shared to greater or lesser
extent by all people.  Each person attending a concert not only
experiences the reality of the event, but also knows that the other
individuals in the hall are experiencing the same event.  It is
a commonly accepted fact that each person experiences the concert
in a somewhat different way.  Some individuals may even fall
asleep and hear only a small portion of the music.  But that is
part of the accepted reality of a concert, and no one doubts,
even the people who fell asleep, that a group of people gathered
in that hall and a concert was performed.

Whatever its philosophical and scientific status, naive
realism is the common mode of experience, even for those who in-
tellectually reject it.  Thus, the people in the hall experience
the music as occurring outside of themselves.  Perhaps because
the music is experienced as occurring outside of ourselves is
what makes it natural to believe that others can directly experience the same reality.  Other experiences, such as thoughts
and daydreams, appear to occur inside of us, and it is true that
other people do not have direct access to our inner thoughts.
But in actual fact, all experiences, whether prompted from without
or within and whether experienced as occurring inside or outside
of us, equally occur inside of our nervous systems.

Each of us, then, constructs everyday reality within our
nervous systems, yet because of a naive realism which seems to be
intrinsic to perception, we experience that reality as outside of
us and shared by everyone.  There are, furthermore, a number of
ways in which we can communicate about that reality.  There is,
first, gesture.  We can point toward things we want another to
look at, convey attitudes by facial expressions, etc.  The development of language in humans, however, has provided for a vastly
more extensive and detailed means of communication.  Language
and gesture both serve the purpose of conveying something about

our experience to other persons and influencing their experience.
Since the topic of stimulus meaning has been approached in this
book primarily by the use of verbal stimuli, I shall focus mainly
on language.

There are two main purposes to language.  The first is to
communicate information about things external to us.  A family
may be sitting down to dinner, for example, and soup brought
from the stove to the table.  The mother may sample the soup and
experience an intense burning sensation.  She then tells the rest
of the family, especially the children, that the soup is too hot
to drink.  The experience of hotness, of course, is a psychological attribute of stimulation.  The mother projects the experience
of hotness to the soup (naive realism) and on that basis believes
that the soup will burn the lips of others if they try it.  In
this instance, the mother is confident that her family will have
similar experiences at this point in time with the soup.  People
generally recognize, however, that there are varying degrees to
which others will have comparable experiences with external
stimuli.  If, for example, the family were trying a new soup, and
the mother sampled the soup for its taste, and found it pleasing,
it is likely that she would tell her family that she thinks they
will like it.  By and large, we are reasonably accurate in the
degree of confidence placed in knowing how similar other person's
experiences will be in regard to the same stimuli.

The second major purpose which language serves is to convey
experiences which are private.  For example, the same mother may
taste the soup and remark to her husband that it reminds her of an
experience with a friend which the husband knows nothing about.
There is a realization, however, that if the husband were to experience an identical taste of the soup, it could not remind him
of an event which is private to her.  Finally, people can also
communicate about private events which are generated internally
with no reference to stimuli in the environment.

Language, then, can be used to communicate thoughts or feelings about the external or private world.  Put in other terms,
people can convey aspects of their personal realities to one
another.

A matter of central theoretical importance is the circumstance
that the physical characteristics of spoken and written language
are arbitrary with respect to the meanings communicated.  It does
not matter what configuration of sound (or sound waves) denotes
hotness.  So long as the speaker and listener share the same
convention, the reality experienced by one person can be communicated to another.  In order for language to work, however,
people must share generally similar personal realities as well

as the same language conventions.  This point is best illustrated
by a comparison of perception of the physical environment to comprehension of language, which is rooted in the human environment.
In the case of the physical environment, the transformations that
occur from the real object to the object of experience prevent us
from directly knowing the nature of the object, or what Kant
called things-in-themselves.  But we can have useful perceptions
of the physical environment, as discussed earlier, on the basis
of the psychological attributes of stimulation.  In order for useful perception to occur there must be invariances in the pattern
of stimulation generated by or reflected from the object.  If
the world were such that the patterns of physical stimulation
associated with objects were arbitrary, then useful perception
would be impossible.  The situation with language is entirely
different.  Whereas it is not possible to know directly the nature
of physical objects, we do know directly the psychological attributes associated with physical attributes of stimulation.  Thus,
all people with normal nervous systems see colors, hear sounds,
have depth perception, and so on.  When people communicate aspects
of conscious experience to one another, they know, more or less,
what the referent is.  Since the characteristics of the physical
stimulation which convey language through speech and writing
constitute a convention created by the brain, then learning that
convention permits communication, but the reason why the convention works is because people share the referents of language.  Of
all the events which occur outside of us, the only things-in-themselves which we do have reasonably accurate knowledge of their
nature are other persons' conscious experiences.  In the case of
objects, in other words, we can never know their nature but only
their structural properties (Russell, 1948);  whereas with another person's consciousness, we can roughly know its nature because
we know from direct experience what consciousness is.

An analogy may be helpful in illustrating the distinction
between perceptions of the physical environment and the comprehension of what other persons communicate to us in language.
When we speak with a friend on the telephone, or watch a television program, there are a series of transformations which occur
from the real object to the object of experience.  These transformations include electrical impulses which traverse copper wires,
in the case of a telephone conversation,  and electromagnetic
waves which travel through the air, when viewing a television
program.  But, in contrast to perceptions of the physical environment, we know the nature of the real object that is on the other
side of the transformations because we either have had (or in
principle could have) the relevant direct experiences.  Thus,
with respect to the physical environment, when people look at an
object, they may not know what its physical nature is, but whatever that may be it is associated with invariant patterns of

stimulation which produce in us similar psychological attributes of perception. When a person says that something is hot, what is communicated is not something about the nature of heat, but rather (whatever heat may be) that the object will generate the experience of hotness if touched. People may not know the nature of objects, but they can communicate about their experiences of objects. The physical characteristics of the word "hot," therefore, can be arbitrary and vary from one language to another because people know what the experience of hotness is. With respect to the private world, when people tell us that they are elated, angry, depressed, in pain, sexually aroused, nauseous, hungry or tired, we have a general understanding of their meaning due to our own acquaintance with these states. Since we share these experiences, the physical characteristics of these words also can be arbitrary. Conscious experiences, as things-in-themselves, are the basic facts of existence for humans. Language permits us to share, teach, discuss and argue about those facts.

Language, therefore, is a vehicle for people to communicate personal reality, whether it pertains to perception, thought, feelings, or whatever.

> Language originates in and has primary reference to everyday life; it refers above all to the reality I experience in wide-awake consciousness... and which I share with others in a taken-for-granted manner. Although language can also be employed to refer to other realities... it even then retains its rootage in the commonsense reality of everyday life (Berger and Luckman, 1966, p.36).

> Language is a means of externalizing and publicizing our own experience (Russell, 1948, p.60).

Since the referent of language is to personal reality, then the investigator must know what the referent is in order to study how the brain's response to words is related to the information they convey. The information words encode can only be understood in terms of conscious experience. For example, the word "red" has as its referent the color red as experienced. Redness occurs, so far as is known, only in conscious experience. It is true that it might be determined that when a person says "red," there often (but not always) are light waves of a certain frequency impinging on his retina, and in that sense a scientist might use the light waves in a gross way as the referent of the word "red" for his purposes. But if one person were to say, "that red looks beautiful over there," while another said, "Oh no, I think it looks ugly," the scientist would be at a loss in determining the referents for beautiful and ugly. Ascertaining the total number

of light wave combinations, in particular settings, at different
ages in a sample of people, which are present when the word
"beautiful" is used (and the same for the sound waves of music
and the patterns of words used by poets and novelists) is not
only an insurmountable task, it would still not provide the relevant information as to what is meant by beautiful.  Most importantly, the meaning of the constant flow of language among people,
with conscious experience of one sort or another its general
referent, would be inaccessible to a scientist who did not share
the personal reality encoded by language.

     A different state of affairs applies when non-language stim-
uli are used, especially the kind of artificial stimuli employed
in most brain research.  In using the latter, it is possible, for
example, to utilize evoked potentials elicited by the stimuli to
trace anatomical pathways, determine which portions of the brain
are activated, draw clinical inferences about the integrity of
specific brain structures, etc.  Depending on the purpose of the
research, the subject can be passive with regard to the stimuli,
or even asleep or anesthetized.  It is possible to give meaning
to the stimuli for the subject by providing instructions which
make the stimuli task relevant.  In these circumstances, the investigator knows the meaning of the stimuli to the subjects because he has given them that meaning as a part of the design of
the experiment.

     Language stimuli could be presented to subjects for the pur-
pose of examining the brain's response to their physical features,
but this would be rather trivial, as the same end could be
achieved with non-language stimuli.  In fact, a critical aspect
of evoked potential experiments which use verbal stimuli is to
insure that the results are not based on purely physical aspects of
the stimuli.  Suppose, for example, subjects were required to
make choice RTs to two words randomly alternated in a block of
trials.  Since it is possible for animals who have no language
comprehension to learn to perform the task on the basis of the
physical features of the two words, the investigator can not know
for sure whether human subjects used the physical or language
aspects of the stimuli to perform the task.  By contrast, if a
series of words were presented and subjects required to make
choice RTs based on whether the stimuli were animal words or
sports-related words, then it would be clear that the physical
features of the stimuli could not by themselves provide the relevant information.  In this way it would be possible to study the
brain's response to the meaning of the words, independent of
their physical characteristics.  Note, however, that the only
way that the investigator could construct an appropriate list
of words, as well as determine whether the subjects made correct
or incorrect responses on individual trials, would be if he knew
the meaning of the words himself.

An effective selection of words used in a given experiment, therefore, depends on which aspect of language meaning the investigator wishes to study. Of course, physical features of the stimuli, such as size, number of letters, total luminance, etc., need to be controlled, but that is for the purpose of eliminating their effects. The actual selection of specific words is mainly determined by their meaning to the experimenter when, as in Thatcher's paper, correct and incorrect responses are essential to the experimental design. The other two experimental reports preceding the present paper were different than Thatcher's in that the subject's responses were not considered as being either correct or incorrect. Nevertheless, in the study by Begleiter, Porjesz and Garozzo, words were selected in such a way as to reflect words ranging from one end to the other along a continuum from pleasant to unpleasant. Chapman's selection of words was based on the work of another psychologist (Osgood) who, in turn, asked subjects to rate words on dimensions known to him and other scientists through their own personal experience. That the physical characteristics of the words are arbitrarily related to the connotative meaning of the words (the focus of the study) is emphasized by Chapman. He points out that differences in morphology of evoked potentials associated with given connotative dimensions could not be due to the physical features of the stimulus words, as those features were randomly distributed across the words selected as members of the connotative dimensions employed.

Having selected words in particular ways, subjects can be asked to rate the words along one (Begleiter et al.) or several (Chapman) dimensions. The reasons why these investigators selected the stimulus words in advance was to optimize the range of responses, from most to least along specific dimensions, in small samples. In principle, large, random samples of stimulus words could have been used. However, the instructions to rate the words along particular dimensions could only be meaningful to the experimenter on the basis of his own experience, as the dimensions employed (for example, pleasantness, evaluative, etc.) have their referents solely in conscious experience.

The study of the brain's responses to language stimuli provides a good basis for summarizing some of the main points made so far in this paper.

    1. Whether abstract or concrete, "stimulus meaning" consists of a transformation which adds something not contained in sensory input.

    2. Stimulus meaning is inextricably tied to conscious experience.

3. The encoding of conscious experience into language constitutes an additional transformation of sensory input, the referent of which is conscious experience.

4. The brain's response to the meaning of language stimuli is necessarily related, directly or indirectly, to brain activities associated with consciousness.

5. The physical attributes of verbal stimuli are arbitrarily related to their meaning, and do not have the kind of invariant correspondence as objects have to the pattern of stimulation associated with them.

6. The brain itself has developed the conventions by which meaning is encoded in language, and this occurs with reference to conscious experience of which the brain forms the necessary substratum.

7. Language can be used to communicate conscious experiences of environmental or private events.

8. The reason why language is effective in communicating with and influencing other persons is because they share reasonably similar conscious experiences.

9. The conscious experiences of other people can be the object of knowledge through language, as in literature and philosophy, and through other human creations, such as music and art.

10. Conscious experience must play a causal role in brain activity in order for these statements to be true.

11. The most important transformation of sensory input pertains not to the generation of isolated perceptions, feelings, ideas or behaviors, but to the construction of personal reality.

12. A fundamental goal of the study of cognition and the brain is to comprehend how the nervous system constructs conscious experience and personal reality, as they constitute the media through which all knowledge of the world is obtained and integrated.

13. The only way in which it could be known that the brain constructs personal reality, with its psychological as opposed to physical attributes, is to have experienced those psychological attributes as elements in a personal reality.

14. Scientists know about and can investigate the brain's construction of personal reality because of their own conscious

experiences.  Whereas some readers may not fully agree with the
last statement, many are likely to agree that experiencing their
own personal reality facilitates the investigation of the means
by which the brain constructs the reality of being human, as well
as how people have knowledge of the world, and that systematic
exclusion of any reference to their own personal reality in
scientific thinking on these matters is done at their own peril.


## BIOPHYSICAL TRANSFORMATIONS

Brain research has identified a number of transformations
which stimulus input undergoes in the nervous system.  In the case
of the visual system, light waves from a light source or reflected
from objects in the environment cause a bleaching action in the
receptors located in the retina.  Thus there are already at least
two transformations from the object to the bleaching.  The object
reflects a pattern of light waves which must have a structural
correspondence with the object in order to convey information about
the object, but the pattern of light waves is not the same as the
object and therefore is a transformation.  (Similar considerations
apply if light waves emanate from a light source:  the light waves
given off by the sun, for example, are not the same as the sun).
The transduction from light waves to bleaching is another transformation, after which follow further transformations to electrical potentials and to the release of neurotransmitter substances.
Different kinds of transformations occur at the receptors of other
sensory systems, perhaps the most fascinating of which is the
series of transformations in the ear.  But whatever the nature of
the energies which impinge upon, or the transformations that occur
at, the receptors of a given sensory system, there are no known
differences among the electrical impulses which travel along the
sensory nerves.  Inside the brain these impulses activate iterative
transformations between electrical activity (consisting of graded
and spike potentials) and chemical activity at synaptic junctions.
At the present time, much research is being conducted investigating
the kinds of structural changes which may be the basis for encoding
information into long-term memories.  Whatever the nature of these
changes, they constitute further transformations of the information
conveyed by electrical impulses and the release of neurotransmitter
substances.

The number of transformations from the object to the percept
(or from Koffka's "distal stimulus" to Neisser's "object of perception") that we know about is quite impressive when the ease and
naturalness of perception is considered.  When listening to music,
for example, we have no sense of sound waves pulsating against
the tympanic membrane, or the knocking of the ossicles against
one another, or the slushing back and forth of the liquid in the

cochlea, and so on, which are interposed between the distal stimulus and the sound we hear.  It is these various transformations,
the circumstance that we do not consciously perceive the stimuli
which actually impinge on the receptors (the light waves, sound
waves, etc.), and that there are no detectable differences among
the electrical impulses of the various sensory nerves, which form
the basis for rejecting naive realism on physiological grounds.
When the electrical impulses of the sensory systems enter the
brain they must undergo differential transformations in order to
form the qualitative differences of the various sensory modalities.

Many investigators of event-related potentials of the brain
work with the assumption that sequential components parallel,
at least in part, stages of information processing.  However, so
far as is known, event-related potential components all have
fundamentally the same biophysical bases (neural activity that
produces dipoles).  There are two possible ways of understanding
this state of affairs.

First, different event-related potential components reflect
different patterns of neural activity, and it is the changes from
one pattern to another which constitutes the transformations of
cognitive psychology.  The contents of consciousness, then, would
also be constituted of certain patterns of neural activity.  I
find the latter a doubtful possibility if neural activity is considered to consist of the classical graded and spike potentials
along with the release of transmitter substances.  Neurons are
physically separate from one another, as are the graded and spike
potentials which occur at their membranes.  The chemicals released
at synaptic junctions by one neuron can come in contact with many
other neurons, but if a large number of neurons are active, as for
example in a perception, then the neurotransmitter substances
released at many synaptic junctions would also be physically
separate from one another.  The electrical and chemical activities
of a complex pattern of neural activity, in other words, are dis-
continuous in space.  Conscious perception, however, is unified.
By way of gross simplification, suppose one neuron was responsive
to a stimulus that was round, and another neuron (about a milli-
meter away) was responsive to when wavelengths of light associated
with redness occurred.  Since the two neurons are physically
separate from one another, it does not seem likely that when the
two fired simultaneously in time they could produce the unified
percept of a red apple.  The same situation applies when there are
many neurons related to a perception.  It is not reasonable in
order to get around this objection, to suggest that all of the
relevant neurons converge their activity onto a single neuron
which, when it is activated, is responsible for generating a
complex percept.  It appears, therefore, that the elements of
classical neurophysiology hold little promise for constituting

the physiological basis of conscious experience.

A second approach to this problem is to consider that certain patterns of neural activity produce additional kinds of transformations which have different properties than those studied in classical neurophysiology.  An example of this sort which is known about is the electrical fields which are generated by neural activity and are the basis for EEG and event-related potential recordings.  These fields were used by Köhler to develop theoretical formulations of electrophysiological processes which underlie perception (e.g., Köhler and Wallach, 1944).  Lashley et al. (1951) examined the theory and found a number of theoretical and empirical weaknesses.  However, it is instructive to note the tone with which they discuss Köhler's formulations.  They remark that it is the "only... theory... which has faced the intricate problems of relational organization which are raised by the phenomena of perception and has suggested an inclusive mechanism for them" (p.123).  They further assert that the theory "deserves a place of honor among the most original and systematic theories that scientific ingenuity has produced" (p.123).  Recently, John (1976) has proposed an analogous theory for conscious experience which relies more on electrical fields generated by glial than neural potentials, and avoids many of the criticisms of Köhler's theory by placing greater weight on centrecephalic than cortical fields.

In regard to the material which follows, I would like to make clear at the outset that I am not advocating the hypothesis that the electrical fields in the brain are the physiological basis of consciousness.  Whereas the hypothesis is an appealing one, my own guess is that neural activity produces energy transformations of which scientists currently have no knowledge, and these transformations form the basis of conscious experience.  In the mean time, however, the electrical fields can be viewed heuristically as an example of a transformation brought about by neural activity which could underlie consciousness.  Whether the empirical evidence confirms or disconfirms the theories of Köhler and John concerning electrical fields, my intent is that some of the principles which can be gleaned from considering the possibility of such transformations would be useful, whatever the actual nature of the transformations associated with consciousness may be.

An important characteristic of electrical fields is that they are continuous and thereby could form the basis of unified perceptions.  In that the fields differ in orientation, geometry and magnitude as a function of the pattern of neural (and glial) activity, this would mean that perception would depend on the particular neurons activated by the various physical parameters of the stimulus.  If the neurons responsive to the particular wavelengths of light, shape and other characteristics of the stimulus

were located in different places in the brain, that would present
no theoretical problem so long as the number and orientation of the
responsive neurons was such as to produce electrical fields of
sufficient magnitude that volume conduction would permit significant overlapping of the various fields.  If the object reflected
light waves of a particular kind, that would result in one configuration of electrical field forces, whereas if the object reflected light waves of a different kind, but was identical in
all other respects, a different configuration would result due
to the change in the pattern of neural activity.  Furthermore, if
the general overall configuration were the critical aspect of perception, then the statistical nature of neural firing (John, 1972)
would also present no theoretical difficulty.  John has pointed
out that most neurons fire most of the time and are only probabi-
listically related to stimulus input.  The specific ensemble of
neurons that respond to a given stimulus, therefore, varied from
one presentation to another.  But the morphology of the event-
related potential waveforms recorded from given locations in the
brain remain essentially the same, so long as the stimulus and
its meaning to the subject remain the same.  Consequently, perception, and the learning and memory that may be associated with
it, can be thought of in terms of the general configuration of
electrical fields generated by given patterns of neural activity,
rather than in terms of the activity of specific neurons and the
building of connections between particular neurons.

      Perhaps the most interesting aspect of electrical fields for
the general topic of this paper is that they may have effects on
the activity of neurons located within their spatial domain.  The
principle here is analogous to electrical generators.  If a copper
wire and an electromagnetic field are moved with respect to one
another, an electric current is generated in the wire.  In the
brain, the expansion and contraction of electrical fields could
similarly affect the electrical activity of individual neurons by
raising or lowering thresholds or generating spike potentials.
The empirical verification of this possibility is at present uncertain, but the initial findings are favorable (Adey, 1975).

      If the electrical fields have effects on neurons, then using
them as a theoretical model for the electrophysiological basis of
consciousness opens some hitherto closed doors.  It provides a
way of conceptualizing how conscious events could have causal
efficacy in the brain.  For some time, I was puzzled by the circumstance that classical neurophysiology seemed to provide a model
which could fully account for the activity of the nervous system
from stimulus to response.  Something was known about what happened
at receptors, the impulses that travel along sensory nerves, the
graded and spike potentials within the brain, how neurons influenced one another at synaptic junctions via chemicals, and finally

how motor neurons conducted impulses to muscles where the release
of chemicals at neuromuscular junctions caused the muscular contractions of behavior.  If these events basically accounted for
the activity of the nervous system, and all that were needed was
to fill in the details, then there would be no need for consciousness and, furthermore, no place for it.  After all, how
could consciousness cause neurons to fire (or raise or lower
their firing thresholds)?  But if for hypothetical purposes it
is assumed that certain electrical fields could constitute consciousness, and that the fields could affect neural activity, then
an answer to the puzzle becomes possible, at least in principle.
Something of the following could then be a rough but plausible
account of the state of affairs in the brain.  Neural activity is
necessary for electrical fields and consciousness to occur in the
first place and, depending on the nature of the stimulation from
the internal or external environment, neural activity would play
a critical role in forming the contents of consciousness by
generating electrical fields with particular kinds of configurations.  Once consciousness occurred, then at least in some portions of the nervous system subsequent neural activity would be a
joint product of two sources:  the effects of neural activity
associated with classical neurophysiology and of the electrical
fields which constitute the basis of consciousness.  Certain
activities of the nervous system would occur without any participation of consciousness (for example, various reflexes and non-psy-
chological processes associated with the regulation of biological
functions), whereas other activities could only occur with the
participation of consciousness (for example, thought and music
and science).

    Another difficulty which becomes at least partially amenable
to understanding is how sustained conscious activities occur, such
as thinking through a problem or composing a piece of music.  How
could there be coherence and logic to these activities if they
were solely determined by processes which have none of the properties of consciousness?  To give an example, if the reader will
observe his thoughts while thinking, or his speech while speaking,
it will become apparent that it is usually not possible to know
in advance what the next thought or word, respectively, will be.
So presumably there are non-conscious processes of the brain which
play a role in generating thoughts, spoken words and their related
logic and grammar.  But if these non-conscious processes really
do not have conscious properties, then it is difficult (if not
impossible) to comprehend how they could by themselves produce
thought and speech, especially since the referents of thought
and speech are to conscious experiences.  But if certain brain
activities are considered to be the joint product of neural action
and conscious events (via the electrical fields), then the coherence of thought and speech would be due to the joint activity of

processes which do and do not have conscious properties. Although we do not know in advance which specific words or syntactic structures we will use in speaking a sentence, we do know what we want to say. This suggests that conscious intentions play a guiding role in subsequent non-conscious processes which subserve thought and speech. In addition, these intentions provide a basis for monitoring the output, as is known from personal experience by everyone. When an inappropriate word is used in speaking, we register that consciously and inform the listener of the mistake. That could only occur, of course, if we knew what we wanted to say and matched the meaning of the spoken words with our intention. There is a hiatus, then, between wanting to say something and hearing the words spoken. But there are similar gaps in much of our experience, such as between wanting to remember something and the entry into consciousness of the sought for material. These gaps presumably reflect the time required for non-conscious processes, which can be directed by conscious intentions, to accomplish their activity.

A final reflection on the usefulness of considering the electrical fields as a possible basis for consciousness pertains to the question of epiphenomenalism. Let us imagine that future research shows that the electrical fields of the brain have no effect on neural activity. If we still entertained the hypothesis that the electrical fields constitute the electrophysiological basis of consciousness, then, since the fields would be epiphenomenal byproducts of neural activity (so far as subsequent neural activity is concerned), we would have an electrophysiological model in which consciousness is an epiphenomenon. In other words, neural activity would generate conscious experience via the electrical fields, but conscious experience could have no causal effect back on neural activity. But what a strange state of affairs would result. The neural activity which created conscious experience via the electrical fields would have no information about (or feedback from) the conscious experiences it generated. The neural activity would, by definition, not have conscious properties, yet it would generate not just discrete, disconnected states of consciousness, but conscious experiences which had coherence over time. Imagine a brain scientist interested in knowing how the brain generates conscious experience. By hypothesis, it would be necessary to believe that his neural processes, which have no information about consciousness, nevertheless constitute the causal basis for conscious thoughts and scientific behaviors concerned with determining how consciousness is generated. The neural activity eventually produces conscious thoughts about electrical fields, then generates behavior that conducts empirical tests which validate the hypothesis that consciousness consists of electrical fields which turn out on further study to be epiphenomenal in nature and have no effect on neural activity. The neural

activity makes all this happen, of course, without any information
as to the conscious ideas it generates and tests.  Clearly, such a
state of affairs could only suggest one conclusion:  if the electrical fields are epiphenomenal byproducts of neural activity,
then they could not constitute the basis of conscious experience.
(However, the converse could be true:  the fields could have
effects on neural activity and not constitute the electrophysiological basis of consciousness).

## Event-Related Potentials

Despite the vast amount of information that has been accumulated about the brain, current research is far from providing
the grounds for comprehending how the brain produces conscious
experience or personal reality.  The study of cognition and the
brain, therefore, is at its very beginnings.  At present, one
strategy for achieving an understanding of how the brain produces
personal reality is to relate specific brain events to conscious
experience.  There are two reasons which make this strategy cogent.
First, it is easier to do.  Conscious experience can be broken
down into a variety of parts and aspects, as for example that
we see color and that wavelengths of light are associated with
the perception of particular colors.  Since conscious experience
is intimately related to personal reality, an accumulation of
knowledge about how particular brain processes are related to
various kinds of conscious experiences is likely to lead to an
understanding of how the brain produces personal reality.

Despite our relative ignorance about how cognition occurs
in the brain, it has been established that electrical impulses
are necessary for input to and output from the brain.  It is
further known that chemical transactions at synaptic junctions
constitute the basis for graded and spike potentials within the
nervous system, thereby permitting neurons to affect one another.
Since event-related potentials are generated by non-random electrical events, this suggests that the electrical activities they
reflect have functional significance for the nervous system.
Furthermore, some of the electrical activities underlying event-
related potentials can be shown to be related to consciousness.
While it is not known how these electrical activities are related
to the transformations necessary for consciousness, they can be
used as indices in time and space of brain events which are step-
ping stones either to or from conscious experience.

Many electrochemical processes in the nervous system, as
for example the bleaching action that occurs in rods and cones,
are necessary for particular conscious events to occur, but not
by themselves sufficient.  Information about receptors and sensory

pathways is naturally crucial for the study of cognition and the brain.  But sensory input does not ordinarily become a part of our personal knowledge of the world unless we become conscious of it.  In an ever fresh chapter, William James (1890) suggested that it is the process of attention which determines whether we become conscious of sensory input.  He pointed out that there are two basic kinds of attention:  active and passive.  By "active" attention is meant voluntary direction of the focus of attention, as when a person decides in advance to read a book, listen to some music, or deliberately tune the world out to concentrate on a train of thought or a favorite fantasy.  By "passive" is meant involuntary attention, such as occurs when a sudden, unexpected stimulus occurs to which our attention is drawn without conscious intent.  Since attention plays such a crucial role in consciousness and cognition, it is helpful that it has been a major focus of research in comtemporary brain research and experimental psychology.

After a variety of unsuccessful attempts in a number of laboratories to identify specific event-related potentials with attention (see Näätänen, 1975, for review), Hillyard and Picton (in press) demonstrated that N100 is associated with what James called active attention.  (N100 is a wave of negative polarity recorded from the scalp with an average peak latency of approximately 100 milliseconds).  The key to their experimental design was to present two or more sources of stimulation (for example, dichotic stimulation) and require subjects to perform a task arranged in such a way that it would be beyond their capacity to simultaneously attend to all the sources of stimulation.  For example, tones of one pitch were presented to one ear and tones of another pitch presented to the other ear;  embedded within the stimuli delivered to each ear were tones of a slightly different pitch which occurred randomly ten percent of the time.  The subjects were required to count the number of infrequent pitch changes that were delivered to one of the two ears, and the stimuli of both ears presented at such a rapid rate that it was not possible to attend to both channels simultaneously.  In effect, an experimental analogue of the "cocktail party phenomenon" was created, where it is feasible to only really listen to one conversation at a time.  Results consistently showed, over a series of experiments, that the amplitude of N100 was larger for the stimuli of the attended than the unattended channels.

The N100 effect just described is related to consciousness in two ways.  When people decide to selectively direct their attention to a particular conversation of interest to them at a cocktail party, they know which conversation they want to hear, but have no awareness of how their nervous system accomplishes the selection.  This is true even if, for example, they realized

that the voices of the people in the attended conversation sounded
different than the voices of the rest of the people in the room
(and could therefore serve as discriminative cues). It is something like the gap between wanting to say something and the actual
production of words and sentences, discussed before. The lack of
awareness in each instance refers to non-conscious processes of
the brain which achieve the desired result. In the case of active attention, these processes analyze stimulus input for particular characteristics prior to awareness of the stimuli which are
selected for conscious perception. We know from personal experience that at a cocktail party we do not first hear all of the
words being spoken at a given moment, and then consciously select
the words that are related to the conversation we want to hear.
It is clear, though, that we have directed those non-conscious
processes to select certain stimuli and not others.

If it is assumed that N100 reflects some or all of the electrical events in the brain related to the selection of particular
stimuli, then one way N100 is related to consciousness is that conscious intentions set in motion the processes of selection which
are reflected in the enhancement of N100 for the stimuli we intend
to listen to. In short, conscious intentions affect the electrical
activity associated with the greater amplitude of N100 found by
Hillyard, Picton and their colleagues for attended over nonattended stimuli.

The other way in which the N100 effect under discussion is
related to consciousness is its relationship to the subsequent
contents of consciousness, that is, the contents which follow in
time the occurrence of an enhanced N100. If what was just said
about the stimulus selection processes which N100 reflects is
true, then the electrical activities which underlie N100 determine
which stimuli in the environment enter the focus of conscious perception. Further discussion of the relationship between N100
and consciousness, along with how other event-related potentials
(such as the CNV and P300) are related to consciousness, can be
found in another paper (Ritter, in press).

I would like to point out that the previous discussion of
N100 depends for its comprehensibility upon personal experiences
shared by the writer and his readers. The only way the selec-
tivity of conscious experience is likely to be known is through
having experienced it. In the absence of that knowledge, it is
just as plausible that all simultaneous stimulation reaches consciousness, that none of it reaches consciousness, or that some
does and some does not on a purely random basis (and that the
portions which do and do not reach consciousness are unrelated
to subsequent thought, feeling, memory and behavior). But we
are confident that conscious experience is selective, and know

quite well that if we are engrossed in a fantasy during a lecture or a talk that we will remember very little of what was said. Furthermore, the interpretations offered concerning N100 and attention, such as the two ways N100 could be related to consciousness, and that stimulus selection is a non-conscious process which occurs prior to conscious perception of the stimulus, essentially make sense because they accord with our own conscious experience.

Reference to one's own experience can be used to make some interpretative comments on the two preceding reports which dealt with the connotative meaning of words. In the first portion of Chapman's paper, subjects were instructed to speak aloud each stimulus word, in order to insure that the words were perceived. It seems likely that the differences in event-related potential morphologies related to the connotative dimensions of the words in this condition are essentially automatic responses, in that it is unlikely that subjects thought of the various connotative meanings of each word as they were perceived and spoken aloud. Introspective reports from the subjects would be helpful in this regard, but in their absence we can infer from our own experience that the differences in event-related potential morphology were automatic in nature and not related to conscious awareness of the connotative meanings of the large number of words presented. The reported morphological differences must be due to previous learning, and might be thought of as being related to associative responses which are available to the person when it is appropriate to experience the connotative meaning of a word. In this sense, the event-related potential effects found by Chapman are indirectly related to prior conscious experiences with the stimulus words.

On the other hand, both the Begleiter et al. and the Chapman studies included a condition where the subjects rated the stimulus words along connotative dimensions. In each study it seems likely that subjects felt few, if any, emotions while rating the words, mainly judging the words through intellectual means. In both studies, however, the effects obtained may be thought of as being related to the conscious intention of rating the words. In the Begleiter et al. experiment, the U curve obtained in the rating condition appears to rule out that the changes in the event-related potential morphology were due to the specific meanings of the words since, as ratings moved to the extremes of pleasantness and unpleasantness, the event-related potential measurement became more similar. In Chapman's report, on the other hand, the results obtained when subjects rated the stimulus words do appear to be related to the specific judgments made in that event-related morphologies were uniquely correlated with the content of the ratings.

## CONCLUSIONS

There is no reason to believe that the brain produces cognition in a manner that is different than how we acquire knowledge of the world in our personal lives and as scientists.  Since all forms of knowledge known to man are mediated by and dependent upon conscious experience, then conscious experience must be central to the cognitive processes of the brain.  Theories that attempt to account for learning and cognition by deliberate exclusion of conscious experience seem seriously misguided because empirical verification of those theories rests upon the very thing that has been denied a role in cognition.

The task of comprehending how the brain is responsible for cognition is a difficult undertaking.  The goal encompasses no less than accounting for how the brain produces and is modified by consciousness, and how conscious experience is woven into an integrated personal reality.  In this complex endeavor we have one fundamental fact to rely upon:  we know what the brain can do, because we experience it every day of our lives.

## REFERENCES

Adey, W.R.  The influences of impressed electrical fields at EEG frequencies on brain and behavior.  In, N. Burch and H.L. Altschuler (Eds.), Behavior and Brain Electrical Activity.  New York: Plenum, 1975.

Berger, P.L. and Luckman, T.  The Social Construction of Reality. New York:  Doubleday, 1966.

Gibson, J.J.  The Senses Considered as Perceptual Systems.  Boston: Houghton Mifflin, 1966.

Henle, M.  On naive realism.  In, R.B. MacLoed and H.L. Pick, Jr. (Eds.), Perception.  Essays in Honor of James J. Gibson.  Ithaca: Cornell University, 1974.

Hillyard, S.A. and Picton, T.W.  Event-related potentials and selective information processing in man.  In, J.E. Desmedt (Ed.), Cerebral Evoked Potentials in Man.  In press.

James, W.  The Principles of Psychology.  New York:  Holt, 1890.

John, E.R.  Switchboard versus statistical theories of learning and memory.  Science, 1972, 177, 850-864.

John, E.R. A model of consciousness.  In, G.E. Schwartz and D.

Shapiro (Eds.), Consciousness and Self-Regulation. Advances in Research. Volume I. New York: Plenum, 1976.

Köhler, W. and Wallach, H. Figural after-effects: An investigation of visual processes. Proceedings of the American Philosophical Society, 1944, 88, 269-357.

Lashley, K.S., Chow, K.L. and Semmes, J. An examination of the electrical field theory of cerebral integration. Psychological Review, 1951, 58, 123-136.

Näätänen, R. Selective attention and evoked potentials in humans - a critical review. Biological Psychology, 1975, 2, 237-307.

Neisser, U. Cognitive Psychology. New York: Appleton-Century-Crofts, 1967.

Ritter, W. The place of consciousness in brain research. In, D. Otto (Ed.), Multidisciplinary Perspectives in Event-Related Brain Potential Research. Washington, D.C.: Government Printing Office, in press.

Russell, B. Human Knowledge: Its Scope and Limits. New York: Schuster, 1948.

Section II

# BRAIN DYSFUNCTION AND EVOKED POTENTIALS

# ELECTROPHYSIOLOGICAL ASSESSMENTS IN MENTALLY RETARDED INDIVIDUALS: FROM BRAINSTEM TO CORTEX*

G.C. Galbraith, N. Squires, D. Altair, and J.B. Gliddon

University of California Neuropsychiatric Institute –

Pacific State Hospital Research Group, Pomona, CA 91766

The problems of mental retardation are complex and can be conceptualized in a number of ways. For example, one can adopt a biomedical model which assumes that basic alterations in the nervous system are the primary cause of mental retardation. Certainly, there are numerous genetic and organic insults to the nervous system that support a biomedical model. In contrast, one may consider mental retardation in socio-cultural terms, with emphases being placed upon developmental impairment in infancy and pre-school years, the deleterious effects of social labeling, poor social-vocational adjustment, etc. Yet, in view of growing evidence that environmental deprivation can markedly impair the anatomical, biochemical and functional development of the nervous system (e.g., Greenough, 1975), it is likely that even individuals diagnosed as mentally retarded on socio-cultural grounds may show patterns of neural activity that deviate from normal. Such abnormal neural activity will be manifest to some degree, it is assumed, in patterns of electroencephalographic activity.

Recent evidence confirms the presence of both gross- and fine-structural abnormalities in the brains of mentally retarded individuals. In Down's syndrome, for example, the brainstem and cerebellum are proportionally smaller (Crome, Cowie & Slater, 1966), and there is generalized cellular agenesis, fibrillary gliosis of cortical neurons and incomplete myelination (Benda, 1969). Also, there is impaired developed of cortical U-fibers which provide

*Supported by USPHS Program Project Grant No. HD-5958, and USPHS Fellowship No. 1F32 NS05725-01 (to N. Squires).

the necessary cortico-cortical connections between association
areas and primary sensory receiving areas. Marin-Padilla (1972)
found microstructural pathology in a Down's syndrome infant consisting of pyramidal neurons which were either severely deprived
of dendritic spines or densely covered with atypically distributed
spines. In cases of profound (non-Down's) retardation, Purpura
(1974) found abnormally long, thin, spines on dendrites of cortical
neurons. Cragg (1975), however, has reported significantly higher
synaptic densities in frontal and temporal neocortex, suggesting
that profound mental retardation may exist without a deficiency of
synaptic development.

Brain damage often results from perinatal asphyxiation, and
the incidence of birth complications with anoxia is elevated among
the mentally retarded (Gottfied, 1973). Several studies indicate
that the auditory relay nuclei of the brainstem are particularly
vulnerable to such anoxic insult. For example, Hall (1963; 1964)
compared the histopathology of neonates who died of perinatal
asphyxia with infants who suffered accidental deaths. A normal
histological and cytological picture was found for both groups in
auditory cortex, medial geniculate body, motor nuclei of the brainstem, and the cochlea. However, the asphyxiated brain series
showed dramatic pathology of the cochlear nucleus, especially the
dorsal cochlear nucleus with a 66 percent cell loss. Cellular
destruction was also present in the superior olivary complex and
inferior colliculus. In view of such selective damage to auditory
structures, it is not surprising that there is an increase in the
incidence of partial deafness among mentally retarded individuals
(Lloyd & Reid, 1967).

Certainly, more research is required in order to clarify the
nature of anatomical differences in the brains of retarded individuals. Nevertheless, the weight of evidence indicates that widespread regions of the brain are involved, ranging from the earliest
synaptic levels of the brainstem to the association cortex. In the
present chapter we report the results of two electrophysiological
techniques that assess neural function from an equally wide range
of brain loci: (1) the short latency (<10 msec) brainstem auditory
evoked response (BAER), which is thought to reflect activity in the
auditory nerve and succesive brainstem nuclei (and associated fiber
pathways) of the auditory system, and (2) the late (>300 msec), positive, event-related potential (termed P300, or P3) which reflects
higher cognitive processing. By means of such diverse procedures we
sought to determine if mentally retarded individuals differ in neuroelectric activity, measured from the very first synaptic levels of
the brainstem to essentially the "last" synapses of higher cortex.

Experiment I.  Effects of Repetition Rate on the BAER of Retarded and Non-retarded Individuals.

## METHOD

Subjects.  Mentally retarded subjects (Ss) were institutionalized residents at Pacific State Hospital.  They were divided into the following two groups: (1) Down's syndrome, which constitutes a relatively homogeneous form of mental retardation that is genetic in origin (N = 8; mean CA = 29.2; mean IQ = 34.3), and (2) a group with mixed, non-genetic, etiologies consisting primarily of individuals diagnosed as asphyxia at birth or uncertain-functional (N = 20; mean CA = 22.7; mean IQ = 43.0).  A nonretarded control group was derived from undergraduate university students enrolled in a special program at the hospital (N = 7; mean CA = 22.0).

Procedures.  BAERs were elicited by 0.1 msec binaural click stimuli delivered through TDH-39 headphones.  Blocks of stimuli at repetition rates of 2, 5, 10, 20 and 50 clicks/sec were presented in a random sequence, with each rate presented twice in the series.  Stimulus intensity was held constant at 64 dB HL.  Ss reclined on a bed in an IAC sound chamber, and were typically asleep throughout most of the experiment.

The EEG was recorded from a vertex scalp electrode referred to left mastoid; the forehead served as subject ground.  Interelectrode resistances were below 4K ohms.  The EEG was amplified by a factor of 500,000 within a bandpass of 60-6K Hz.  Averaging of the BAER was performed on a CAT 400B Computer and then graphed on an X-Y plotter for subsequent manual analyses of amplitude and latency of BAER waves.  Typically, 1,500 clicks were delivered at each repetion rate.  For four Ss it was necessary to extend the recording session over two days (1 hour each day).

Calibration of the graphic plots was accomplished by averaging and graphing a 1K Hz sine wave of known amplitude.  BAER voltages were measured from each positive component peak to the subsequent negative trough, except for wave IV, where the negative trough used was that following wave V.  The values for the two replications at each stimulus rate were averaged.

A separate repeated measures analysis of variance (Weiner, 1962) was performed for each BAER wave, with repetition rate serving as the repeated dimension.

## RESULTS

Figure 1 illustrates BAER recordings obtained from one S in each group.  However, equally good recordings were obtained from

the remaining sample of retarded and nonretarded individuals.  It
was thus possible to consistently define the sequence of BAER waves
in all Ss.

The effects of repetition rate on the group data are shown in
Figure 2.  Overall amplitudes and latencies for the three groups
differed consistently. Amplitudes were largest for the normal group,
intermediate for the mixed group, and smallest for the Down's group.
These effects were reflected in significant ($p < .01$) Group F-values
for each of the five BAER waves.  Repetition rate also had a pronounced effect upon BAER amplitudes.  For waves I–IV there was a
consistent reduction in amplitude with increasing click rates ($p < .01$).  However, the amount of amplitude reduction varied with the
different groups.  Thus, the normal group showed the greatest degree
of change, and the Down's group showed the least. This latter effect
resulted in significant ($p < .01$) Group x Rate interaction terms for
waves I, II and IV.  (Although the wave V interaction term was also
significant, this was due primarily to the V-shaped pattern of the
normal group.

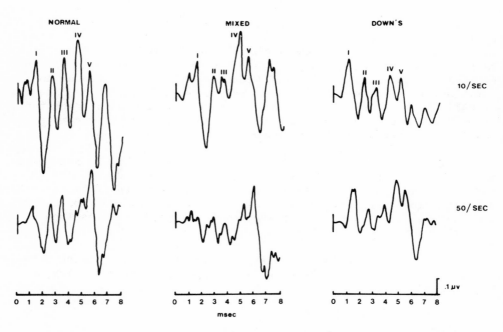

Figure 1.  Individual BAERs recorded from a single subject in
each group at click rates of 10/sec and 50/sec.  Abscissae are in
msec; voltage calibration is 0.1 μV, positive up.

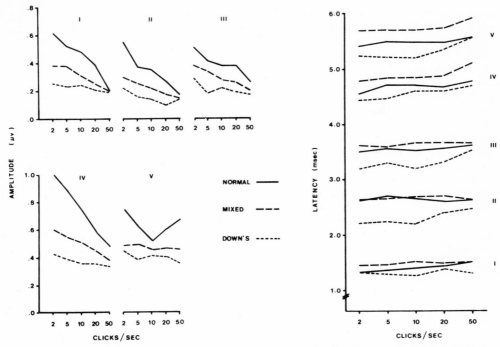

Figure 2. Effect of repetition rate upon BAER amplitude (left) and BAER latency (right). Data are group means, presented separately for waves I-V. Repetition rate appears on abscissae (in clicks/sec); amplitude (in tenths of μV) appears on left ordinate, latency (in msec) appears on right ordinate.

The latency data also showed significant overall group effects. Latencies for the Down's syndrome group were consistently shorter than latencies for the other groups. This was the case for all rates and for all waves, although it was most pronounced for waves II and III. The mixed group, on the other hand, had latencies quite similar to the normal group for early waves, but progressively longer latencies for waves IV and V. There was no overall effect of repetition rate on waves I or II, although a significant ($p<.05$) Group x Rate interaction term resulted for wave II due to the increased latencies for the Down's syndrome group at the higher rates of stimulation. Waves III, IV and V showed a significant ($p<.01$) increase in latency with increasing repetition rate.

## DISCUSSION OF EXPERIMENT I

The present results are generally consistent with previous studies of repetition rate upon BAER amplitude and latency. Thus, amplitudes decreased (cf. Hyde et al., 1976; Pratt & Sohmer, 1976) and latencies of later waves increased (cf. Hyde et al., 1976; Pratt & Sohmer, 1976; Don et al., 1977) with increasing repetition rate. However, the significant Group x Rate interaction terms indicate that group differences exist in auditory information processing.

The amplitude data show similar results at the fastest rate of auditory stimulation (50/sec), but as the repetition rate is reduced to the slowest rate (2/sec) there is a progressive separation in the amplitude curves. At 2 clicks/sec the normal group shows the largest amplitudes, suggesting greater auditory recovery, while the Down's syndrome group shows the smallest amplitudes, suggesting the least degree of recovery to repetitious auditory stimulation. However, since none of the amplitude functions appear to be asymptotic, it is not possible to state whether the BAERs of mentally retarded individuals have lower asymptotic amplitudes at slow rates of stimulation or whether their recovery cycles are prolonged. Nor is it clear how slight differences in hearing ability might affect the data. Based upon BAER amplitudes at slow rates of stimulation it might be concluded that normal Ss hear clicks that are subjectively louder than do Down's syndrome individuals. This result is diametrically opposed to the findings from evoked response studies evaluating components in the 100–300 msec range. In these studies Down's syndrome individuals consistently yield larger evoked response amplitudes to auditory, visual and somatosensory stimuli (Bigum, Dustman & Beck, 1970; Gliddon, Busk & Galbraith, 1975). The final resolution of this question will probably depend upon a psychophysical comparison of sensory magnitudes in mentally retarded and nonretarded individuals.

The latency data showed patterns that differed from those of the amplitude data. For example, the effects of repetition rate were not visible until wave III and beyond. Thus, unlike the amplitude data, the latency differences that derive from repetition rate appear to develop in more central brainstem nuclei rather than in the periphery of the auditory system. Also, since there were no significant Group x Rate interaction terms for these later waves, the latency data do not suggest that subjective loudness differentially changed in the three groups as a function of repetition rate. The possible single exception was the Down's syndrome data for wave II, which showed significantly longer latencies at faster rates of stimulation.

Overall latencies of the two mentally retarded groups showed an interesting contradiction with the amplitude data, as compared with the normal group. Thus, the mixed group showed, for later waves, both smaller amplitudes and longer latencies. The simplest explanation of this BAER pattern is that the mixed group had a relatively mild hearing loss. However, such an explanation is unable to account

for the Down's syndrome group, which paradoxically had the smallest
amplitudes as well as the shortest latencies.  (Shorter BAER latencies in a group of Down's syndrome individuals have previously been
reported in our laboratory (Gliddon, Galbraith & Kuester, 1975)).
Although both brainstem pathology and hearing deficits are known to
result in longer latencies, we believe the present finding in the
Down's syndrome group is the first indication of a condition resulting in shorter BAER latencies. The cause of these shorter latencies
is not clear.  It may be due to the smaller brainstems in Down's
syndrome individuals (Crome et al., 1966), which would imply shorter
conduction pathways.  However, in normals, adult-level latencies are
reached as early as 12-18 months of age (Hecox & Galambos, 1974;
Hecox, 1975), even though the brainstem at this age has still not
reached it's ultimate adult size.

In summary, the present results agree with previous studies concerning the overall effects of stimulus repetition rate.  All groups
showed reduced amplitudes and longer latencies as a function of faster click rates.  However, the specific amplitude and latency trends
for the different groups indicate differences in sensory processing
at the very first stages of synaptic input in the auditory brainstem
nuclei.  Moreover, these differences appear to differentiate not only
between nonretarded and retarded individuals, but also between different groups of mentally retarded individuals.

Experiment II.  Event-related Potentials in Mentally Retarded Individuals.

In the present study we are concerned primarily with the positive voltage component that occurs in a time-window of approximately 300-500 msec following the onset of a stimulus event.  This
component is typically referred to as the "P300" or "P3" wave, and
is thought to reflect endogenous, modality non-specific brain processes since a P3 is elicited by unexpected stimuli in any sensory
modality (e.g., Simson, Vaughan & Ritter, 1977) as well as by the
unexpected omission of a stimulus event (Picton, Hillyard & Galambos,
1974; Simson, Vaughan & Ritter, 1976; Ruchkin & Sutton, in press;
Squires, Squires & Hillyard, in press).  P3 latency, amplitude and
scalp distribution are known to correlate with different psychological processes.  Thus, P3 latency increases as the discrimination
between expected and unexpected stimuli becomes more difficult
(Ritter, Simson & Vaughan, 1972; Ford, Roth & Kopell, 1976a, b;
Squires, Donchin & Grossberg, 1977), or as the task requires greater complexity in processing the stimuli (Kutas, McCarthy & Donchin,
1977).  P3 amplitude, however, varies with S's subjective expectancies about the likelihood of a stimulus occurring, the amplitude
being larger for unexpected stimuli (Sutton, Braren, Zubin & John,

1965; Tueting, Sutton & Zubin, 1970; Squires, Wickens, Squires & Donchin, 1976).

Since a P3 component is elicited only by events to which S is attending (Squires et al., 1975; Ford et al., 1976b), P3 has also been used as a measure of attention. Squires et al. (1976) also showed that, in a random series of events, S's expectancies (and thus P3 amplitude) varied with the particular sequence of stimulus events. P3 amplitude on a given trial depended upon the immediately preceding history of stimulation, extending backwards 7-10 stimuli. When analyzed in this manner, the extent of effect of prior stimulation upon P3 amplitude may provide a quantitative measure of memory span.

From the fact that a particular stimulus evokes a P3 we may infer the following: (1) S is attending to the eliciting events, (2) S can discriminate between expected and unexpected events, (3) S has a memory for prior events, and (4) S is forming expectancies based upon those prior events. Cognitive theories of mental retardation have implicated processes of attention (Zeaman, 1973; Bower, 1974; Lindsley, 1976; Wilhelm & Lovaas, 1976), sensory processes and discriminability (Deich, 1968; Niswander & Kelley, 1976), memory (Spitz, 1973; Miranda & Fantz, 1974) and expectancy formation (Gosling & Jenness, 1974; Silverman, 1975; Kirby, Nettelbeck & Tiggeman, 1977). Thus, the properties of P3 offer considerable promise in many important areas of mental retardartion research. This is especially the case since P3 variations appear to be independent of output or motor processes (Squires et al., 1977), and mentally retarded individuals frequently suffer from motor impairments.

Although many studies have evaluated evoked response components in the range of 50-250 msec in mentally retarded individuals, there are few studies dealing with later components, especially in experimental paradigms specifically designed to elicit P3. The available evidence indicates longer P3 latencies among mentally retarded Ss (Brown, 1968; Karrer & Ivins, 1976). There is no evidence, however, concerning stimulus discriminability or memory. Moreover, the mentally retarded Ss in past studies have been relatively high functioning individuals. In the present study we sought to investigate P3 in greater detail in a group of severely and profoundly retarded individuals.

METHOD

Subjects. Ten mentally retarded Ss were chosen from a project in non-vocal communication. Ss ranged in age from 10 to 14 years (mean = 12.4), and in IQ from 9-45 (mean = 22.6). IQ scores were obtained by either a Kuhlman-Binet or Leiter, administered within two

months of the EEG recording.  In addition, three young adult normal
Ss were run to verify the P3 paradigm.

   Procedures - The stimuli, which depicted certain symbols used
in the non-vocal language program, were in the form of color slides
projected at a rate of once each 1.5 sec.  The slides subtended a
visual angle of 4.5 degrees.  Luminance was 11.2 ft. L.  Additional
slides were red (33.7 ft. L.) or blue (7.2 ft. L.) only, without a
language symbol.  Stimuli were presented in blocks of 20, with each
block consisting of one of the following pairs: (1) easy form discrimination, (2) difficult form discrimination, or (3) color discrimination.  In each pair there was a frequent (p = .75) and infrequent (p = .25) stimulus.  The first stimulus of each block was the
frequent stimulus, and it remained visible for 20 sec in order to
enhance the expectation for that particular stimulus.  Verbal praise
and a candy reward were given at the end of a block if S's behavior
was appropriate.

   The EEG was recorded from the vertex, and from over Wernicke's
and Broca's areas of the left hemisphere and homotopic placements
over the right hemisphere. An electrode above the outer canthus of
the right eye was used to monitor eye movements.  All electrodes
were referenced, in a monopolar derivation, to linked earlobes.
Signals were amplified by Grass P5 amplifiers (bandpass .1 to 100
Hz).  An on-line data acquisition system digitized the signals at
200 samples/sec and stored the results on magnetic tape for later,
off-line, computer analysis.  One experimenter observed the EEG and
eye movement signals, while a second experimenter observed S's behavior.  Trials contaminated with artifacts or inattention to the
task were identified and deleted in subsequent computer analyses.

   Objective measurement of amplitude and latency was performed
by computer.  N1 latency was chosen as the most negative deflection
between 50 and 150 msec, P2 as the most positive deflection between
100 and 300 msec, N2 as the most negative deflection between 200 and
400 msec, and P3 as the most positive deflection between 300 and 800
msec.  However, in the case of P3 a mean latency was computed if two
peaks were detected within the 300-800 msec time window that differed in amplitude by as little as 5 μV.  Amplitudes were measured from
a baseline consisting of the average voltage of the initial 30 msec
(6 data points) of the waveform.

## RESULTS

   Figure 3 presents the evoked response data for mentally retarded
Ss to frequent and infrequent stimuli, averaged across the different
stimulus pairs.  The plots are presented according to IQ, with the
cross-hatched area in each plot representing greater positivity to
the infrequent stimuli.  It is clear from Figure 3 that all mentally

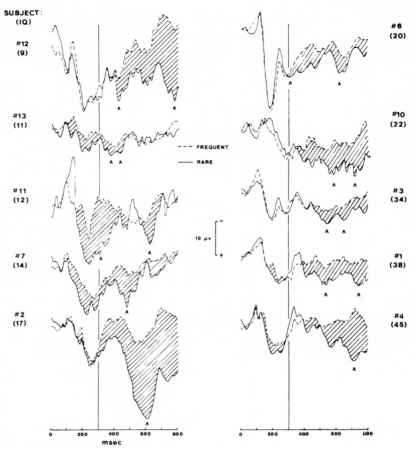

Figure 3.   P3 potentials to frequent (broken line) and infrequent (solid line) visual stimuli.   The cross-hatched area defines
greater positivity to infrequent stimuli.   Plots are ordered from
low (top left) to high (lower right) IQ scores.   The arrow pointers
in each plot indicate the P3 latency automatically selected by the
computer (where two pointers appear P3 latency is taken as the mid-
point).   Abscissae are in msec (vertical time line is at 300 msec);
voltage calibration is 10 μV, positive down.

retarded Ss in our sample showed late positivity to the infrequent
stimuli.

     Mean P3 amplitude in the mentally  retarded group was 13 μV
(range = 7–26 μV) as compared to a mean of 10 μV (range = 3–14 μV)
in the normal group (t = 0.68, N.S.).   Mean P3 latency was 577 msec
(range = 420–705 msec) in the mentally retarded group as compared

with 397 msec (range = 365-450 msec) in the normal group (t = 3.13, p< 01). The latencies of earlier components did not differ. For example, N1 latencies were 118 and 115 msec, and P2 latencies were 225 and 228 msec, in the mentally retarded and normal groups, respectively.

The effect of difficulty of discrimination on P3 was assessed within each group by comparing the amplitudes and latencies for the easy and difficult trial blocks. Amplitudes were not significantly different in either group. However, latencies were shorter for both groups during the easy discrimination trials (550 vs. 596 msec for the mentally retarded group; 377 vs. 405 msec for the normal group), although only the results for the normal group reached statistical significance (p< 05, one-tail test).

Figure 4 illustrates group differences in P3 asymmetry recorded from the electrodes placed over left and right hemispheres. Amplitude of P3 is typically maximal over posterior regions of the head. The degree of posterior positivity is represented in Fig. 4 by the cross-hatched areas in the separate plots. All normal Ss showed a similar degree of posterior positivity over left and right hemispheres, i.e., there was minimal asymmetry of P3 activity. Mentally retarded Ss, however, responded with quite different patterns of P3 asymmetry. Of the nine Ss for whom there was complete data, two showed essentially a normal pattern, two showed no tendency towards a posterior distribution of P3, while five showed posterior positivity only over one hemisphere, i.e., there was marked P3 asymmetry.

## DISCUSSION OF EXPERIMENT II

Although event-related potentials have been studied extensively in adults, few studies have examined such potentials in normal children. Courchesne (1977) and Shelburne (1973) found that P3 latency is longer in children than adults, while Symmes & Eisengart (1971) did not find a P3 in their sample of children. However, the data of Goodin, Squires, Henderson & Starr (in press) indicate that the group age differences in the present study (12.4 vs. 22.6 yr.), at least for nonretarded Ss, should not result in appreciable differences in P3 latency. Of course, there is little evidence concerning P3 activity in mentally retarded individuals. Brown (1968) reported longer latencies; Karrer & Ivins also reported late positivity, but their experiment was not specifically designed to assess P3 activity. Further evidence obtained in our laboratory (not presented here) comparing age-matched retarded and nonretarded adults demonstrates significantly longer P3 latencies in mentally retarded individuals. In the present experiment we demonstrate reliable P3 waves in profoundly retarded children which occur at significantly longer latencies than for nonretarded individuals. Yet, latencies

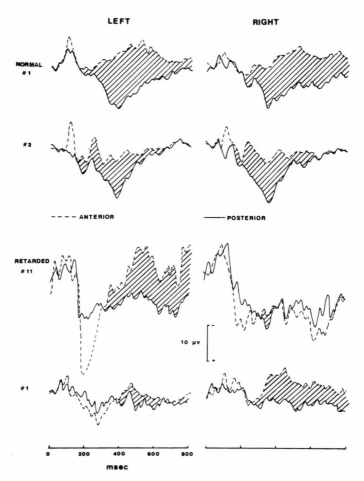

Figure 4. P3 activity recorded over left and right hemisphere in two normal (top two pairs of plots) and two mentally retarded (bottom two pairs of plots) individuals. Recordings are from anterior (broken line) and posterior (solid line) electrode placements. The cross-hatched area defines greater posterior positivity. Abscissae are in msec; voltage calibration is 10 μV, positive down.

of earlier evoked response components did not differ between the two groups. Since early evoked response components are considered to reflect sensory mechansims, while late components are known to reflect higher decision processes, we are led to conclude that P3 may provide a reliable indication of retarded cognitive development in mentally retarded individuals. This appears to be the case, moreover, even if sensory mechanisms do not differ from the nonretarded.

Because reliable P3 waves were recorded in all mentally retarded Ss, it is assumed that they discriminated between the frequent and rare stimuli. Studies with normal Ss have shown that P3 latencies are shorter for easy discriminations and longer for more difficult discriminations (Ford et al., 1976a; Squires et al., 1977). The present results were in the predicted direction for both groups, but only the data for the nonretarded group reached statistical significance. The trend in the data for the mentally retarded group indicates, nevertheless, that they were also responding to the easy and difficult discriminations. In many cases of profound mental retardation it is difficult to determine whether or not the individual can reliably discriminate between two stimuli. P3 latency appears to provide a technique whereby perceptual discriminations in mentally retarded individuals may be objectively assessed. Such information could prove useful in rehabilitative and training programs.

The results shown in Fig. 4 indicate interesting asymmetry differences in the late P3 wave. Typically, larger P3 amplitudes are recorded from posterior electrode placements. The cross-hatched areas in Fig. 4 reflect this greater posterior positivity. However, in Fig. 4 these anterior-posterior comparisons were made over the left and right hemispheres. The results for nonretarded individuals showed essentially equal anterior-posterior patterns over left and right hemispheres. However, our sample of mentally retarded individuals showed marked hemispheric asymmetry that did not appear to favor one particular hemisphere. Once again, the results for late event-related potentials differ from that found for earlier evoked response components, where hemispheric asymmetry is more characteristically found in nonretarded individuals (Bigum, Dustman & Beck, 1970; Gliddon, Busk & Galbraith, 1975). Indeed, Bigum et al. (1970) suggest that evoked response asymmetry is greater in those individuals with higher intelligence. However, since event-related potentials are more clearly related to cognitive processing than are earlier evoked response components, one might reasonably expect P3 asymmetry to more accurately reflect intellectual level. If so, then the present results suggest that individuals with lower intelligence show greater asymmetries in anterior-posterior P3 activity.


FINAL STATEMENT

It is clear that a comparison of mentally retarded and nonretarded individuals yields marked differences in patterns of electrical activity of the nervous system. The present studies demonstrate that these differences can be found as early as the first synaptic levels of the brainstem, as well as the "highest" reaches of the nervous system responsible for decision-making and discrimination. With improved refinement and utilization, these electrophysiological pattern differences may prove to be a valuable assessment tool for

the clinician and practitioner involved in the diagnosis and treatment of mentally retarded individuals.


REFERENCES

Achor, L. J. Field analysis of auditory brainstem responses.
     Neurosci. Abstr., 1976, 2, 12.
Benda, C. E. Down's syndrome. New York: Grune & Stratton, 1969.
Bigum, H. B., Dustman, R. E. & Beck, E. C. Visual and somato-
     sensory evoked responses from mongoloid and normal children.
     Electroenceph. clin. Neurophysiol., 1970, 28, 576-585.
Bower, A. C. Autonomic correlates of anticipation and feedback
     in retarded adolescents. J. ment. Defic. Res., 1974, 18,
     31-39.
Brown, W. S. Evoked potential correlates of information delivery
     and responsiveness in mongoloid and normal children. Unpub-
     lished Master's thesis, Univ. So. Calif., 1968.
Buchwald, J. S. & Huang, C. M. Far-field acoustic response:
     origins in the cat. Science, 1975, 189, 382-384.
Courchesne, E. Event-related brain potentials: Comparison between
     children and adults. Science, 1977, 197, 589-592.
Cragg, B. G. The density of synapses and neurons in normal, mental-
     ly defective and ageing human brains. Brain, 1975, 98, 81-90.
Crome, L., Cowie, V. & Slater, E. A statistical note on cerebellar
     and brain-stem weight in mongolism. J. ment. Defic. Res., 1966,
     10, 69-72.
Deich, R. Reproduction and recognition as indices of perceptual
     impairment. Amer. J. ment. Defic., 1968, 73, 9-12.
Don, M., Allen, A. R. & Starr, A. Effect of click rate on the
     latency of auditory brain stem responses in humans. Arch.
     Otol., Rhin. and Laryngol., 1977, 86, 186-195.
Ford, J., Roth, T. & Kopell, B. Auditory evoked potentials to
     unpredictable shifts in pitch. Psychophysiol., 1976, 13,
     32-39 (a).
Ford, J., Roth, W. & Kopell, B. Attention effects on auditory
     evoked potentials to infrequent events. Biological Psy.,
     1976, 4, 65-77 (b).
Gliddon, J. B., Galbraith, G. C. & Kuester, D. Effects of stim-
     ulation rate on short latency far-field responses in the
     mentally retarded. Annual meeting of the American Association
     on Mental Deficiency, Chicago, May 30-June 2, 1976.
Gliddon, J. B., Busk, J. & Galbraith, G. C. Visual evoked re-
     sponses as a function of light intensity in Down's syndrome
     and nonretarded subjects. Psychophysiol., 1975, 12, 416-422.
Goodin, D. S., Squires, K. C., Henderson, B. H. & Starr, A. Age-
     related variations in evoked potentials to auditory stimuli
     in normal human subjects. Electroenceph. clin. Neurophysiol.,
     in press.

Gosling, H. & Jenness, D.  Temporal variables in simple reaction
    time of mentally retarded boys. Amer. J. ment. Defic., 1974,
    79, 214-224.
Gottfied, A. W.  Intellectual consequences of perinatal anoxia.
    Psychol. Bull., 1973, 80, 231-242.
Greenough, W. T.  Experiential modification of the developing brain.
    Amer. Sci., 1975, 63, 37-46.
Hall, J. G.  On the neuropathological changes in the central nervous
    system following neonatal asphyxia. With special reference to
    the auditory system. Acta Oto-Laryngol. Suppl., 1963, 188,
    331-338.
Hall, J. G.  The cochlea and cochlear nuclei in neonatal asphyxia.
    A histological study. Acta Oto-Laryngol. Suppl., 1964, 194,
    6-93.
Hecox, K. Electrophysiological correlates of human auditory develop-
    ment.  In: Cohen & Salapater (Eds.), Infant Perception: From
    Sensation to Cognition, Vol. II, New York: Academic Press, 1975,
    pp. 151-191.
Hecox, K. & Galambos, R.  Brainstem auditory evoked responses in
    human infants and adults. Arch. Otolaryngol., 1974, 99, 30-33.
Huang, C.-M. and Buchwald, J. S.  Interpretation of the vertex short-
    latency acoustic response: A study of single neurons in the
    brainstem. Brain Res. (in press).
Hyde, M. L., Stephens, S. D. G. & Thornton, A. R. D.  Stimulus
    repetition rate and the early brainstem responses. Brit. J.
    Audiol., 1976, 10, 41-50.
Jewett, D. L.  Volume conducted potentials in response to auditory
    stimuli as detected by averaging in the cat. Electroenceph.
    clin. Neurophysiol., 1970, 28, 609-618.
Jewett, D. L. & Williston, J. S.  Auditory evoked far fields
    averaged from the scalp of humans. Brain, 1971, 94, 681-696.
Karrer, R. & Ivins, J.  Steady potentials accompanying perception
    and response in mentally retarded and normal children.  In:
    Karrer, R. (Ed.), Developmental Psychobiology of Mental
    Retardation.  Springfield: Thomas, 1976, pp. 361-417.
Kirby, N. H., Nettlebeck, T. & Tiggeman, M.  Reaction time in
    retarded and non-retarded young adults: sequential effects
    and response organization. Amer. J. ment. Defic., 1977, 81,
    492-498.
Kutas, M., McCarthy, G. & Donchin, E.  Augmenting mental chronom-
    etry:  the P300 as a measure of stimulus evaluation time.
    Science, 1977, 197, 792-795.
Lev, A. & Sohmer, H.  Sources of averaged neural responses record-
    ed in animal and human subjects during cochlear audiometry
    (electrocochleogram). Arch. klin. Exp. Ohren Nasen Kehl-
    kopfheilkd., 1972, 201, 79-90.
Lindsley, D. B.  Mental retardation: Historical and psychophysiolog-
    cal perspective.  In: Karrer, R. (Ed.), Developmental Psycho-
    physiology of Mental Retardation, Springfield: Thomas, 1976
    pp. 3-38.

Lloyd, L. L. & Reid, M. J.   The incidence of hearing impairment in an institutionalized mentally retarded population. Amer. J. ment. Defic., 1967, 71, 746-763.

Marin-Padilla, M.   Structural abnormalities of the cerebral cortex in human chromosomal aberrations: A Golgi study. Brain Res., 1972, 44, 625-629.

Miranda, S. B. & Fantz, R. L.   Recognition memory in Down's syndrome and normal infants. Child Develop., 1974, 45, 651-660.

Niswander, P. & Kelly, L.   Comparison of speech discrimination in nonretarded and retarded listeners. Amer. J. ment. Defic., 1976, 80, 217-222.

Picton, T. W., Hillyard, S. A. & Galambos, R.   Cortical evoked responses to omitted stimuli. In: Livanov, M. N. (Ed.), Major Problems of Brain Electrophysiology, USSR Acadamey of Sciences, 1974, pp. 302-311.

Pratt, H. & Sohmer, H.   Intensity and rate functions of cochlear and brainstem evoked responses to click stimuli in man. Arch. Oto-Rhino-Laryng., 1976, 212, 85-92.

Purpura, D. P.   Dendritic spine "dysgenesis" and mental retardation. Science, 1974, 186, 1126-1128.

Ritter, W., Simson, R. & Vaughan, H. G.   Association cortex potentials and reaction time in auditory discrimination. Electroenceph. clin. Neurophysiol., 1972, 33, 547-555.

Ruchkin, D. & Sutton, S.   Latency characteristics and trial-by-trial variation of emitted potentials. In: Desmedt, J. E. (Ed.), Cerebral Evoked Potentials in Man, Brussels, in press.

Shelburne, S. A.   Visual evoked responses to language stimuli in normal children. Electroenceph. clin. Neurophysiol., 1973, 34, 135-143.

Silverman, W.   Utilization of redundant information by EMR and non-retarded adults. Amer. J. ment. Defic., 1975, 80, 197-201.

Simson, R., Vaughan, H. G. & Ritter, W.   The scalp topography of potentials associated with missing visual or auditory stimuli. Electroenceph. clin. Neurophysiol., 1976, 40, 33-42.

Simson, R., Vaughan, H. G. & Ritter, W.   The scalp topography of potentials in auditory and visual discrimination tasks. Electroencephalog. clin. Neurophysiol. 1977, 42, 528-535.

Sohmer, H. & Feinmesser, M.   Routine use of electrocochleography (cochlear audiometry) on human subjects. Audiol., 1973, 12, 167-173.

Spitz, H. H.   The channel capacity of educable mental retardates. In: Routh, D. K. (Ed.), The Experimental Psychology of Mental Retardation, Chicago: Aldine, 1973, pp. 133-156.

Squires, K. C., Wickens, C., Squires, N. K. & Donchin E.   The effect of stimulus sequence on the waveform of the cortical event-related potential. Science, 1976, 193, 1142-1146.

Squires, N. K., Donchin, E., Squires, K. C. and Grossberg, S.   Bi-sensory stimulation: Inferring decision-related processes from the P300 component. J. exp. Psychol.:HPP, 1977, 3, 299-315.

Squires, N., Squires, K. C. & Hillyard, S.   Two varieties of long-
    latency positive waves evoked by unpredictable auditory stim-
    uli in man.   Electroenceph. clin. Neurophysio., 1975, 38,
    387–401.
Squires, N. K., Squires, K. C. & Hillyard, S.   On the functional
    equivalence of signal–present, signal–absent, and threshold-
    detect P3.   In: Otto, D. (Ed.), New Perspectives in Event-
    related Potential (ERP) Research, Washington, D. C.: U. S.
    Government Printing Office, in press.
Starr, A.   Auditory brainstem responses in brain death.   Brain,
    1976, 99, 1543–1554.
Starr, A. & Achor, J.   Auditory brain stem responses in neurologi-
    cal disease.   Arch. Neurol., 1975, 32, 761–768.
Stockard, J. J. & Rossiter, V. S.   Clinical and pathologic corr-
    elates of brain stem auditory response abnormalities.   Neurol.,
    1977, 27, 316–325.
Sutton, S., Braren, M., Zubin, J. & John, E. R.   Evoked potential
    correlates of stimulus uncertainty.   Science, 1965, 150, 1187–
    1188.
Tueting, P., Sutton, S. & Zubin, J.   Quantitative evoked potential
    correlates of the probability of events.   Psychophysiol., 1970
    7, 385–394.
Weiner, B. J.   Statistical Principles in Experimental Design.   New
    York: McGraw-Hill, 1962.
Wilhelm, H. & Lovaas, O. I.   Stimulus overselectivity: A common
    feature in autism and mental retardation.   Amer. J. ment. Defic.
    1976, 81, 26–31.
Zeaman, D.   One programmatic approach to retardation.   In: Rauth, D.
    K. (Ed.), The Experimental Psychology of Mental Retardation.
    Chicago: Aldine, 1973, pp. 78–132.

# THE USE OF EVOKED RESPONSE PROCEDURES IN STUDIES OF READING DISABILITY

Malcolm S. Preston

Department of Pediatrics, Johns Hopkins University
School of Medicine, Baltimore, Maryland 21205

## INTRODUCTION

This paper defines the concept of specific reading disability, discusses its genetic and neurologic bases, and examines the results of eight evoked response studies which have appeared in the literature. While testing and analysis procedures vary in these reports, there is some evidence to suggest that evoked potential differences between normal and disabled readers may exist, particularly when recordings are made from parietal areas, and when linguistic stimuli are used. The suggestion is offered that the heterogeneity of the disorder may tend to obscure differences between normal and disabled readers when comparisons are made between group means. An approach employing the genetic method as used in the study of inherited conditions in families may help to isolate different subtypes of the disorder. This approach initially requires the establishment of the range and limits of normal response. Some data exploring laterality effects in normal readers using linguistic stimuli are presented and discussed in terms of this approach.

## Specific Reading Disability

Some children experience great difficulty in learning to read. The acquisition of reading skills is affected by factors such as low intelligence level, poor oral language development, impoverished home and cultural backgrounds, inadequate reading instruction, and

presence of emotional problems. However, some children still experience great difficulty in learning to read in spite of the absence
of all of these factors. Such children are said to have developmental dyslexia, or specific reading disability.

The existence of specific reading disability is supported by the
results of several recent studies (Symmes and Rapoport, 1972; Rutter and Yule, 1975). For example, in the Symmes and Rapoport
study, 108 children (aged 7-13) with reading problems were identified. Of these, the investigators excluded 54 who were found to
have a primary neurological, psychiatric, or other handicap sufficient to account for retardation in the reading process. The remaining 54 children were said to have an unexplained reading failure. They had a mean WISC IQ of 113, demonstrated a high incidence of reading and learning disabilities in their immediate families,
included only one girl, and were described as emotionally stable.

This study clearly indicates the existence of a specific disability in reading in contrast to poor reading ability of known etiology. It is important to note, however, that it does not suggest
that that specific reading disability is a unitary syndrome. In fact,
other studies (Ingram, Mason, and Blackburn, 1970; Boder, 1973)
suggest that there may be several distinct subtypes of the disorder.
For example, Boder (1973) postulates three types: 1) dysphonetic
dyslexia in which the underlying deficit lies in the ability to relate
graphemes to their corresponding phonetic sound values, 2) dys-
eidetic dyslexia in which the deficit lies in the formation of adequate visual configurations for words and letters, and 3) mixed
dyslexia in which both visual and sound-symbol deficits are present.

## Genetic Bases of Specific Reading Disability

The disproportionate number of males who are affected by specific reading disability (Critchley, 1970) suggests that the disorder
may have a biologic origin. Twin studies lend strong support to the
genetic hypothesis. Zerbin-Rudin (1967) summarized the results of
three investigations in which all 17 MZ twin pairs studied were con-
cordant for reading disability while only 12 of 34 DZ twin pairs
showed concordance. Family studies of reading disability also
point to a genetic basis for the disorder. Hallgren (1950), in his
study of 112 families, found that in the 90 families in which one
parent was affected, the proportion of affected children was consistent with an autosomal dominant mode of inheritance.

Finucci, Guthrie, Childs, Abbey, and Childs (1976) studied nearly every first-degree relative of the index cases in 20 families. A carefully-selected battery of reading and IQ tests was used to classify subjects as normal or disabled readers. The results of this study showed that 45% of the first-degree relatives were disabled: 56% of the males and 33% of the females. No consistent pattern of genetic transmission emerged from an examination of the family pedigrees, although some were consistent with a single gene effect manifested as dominant in males and recessive in females. One explanation that may account for these findings is that the disorder is genetically heterogeneous; that is, there may be several genetically distinct subtypes. Some sort of multigenic inheritance is also a possibility. In general, the results of these studies clearly point towards a genetic basis for specific reading disability, although the precise nature of genetic transmission and the manner in which possible genetic mechanisms affect the functioning of the brain during the reading process remain to be discovered.

## Neurologic Bases of Specific Reading Disability

There has been much speculation about the neurologic basis of this disorder. Benton (1975), for example, outlines several theoretical approaches. One of these attributes specific reading disability to a focal maldevelopment or a delay in development of some particular area of the brain. According to this view, one form of which has been advanced by Satz and Sparrow (1970), the affected area most likely lies in the region of the left angular gyrus, a region known to be important in reading from studies of alexia (Benson, 1976). However, because of the ease with which language functions can be transferred from one hemisphere to another in young children following injury, it seems more likely that defects in both parietal lobes would be necessary to produce a deficit.

Another approach holds that specific reading disability results from a deficit in the overall organization of cerebral function. This theory was originally introduced by Orton (1937). Briefly, he suggested that the two hemispheres are functionally equivalent in the analysis of visual information in the striate and parastriate regions. However, at higher levels of visual analysis, such as that required in recognition of symbolic stimuli, which is presumably handled in the parietal regions, efficient operation requires that only one hemisphere be active in information processing, suppression of the other being necessary to prevent interference. Failure to suppress the

non-dominant hemisphere results in an impaired ability to perceive
visual symbols and consequently an impairment in associating the
symbols with appropriate phonetic sound values.

A more recent neurological theory has been proposed by Witelson
(1977) based on an interpretation of the results of a study employing
dichotic listening, visual hemifield, and dichhaptic techniques. She
hypothesizes that in males, reading disability is a consequence of
bilateral representation of spatial perception coupled with left hemisphere deficit in language function. In females, only one factor is
involved: deficient left hemisphere function. Still another theory attributes the disorder to cerebellar-vestibular dysfunction (Frank and
Levinson, 1973). According to this approach, the cerebellar-vestibular defect produces ocular fixation and sequential scanning difficulties which in turn interfere with the cortical processing of spatial
relationships affecting the identification of letters and words.

However plausible these various neurological theories may be,
there is little direct evidence to support any of them. This may be
a result partly of the heterogeneous nature of the disorder and partly
a result of the indirect and imprecise nature of the behavioral techniques such as visual hemifield, dichotic listening, or dichhaptic
presentation used most often in the study of human brain function.
Only in the past few years have more direct measures of brain activity such as visual evoked response been used with reading disabled
subjects. The few such studies that have been carried out have been
both disappointing and encouraging: disappointing because of certain
errors in design or technique, but encouraging for the most part in
suggesting that the pareital region is a likely area to show differences
between normal and disabled readers.

Evoked Potential Studies of Specific Reading Disability

Initial studies employed non-linguistic stimuli such as light
flashes or clicks. For example, Shipley and Jones (1969) were interested in comparing the effects of simultaneous auditory and visual
stimulation with results for each modality separately in normal and
disabled readers, although data are reported only for 10 disabled subjects (8-14 year-old males). They used light flashes and clicks as
stimuli. The subject's task was to count the stimuli silently.
Evoked responses were recorded from two bipolar arrangements. In
one of these, one electrode was located 4 cm to the left of $C_z$ and
2 cm anterior, while the other electrode was located 4 cm posterior

to the first. In the other arrangement, one electrode was located at
the occipital pole and the other 8 cm anterior along the midline. Averages consisted of 32 presentations with a 500 msec sweep time.

The results consisted of difference curves for each of the bipolar
arrangements obtained by adding together the evoked response waveforms for auditory and visual stimuli presented separately and subtracting the result from the waveform obtained with simultaneous presentation. Positive values along the resultant difference curve were
considered physiological indices of "arousal" while negative values
were considered indices of "inhibition." A ratio (E) of positive to
negative area (multiplied by 100) along the difference curve was obtained for each bipolar arrangement. The mean E for the ten subjects
was 80, indicating a tendency towards "inhibition." However, since
no data for normals were presented, it is impossible to tell if this
was an abnormal finding.

Ross, Childers, and Perry (1973) carried out a visual evoked
response study with 30 disabled children ranging in age from 6 to 14
years. Five electrodes were attached in the form of a cross with the
center electrode located 5 cm above the inion on the midline. The
other four were located 5 cm from the center electrode which served
as reference. Stimuli consisted of 80 flashes of colored light presented at 2 per second under three separate conditions: binocular
red, binocular green, and dichcoptic (left eye red, right eye green).
The subject's task was not reported.

According to the authors, the most striking finding was that the
right occipital waveforms were inverted (phase reversed) compared to
posterior midline waveforms in 20 out of 30 disabled subjects tested
in contrast to an unstated number of control subjects who showed no
such inversion. However, since there was no indication of sweep
time, no measurements of specific components made, and no waveforms presented, it is difficult for the reader to make any meaningful
interpretations of these findings.

The work of Conners (1970) greatly increased expectations that
it might be possible to identify evoked response correlates of reading
disability. Conners investigated similarities and differences in visual
evoked response waveforms in a family with five of six members affected by reading disability and also examined several groups of disabled readers differing in severity of the disorder. Testing procedures
involved the presentation of light flashes with eyes closed. About
20% of the flashes were less bright than the others. The subject's

task was to press a telegraph key whenever a dim flash occurred.
Averages were computed for the bright flashes only (n = 64, sweep
time = 512 msec, interstimulus interval = 1.6 sec). Electrodes were
attached to $O_1$, $O_2$, $P_3$, and $P_4$, all referenced to $C_z$, which makes
interpretation of the waveforms difficult since $C_z$ is an active location (Kooi, 1972; Conners, 1972). The waveforms for the six family
members were presented in graphic form. The remaining data were
analyzed by identifying a positive peak around 140 msec (P140) and
a negative peak around 200 msec (N200). Latencies, baseline-to-
peak, and peak-to-peak measures were then obtained.

With respect to the family data, Conners states that the waveform for the $P_3$ electrode is "noticeably attenuated in the late components" for the index case (a male, $11\frac{1}{2}$ years old) compared to the
$P_4$, $O_1$, and $O_2$ electrodes. He notes similar findings in three other
siblings also affected by reading disability, but not in the normal
reading mother or in the disabled father, the latter showing fewer
oscillations in the components prior to 200 msec on the $P_3$ electrode.
I am not sure all readers would agree with these observations. By
my estimation, for example, the data reveal a considerable flattening
across the entire waveform on the $P_3$ electrode in the index case and
one sib (15-year-old sister). Two other sibs and the mother show
lesser degrees of attenuation in the $P_3$ electrode.

A second finding in Conners' paper concerns some correlations
between evoked response measures and reading achievement in a
group of 27 disabled children with a mean age of 9.9 years. Significant correlations of .61 and .57 occurred on the $P_3$ electrode between amplitude from baseline for N200 and scores on the Wide
Range Achievement Spelling and Reading Subtests. Slightly lower
correlations on the same electrode were noted for peak-to-peak P140-
N200. Retesting six weeks later also showed the same results. A
third finding revealed a significant difference in amplitude on the $P_3$
electrode for N200 between a mildly disabled group of ten male subjects (mean age = 11.9) and a more severely disabled group of the
same size and sex (mean age = 11.9). The mild group showed greater
amplitude from baseline using a one-tailed test.

Besides the unfortunate choice of electrode for reference and the
fact that no direct comparisons between corresponding electrodes for
each hemisphere were made, another major problem with Conners'
studies is the fact that no normal reading controls were tested. However, in spite of these difficulties, these findings are at least mildly
suggestive that differences between good and poor readers are likely

to be evident on the $P_3$ electrode.

Sobotka and May (1977) used a testing procedure very similar to Conners (1970) with 24 normal and 24 disabled readers, six in each group at 7, 9, 11, and 13 years of age. Subjects pressed a response key whenever a dim flash occurred in an eyes-closed condition. Electrodes were attached to $O_1$, $O_2$, $P_3$, and $P_4$, all referenced to $C_z$. Averages were computed over 64 presentations with sweep time at 409 msec. Three peaks were identified in each waveform corresponding approximately to P140, N210, and P300. Peak-to-peak measures for P140-N210 and N210-P300 as well as latencies for all three peaks were obtained. Both groups showed significantly greater N210-P300 amplitudes on the right side for the parietal and occipital leads with no difference between groups. Group differences did emerge, however, when data was combined over hemispheres. In this case, the disabled subjects showed greater P140-N210 and N210-P300 amplitudes on the parietal and occipital leads, respectively.

Although the testing procedure used by Sobotka and May was very similar to that used by Conners (1970), the findings of these two studies were not entirely comparable because the Sobotka and May study did not employ baseline-to-peak measures. The most that can be said is that Conners' work suggests a lower amplitude of response is associated with reading disability for the N200 component on the $P_3$ electrode, while the Sobotka and May study suggests a higher amplitude of response can be found for disabled readers for the P140-N210 component on both parietal leads and for the N210-P300 component on both occipital leads.

Weber and Omenn (1977) investigated the flattening of the visual evoked response in disabled readers noted by Conners (1970) in three large families containing both normal and disabled readers. Data is also reported on 18 additional disabled children aged 8 to 17 years. Subjects were presented with 64 light flashes and 64 bursts of white noise through head phones. The visual and auditory stimuli were randomly intermixed (mean interstimulus interval = 3.7 sec) and subjects were asked to press a button in response to either the light flash or the noise burst at the beginning of the test run, a major defect in design since the motor activity may have affected the evoked responses under study. Electrodes were attached over the parietal region of both hemispheres (no mention of 10-20 System) and both were referenced to linked mastoids. Separate averages were obtained for the visual and auditory stimuli. Peak-to-peak amplitude was measured for N150-P190 for the light flashes and N100-P200 for the white noise bursts.

Results for 11 disabled subjects and 9 normals from the three families showed no significant differences between hemispheres for either group, and also no significant difference between groups for the two evoked response measures. When the data for the eldest child in each family were combined with the data for the additional 18 disabled children, there were again no significant differences between hemispheres for either evoked response measure. Since the reference employed in this study was relatively inactive, these hemispheric findings may be considered more meaningful than those observed in the previous studies employing bipolar arrangements. However, it would have been preferable if data for normal readers from normal-reading families had been presented to ascertain whether the lack of asymmetry noted for the disabled subjects was a normal or abnormal finding.

All of the evoked response studies reviewed so far used light flashes of some kind for visual stimuli with varying degrees of attention required by the subject. Four of the five used bipolar recording techniques and only one of the five reported data obtained from a suitable normal control group. It seems reasonable that if differences exist between normal and disabled readers, they are more likely to be found if the subject is presented with linguistic stimuli and asked to process the information in some way. Furthermore, since cortical areas are of interest, particularly hemispheric differences in the parietal region, monopolar arrangements with a common reference should be favored over bipolar montages.

Symann-Lovett, Gascon, Matsumiya, and Lombroso (1977) used three- and four-letter words which were either the names of animals or body parts as stimuli in a visual evoked response study of 12 normal and 10 disabled readers, median age 12.0 and 12.6, respectively. No discrimination task was imposed, but subjects were told they would be questioned about the words at the end of the experiment. In addition, they were required to press a key in response to a question mark which appeared two seconds after each stimulus was presented. Two seconds later the next stimulus occurred. Electrodes were attached at $C_z$, $O_1$, $O_2$, $P_3$, and $P_4$, as well as over Wernicke's area on both sides ($W_1$ and $W_2$). All electrodes were referred to linked ear lobes. Averages were computed over 100 stimuli with sweep time equal to 512 msec. The analysis of the data consisted of counting the number of waves whose amplitude exceed the previous peak by 2.5 $\mu v$ either before (early) or after (late) 200 msec. Significant differences between groups occurred on the $P_3$ and $W_1$ electrodes for the early measures with the normal readers showing more waves than the disabled readers.

Intrigued by Conners' (1970) study, a group of us at Johns Hopkins, including John Guthrie, Barton Childs, and myself, began our evoked response studies of reading disability by testing a group of nine disabled readers with a mean age of 9.8 and two groups of normals containing nine subjects each with mean ages of 10.1 and 7.5, respectively (Preston, Guthrie, and Childs, 1974). The young normal group was reading at the same level as the disabled group, as determined by the Gates-MacGinitie Reading Test, and all three groups had comparable IQs. It was assumed that if the results showed that the two control groups differed from the disabled group, but not from each other, then reading level as well as age and IQ could be ruled out as factors, leaving neurologic dysfunction as the most likely explanation. Electrodes were attached to $C_z$, $O_1$, $O_2$, $P_3$, and $P_4$, all referenced to left mastoid. Stimuli consisted of two runs of 50 presentations of a flash of light and two runs of the same number of presentations of the word "cat" with interstimulus interval and sweep time both set at one second. The subjects were asked simply to observe the stimuli.

Being our first attempt at gathering evoked response data, we were beset with some technical problems and felt confident only with the data from the $P_3$ electrode. Inspection of that data showed two components evident in almost all the records: a negative wave peaking at about 180 msec and a positive wave at about 600 msec. Accordingly, baseline-to-peak measures were made at these two latencies. The results for N180 showed that the two normal groups exhibited significantly greater amplitude for both the flash and "cat" stimuli at this latency than the disabled group with no difference noted between the two sets of normals. The main effect for replication was not significant. All three groups showed significantly greater amplitude to "cat" than flash. Group and stimulus condition effects were not significant at 600 msec.

Although our referencing system was different from that of Conners (1970), we thought our initial work tended to confirm his finding of a reduced amplitude for components in the 200 msec range in more severely disabled readers from the $P_3$ electrode. In our second investigation (Preston, Guthrie, Kirsch, Gertman, and Childs, 1977), we looked for differences between normal and disabled adult readers. The disabled adults (mean age = 40.1) were the mothers or fathers of at least one reading disabled child. The normal adults (mean age = 36.2) were parents of normal reading children. Electrodes were attached to $O_1$, $O_2$, $P_3$, and $P_4$, all referenced to linked mastoids. Each subject was tested under two conditions: light flashes and words.

In the flash condition, subjects were asked simply to look at the
flashes. In the word condition, subjects counted silently a target
word which occurred about 20% of the time and reported the total at
the end of the test run. This was an easy task for all subjects, since
only two (one in each group) gave incorrect counts. Averages were
computed over 32 stimuli in each run with an interstimulus interval of two seconds and sweep time of one second. In the word runs,
the average included both targets and non-targets.

In the analysis, four measures of amplitude were made: peak-
to-peak for P100-N140 and N140-P200, P200 from baseline, and a
late positive component (LPC) consisting of the average of the amplitudes from baseline for latencies at 250, 350, 450, and 550 msec.
An analysis of variance showed no significant main effects for groups
on any of the four evoked potential measures. However, an interaction for the P200 and LPC components between groups, stimuli and
electrode placements was significant. This interaction is best illustrated by noting the difference in amplitude in each group between
the word and flash condition at each of the four electrode positions
and then comparing the two groups on each electrode. When this was
done, the only electrode to show a significant difference between
groups for both P200 and the LPC was $P_3$, with the normal group
showing a larger difference between words and flashes than the disabled group. Figure 1 shows the results for the LPC. Since performance on the word task was nearly perfect in both groups, we concluded that these results might reflect some neurophysiological difference in the way normals and disabled readers process written
material.

## Evoked Potentials and the Establishment of Subtypes

It is obvious that if evoked responses are to be useful in the
study of reading disability, it is necessary to show that some component or components of the evoked response differentiate normal from
disabled readers. The most traditional approach has been to look for
statistically significant differences between group means. However,
as indicated earlier, there may be several distinctly different subtypes
of the disorder. If this is so, then a feature of the evoked response
which characterizes a particular subgroup may not, in fact, be discovered by simply comparing the means of groups of normal and disabled readers. The characteristic may not be present in sufficient
numbers of disabled readers to produce consistently significant differences between groups and, therefore, may escape detection by the

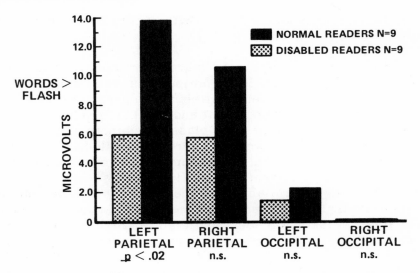

Figure 1:   Mean LPC amplitudes on the word-minus-flash measure
            for normal and disabled readers.  The only significant
            difference between groups occurred on the left parietal
            electrode.

researcher.  On the other hand, if the characteristic is present in
many disabled readers and does result in a significant group difference, there is still no assurance that the "abnormal" scorers in
the disabled group form a subgroup unless it can be shown that they
are differentiated from the other disabled readers on the basis of some
other theoretically important variable, such as a genetically meaningful pattern of inheritance.

     The combination of the genetic method as applied in the study of
inherited disorders in families and the use of evoked potential measures of brain function may prove to be a fruitful research strategy.
The basic principal here is that if reading disability is associated
with the possession of one or more genes, and if certain first-degree
relatives share such genes, all such relatives should show the same
phenotype.  If there are several variant phenotypes in the population
whose expressions are always consistent within families, but different between families, the inference is that the variants must be associated with different genetic mechanism; that is, there may be spe-

cifically definable genetic subtypes with unique evoked response
characteristics.

The limitations of this approach are determined primarily by the
reliability of the evoked response components under study, the likelihood that the components are sufficiently sensitive to reflect differences in brain function in normal and disabled readers, and the
accuracy of the procedure used to classify subjects as normal or
disabled readers. This approach requires the collection of data on
different test days from a sufficient number of normal readers (children and adults of both sexes) whose first-degree relatives are not
reading disabled. The reliability of the data may then be determined
as well as the limits of normal response for each component under
investigation. Disabled readers and their families may then be tested
and responses for each component classified as normal or abnormal
by comparison with the appropriate age and sex distributions for normals. A search can then be made in affected families for consistent
patterns of response reflecting a particular subtype of specific reading
disability.

## Laterality Effects in Normal Readers

The particular approach described above is the one we are pur-
suing at Johns Hopkins in our studies of the neurologic and genetic
bases of specific reading disability. To achieve these aims, we have
begun to collect evoked response data from normal readers in order to
determine what sorts of evoked waveforms or patterns of response may
be expected in these readers when the stimuli are either linguistic or
non-linguistic, and when the task requires the subject to process both
types of stimuli in some fashion.

One question we are interested in is whether evoked response
procedures can be used to demonstrate laterality effects. Although
recent studies using auditory stimuli have not been encouraging (Galambos, Benson, Shulman-Galambos, and Osier, 1975; Friedman, Simson, Ritter, and Rapin, 1975), a separate analysis of the normal data
in the Preston et al (1977) study suggested that further exploration of
the assessment of the cerebral lateralization of linguistic function by
visual evoked response procedures would be of value. In this analysis, the normal readers showed significantly greater amplitude for the
LPC on the left side for word stimuli, but not for flash stimuli. The
disabled subjects did not show any difference for either type of stimuli.
The following study with 20 normal readers confirms the hemispheric

differences noted in our previous work, but also demonstrates the possible limitations of this approach.

## METHOD

### Subjects

The subjects were selected from the members of six families of normal readers consisting of a total of 36 individuals. The data reported here were obtained from the first 20 individuals tested, ranging in age from 9.8 to 55.4 years. All 36 subjects were administered the following psychometric tests: WISC-R or WAIS, Gray Oral Reading Test (Gray, 1963), the Wide Range Achievement Test (WRAT): Spelling and Reading Subtests (Jastak and Jastak, 1965), and three special reading tests obtained from Finucci et al (1976). The criteria used for classification of subjects as normal readers were the same used in the Finucci et al study. Briefly, a subject was classified as a normal reader if his performance on the Gray Oral, WRAT Spelling Subtest and the three special tests fell at or above the levels expected on the basis of education. All 36 subjects were classified as normal readers. Characteristics of the 20 subjects tested with evoked response procedures are given in Table 1. There were 12 males and 8 females. All but two were right-handed, as determined by preferred writing hand. Full scale IQ, with the exception of one subject who obtained a score of 82, ranged from 100 to 143.

### Instrumentation

The subjects were seated in a dental chair located in a shielded, dimly-lighted, double-walled IAC chamber about five feet from a black panel with a white screen (3 x 1 3/4 inches). Stimuli were projected from outside the test room by a Carousel projector. The stimuli subtended lateral and vertical visual angles no greater than $2°52'$ and $1°40'$, respectively. Electrodes were attached to $O_1$, $O_2$, $P_3$, and $P_4$. $O_1$ and $P_3$ were referenced to the left mastoid, while the $O_2$ and $P_4$ were referenced to the right mastoid. A forehead electrode served as ground while two other electrodes were attached near the outer canthii of the eyes to monitor lateral eye movements.

The evoked potentials were amplified by an eight channel Beckman type RM dynograph recorder (band width 0.16 to 45.46 Hz), averaged on line and saved on DEC tape by a PDP-12A computer. To calibrate the system on each chanel prior to testing, a series of 32

Table 1.  CHARACTERISTICS OF SUBJECTS

| Subject | Sex | Hand | Age | Education[a] | FSIQ[b] | VIQ[b] | PIQ[b] | WRAT Spelling[c] | WRAT Reading[c] | Family SES[d] |
|---|---|---|---|---|---|---|---|---|---|---|
| 1 | M | R | 9.75 | 4.9 | 117 | 117 | 112 | 109 | 113 | 2 |
| 2 | M | R | 12.50 | 7.9 | 112 | 114 | 106 | 104 | 106 | 3 |
| 3 | M | R | 12.83 | 7.9 | 100 | 100 | 101 | 116 | 125 | 2 |
| 4 | M | R | 12.83 | 8.0 | 115 | 111 | 117 | 100 | 110 | 1 |
| 5 | M | R | 15.75 | 10.9 | 118 | 118 | 114 | 111 | 105 | 1 |
| 6 | M | R | 16.50 | 11.0 | 82 | 94 | 73 | 110 | 104 | 1 |
| 7 | M | R | 18.92 | 14.0 | 116 | 119 | 110 | 106 | 128 | 3 |
| 8 | M | R | 21.25 | 13.5 | 109 | 104 | 114 | 105 | 107 | 2 |
| 9 | M | R | 33.17 | 16.0 | 141 | 140 | 137 | 137 | 141 | 3 |
| 10 | M | R | 37.25 | 17.0 | 124 | 125 | 120 | 107 | 129 | 2 |
| 11 | M | R | 47.67 | 18.0 | 143 | 140 | 140 | 137 | 155 | 1 |
| 12 | M | R | 55.42 | 17.0 | 127 | 126 | 125 | 130 | 131 | 2 |
| 13 | F | R | 12.33 | 6.9 | 116 | 113 | 115 | 112 | 102 | 2 |
| 14 | F | L | 15.00 | 9.9 | 113 | 102 | 124 | 111 | 107 | 2 |
| 15 | F | R | 15.42 | 10.0 | 113 | 103 | 123 | 107 | 111 | 1 |
| 16 | F | L | 17.42 | 12.0 | 122 | 121 | 120 | 112 | 122 | 1 |
| 17 | F | R | 18.75 | 14.5 | 110 | 116 | 99 | 122 | 115 | 2 |
| 18 | F | R | 33.50 | 13.5 | 110 | 110 | 110 | 123 | 138 | 3 |
| 19 | F | R | 35.67 | 13.0 | 125 | 125 | 122 | 122 | 134 | 2 |
| 20 | F | R | 53.92 | 13.5 | 115 | 118 | 110 | 135 | 130 | 2 |
| Mean | | | 24.79 | | 116.4 | 115.8 | 114.6 | 115.8 | 120.7 | |
| S.D. | | | 14.55 | | 13.0 | 12.1 | 14.2 | 11.5 | 14.8 | |

a = Grade equivalent.  Thus, 4.9 would indicate a subject who has completed the ninth month of fourth grade.  b = WISC–R or WAIS.  c = Standard score.  d = Hollingshead and Redlich (1957) Index of Social Economic Status.  Lower score signifies higher SES.

ten microvolt pulses (produced by a custom built pulse generator) were fed through the electrode board next to the subject and averaged by the computer. During testing, one experimenter remained in the test room with the subject and another operated the equipment outside the test room. Lateral eyemovements were monitored continuously during testing on an oscilloscope. If a subject made an eyemovement during a test run, it was terminated immediately, the subject cautioned, and the run started over from the beginning. This occurred two times, once each with two younger subjects.

## Procedure

Each subject was tested twice under two conditions. In the word condition, a run consisted of a series of three-letter words (illuminated letters, black background) presented one at a time for 100 msec with an interstimulus interval of 2.15 sec. The words used were din, bin, bit, pin, and bid. The letters were all lower case. In the word runs, each word occurred from four to seven times in a pseudo-random order. In both word runs ($W_1$ and $W_2$), the subjects' task was to keep mental count of the number of times the word bin flashed and to report the count at the end of the run. A run consisted of 34 or 35 stimuli. In the first run, the target word occurred seven times, and in the second, six times. A waveform consisted of the average of the first 32 stimuli and thus included both targets and non-targets.

In the second condition (designated Flash), the stimuli consisted of a series of nonsense patterns created by slicing up the letters of each word used in the word runs and distributing the pieces of the letters over the same area occupied by the word. The two orders of stimuli in the flash runs ($F_1$ and $F_2$) corresponded to the two orders of the stimuli in the word runs ($W_1$ and $W_2$). This was designed to keep the amount of light constánt between the two conditions. The subjects' task was to count (mentally) the total number of flash stimuli in a run and report the total at the end of the run. As with the word runs, a waveform consisted of the average of the first 32 stimuli in each run. Half of the subjects received the two word runs first followed by the two flash runs. The order was reversed for the other half. All subjects counted correctly the number of target words and the number of flash stimuli presented.

## Data Analysis

The averaging program commenced sampling on each of the four channels 100 msec prior to the stimulus presentation. The sample

rate for each channel was 256 Hz. After each run, the evoked response waveform for each channel was stored on DEC tape. A waveform analysis program (Willey, 1973) was then used to examine the
data after fitting each waveform with a baseline derived from the 100
msec prestimulus period. The latency window from 348 to 508 msec
following stimulus onset was selected for study in order to reduce
confusion with earlier components which may reflect activity not
specifically originating in the parietal lobes, areas of interest in
the present study.

A measure designated the LPC was defined as the average amplitude from baseline starting with a latency of 348 msec and including
11 sample points 16 msec apart up to and including 508 msec. Having
derived the LPC measures for each electrode for each run for each subject, the data was subjected to a four-way analysis of variance (BMDP-
2V) with Testing ($W_1$, $F_1$ vs $W_2$, $F_2$), Hemispheres (Left vs Right),
Placement (Parietal vs Occipital) and Stimuli (Words vs Flashes).
Interactions were explored with two-tailed $\underline{t}$ tests when justified.
The .05 level was adopted as the criterion for significance.


## RESULTS AND DISCUSSION

The Stimuli, Placement, and Hemisphere main effects were significant, while Testing was not. In general, words produced greater LPC
amplitude than flashes, parietal leads showed greater amplitudes than
occipital leads, and the left hemisphere produced greater amplitudes
than the right hemisphere. There were, however, several significant
interactions between these variables. Table 2, which presents the
details of the Placement x Testing interaction, shows a significant
difference between testings on the occipital leads only. This table
also demonstrates that LPC amplitudes are more positive on the parietal leads compared to occipital leads with the effect more pronounced
on Testing 2. Table 2 also presents the details for the Placement x
Stimuli interaction which reveals that only for the word stimuli is the
LPC amplitude significantly greater on the parietal leads compared
to the occipital leads. In addition, the table shows that the difference between words and flashes is evident on both parietal and
occipital electrodes with the difference greater on the parietal leads.

The triple interaction (Placement x Hemisphere x Stimuli) is illustrated in Figure 2. In probing this interaction with $\underline{t}$-tests, the

Table 2.   LPC INTERACTIONS
(Mean amplitudes and standard deviations in microvolts)

| | Placement x Stimuli | | Mean | |
| | Parietal | Occipital | Difference | S.D.[†] |
|---|---|---|---|---|
| Words | 4.5 | 1.9 | 2.6* | 2.9 |
| Flashes | -1.5 | -1.4 | -0.1 | 2.6 |
| Mean difference | 6.0* | 3.3* | | |
| S.D.[†] | 3.9 | 2.5 | | |

| | Placement x Testing | | | |
|---|---|---|---|---|
| Testing 1 | 1.5 | 0.7 | 0.8 | 2.1 |
| Testing 2 | 1.5 | -0.2 | 1.7* | 2.8 |
| Mean difference | 0 | 0.9* | | |
| S.D.[†] | 2.0 | 1.3 | | |

*Significant at the .01 level.     [†]Standard deviation of difference.

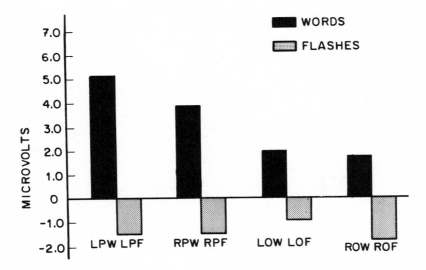

Figure 2.   Mean LPC amplitudes for the four electrodes.  The following comparisons were significant by $\underline{t}$-test (.05 level
or better).  Hemispheres:  LPW vs RPW;  Placement:
LPW vs LOW, RPW vs ROW;  Stimuli:  LPW vs LPF, RPW
vs RPF, LOW vs LOF, ROW vs ROF.
Key:  L = left, R = right, P = parietal, O = occipital,
W = words, F = flashes.

following results became evident:   (1) there were no significant differences between any of the four electrodes under the flash condition;
(2) under the word condition, there was a significantly greater LPC
amplitude on the left parietal electrode compared to the right parietal
electrode with no hemispheric differences on the occipital leads; (3)
under the word condition, the parietal leads showed significantly
greater amplitude than the occipital leads on both hemispheres.

To explore more fully the hemispheric differences at the parietal
locations, a series of t-tests between hemispheres was carried out
for the eleven sample points between the latencies of 348 and 508
msec which defined the limits of the LPC as used in this study.  These
results are presented in Figure 3 along with comparisons between
hemispheres made at latencies of 300, 316, and 332 msec.  Figure 3
shows significant differences between hemispheres beginning at 348
msec and ending at 476 msec with one exception at 380 msec.  Table
3 presents correlations between each of the eight LPC measures and
Full Scale IQ, Verbal IQ, Performance IQ, WRAT Spelling, and WRAT
Reading.  In general, while most are positive, only a few of these
correlations reach significance.  No strong pattern emerges, although
there is a tendency for high correlations on the right occipital electrode under the flash condition.

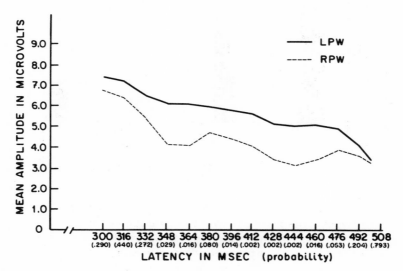

Figure 3.   Mean amplitudes and p-values (in parenthesis) for t-
            tests between left parietal words (LPW) and right parietal
            words (RPW) at latencies between 300 and 508 msec fol-
            lowing stimulus onset.

Table 3.  CORRELATIONS BETWEEN SUBJECT CHARACTERISTICS
          AND LPC MEASURES (Decimals omitted)

|                  | LPW | RPW | LOW | ROW | LPF | RPF | LOF | ROF |
|------------------|-----|-----|-----|-----|-----|-----|-----|-----|
| Age              | 15  | 24  | 34  | 43  | 26  | 01  | 28  | 51* |
| FSIQ             | 18  | 16  | 36  | 32  | 18  | 23  | 34  | 46* |
| VIQ              | 23  | 19  | 47* | 38  | 29  | 27  | 27  | 56* |
| PIQ              | 07  | 09  | 19  | 24  | 06  | 12  | 37  | 32  |
| WRAT Spelling    | 38  | 43  | 53* | 54* | 36  | 15  | 31  | 50* |
| WRAT Reading     | 17  | 24  | 37  | 39  | 09  | -17 | 19  | 42  |

*Significant at .05 level.

In order to examine whether there were any differences between
males and females, a separate analysis of variance was carried out
on the LPC measure combined over testings. The variables were Sex,
Placement, Hemispheres, and Stimuli. No main effect for sex was
noted, and none of the interactions of sex with any of the other variables were significant. The data were also examined for possible
differences between the 18 right-handers and the two left-handers.
Both of the latter showed greater LPC amplitudes on the left side
under the word condition for the parietal leads. In addition, a t-
test between hemispheres on the parietal leads under the word condition for the 18 right-handers showed the left hemisphere advantage
was still significant (p < .02). Finally, within session test-retest
correlations were computed. They ranged from .62 to .81, and all
were significant.

In spite of the extended age range, use of both sexes, and inclusion of two left-handers, the results of the LPC demonstrated a
significant left-sided superiority on the parietal leads for word stimuli only. However, the distribution of difference scores (left parietal minus right parietal) showed that only 14 of the 20 subjects exhibited the left-sided effect. The scores ranged from 1.4 microvolts
(right greater than left) to 5.6 microvolts (left greater than right).
The mean difference was 2.6 microvolts in favor of the left hemisphere. Thus, although useful for showing differences between
group means, this particular evoked response measure is not suitable
for individual assessment of the lateralization of linguistic function.

While some researchers have expressed doubt that evoked response methods are sensitive enough to reflect hemispheric specialization in individual subjects, few if any studies have used testing procedures that require subjects to treat the stimuli presented in an exclusively linguistic manner. The procedure used in the present study (counting the occurrence of a particular pre-designated target word) is obviously not sufficient. A better procedure, and one we are planning to use in future studies, might be to present a series of words with each word a member of a particular semantic category, and ask the subject to count the number of times words belonging to a given category appear while computing averages over target and non-target words separately.

In the preceding pages is outlined the work that has been done so far in looking for evoked potential correlates of specific reading disability. Some studies have demonstrated interesting group differences although none have yet shown evoked response procedures can be used reliably for individual assessment. Future work might be best directed towards first establishing the normal range of response for stimuli and tasks requiring full linguistic processing.

## REFERENCES

Benson, D.F. Alexia. In Aspects of Reading Acquisition, edited by J.T. Guthrie. Baltimore: Johns Hopkins Press, 1976, 7-36.

Benton, A.L. Developmental dyslexia: neurological aspects. In Advances in Neurology, vol. 7, edited by W.J. Friedlander. New York: Raven Press, 1975, 1-47.

Boder, E. Developmental dyslexia: a diagnostic approach based on three atypical reading-spelling patterns. Developmental Medicine and Child Neurology, 1973, 15, 663-687.

Conners, C.K. Cortical visual evoked response in children with learning disorders. Psychophysiology, 1970, 7, 418-428.

Conners, C.K. Letter to the editor. Psychophysiology, 1972, 9, 473.

Critchley, M. The Dyslexic Child. Springfield, Ill.: Charles C. Thomas, 1970.

Finucci, J.M., Guthrie, J.T., Childs, A.L., Abbey, H., and Childs, B. The genetics of specific reading disability. Annals of Human Genetics, London, 1976, 40, 1-23.

Frank, J. and Levison, H. Dysmetric dyslexia and dyspraxia: hypothesis and study. Journal of Child Psychiatry, 1973, 12, 690-701.

Friedman, D., Simson, R., Ritter, W., and Rapin, I. Cortical evoked potentials elicited by real speech words and human sounds. *Electroencephalography and Clinical Neurophysiology*, 1975, 38, 13-19.

Galambos, R., Benson, P., Smith, T.S., Shulman-Galambos, C., and Osier, H. On hemispheric differences in evoked potentials to speech stimuli. *Electroencephalography and Clinical Neurophysiology*, 1975, 39, 279-283.

Gray, W. *Gray Oral Reading Tests*. Indianapolis: Bobbs-Merrill, 1963.

Hallgren, B. Specific dyslexia: a clinical and genetic study. *Acta Psychiatrica Neurologica*, 1950, supplement 65.

Hollingshead, A. and Redlich, F. *Two Factor Index of Social Position*. New Haven, Conn.: Published by authors, 1957.

Ingram, T.T.S., Mason, A.W., and Blackburn, I. A retrospective study of 82 children with reading disability. *Developmental Medicine and Child Neurology*, 1970, 12, 271-281.

Jastak, J.F. and Jastak, S.R. *The Wide Range Achievement Test*. Wilmington: Guidance Associates, 1965.

Kooi, K.A. Letter to the editor. *Psychophysiology*, 1972, 9, 154.

Orton, S.T. *Reading, Writing and Speech Problems in Children*. New York: Norton, 1937.

Preston, M.S., Guthrie, J.T., and Childs, B. Visual evoked responses (VERs) in normal and disabled readers. *Psychophysiology*, 1974, 11, 452-457.

Preston, M.S., Guthrie, J.T., Kirsch, I., Gertman, D., and Childs, B. VERs in normal and disabled adult readers. *Psychophysiology*, 1977, 14, 8-14.

Ross, J.J., Childers, D.G., and Perry, N.W. The natural history and electrophysiological characteristics of familial language dysfunction. In *The Disabled Learner: Early Detection and Intervention*, edited by P. Satz and J.J. Ross. Rotterdam: University of Rotterdam Press, 1973, 149-174.

Rutter, M. and Yule, W. The concept of specific reading retardation. *Journal of Child Psychology and Psychiatry*, 1975, 16(3), 181-197.

Satz, P. and Sparrow, S. Specific developmental dyslexia: a theoretical reformulation. In *Specific Reading Disability: Advances in Theory and Method*, edited by D. J. Bakker and P. Satz. Rotterdam: University of Rotterdam Press, 1970, 17-40.

Shipley, T. and Jones, R.W. Initial observations on sensory interaction and the theory of dyslexia. *Journal of Communication Disorders*, 1969, 2, 295-311.

Sobotka, K.R. and May, J.G. Visual evoked potentials and reaction time in normal and dyslexic children. Psychophysiology, 1977, 14, 18-24.

Symann-Louett, N., Gascon, G.G., Matsumiya, Y., and Lombroso, C.T. Waveform differences in visual evoked responses between normal and reading disabled children. Neurology, 1977, 27, 156-159.

Symmes, J. and Rapoport, J. Unexpected reading failure. American Journal of Orthopsychiatry, 1972, 42, 82-91.

Weber, B.A. and Omenn, G.S. Auditory and visual evoked responses in children with familial learning disabilities. Journal of Learning Disabilities, 1977, 10, 32-158.

Willey, T.J. Waveform: evoked potential analysis. Decus Program Library, No. 12-126, 1973

Witelson, S.F. Neural and cognitive correlates of developmental dyslexia: age and sex differences. In Psychopathology and Brain Dysfunction, edited by S. Gershon and C. Shagass. New York: Raven Press, 1977.

Zerbin-Rudin, E. Congenital word blindness. Bulletin of the Orton Society, 1967, 17, 47-54.


This work was supported in part by USPHS research grant HD 00486 and a grant from the Thomas Wilson Foundation. The author gratefully acknowledges the assistance of Sister Jane Francis, principal of St. Mary School in Baltimore, as well as the families who participated in this study.

BRAIN DYSFUNCTION AND EVOKED POTENTIALS


Discussant:  Edward C. Beck

Veterans Administration Hospital and University of Utah

Salt Lake City, UT   84148


Before discussing these three very interesting presentations,
allow me to generalize on certain aspects of the conference, to
reminisce about how we have come so far and to speculate about
where I feel we should be headed.

Yesterday we heard six excellent papers.  We were greatly
impressed, if occasionally baffled, by the complexities of some
of the new and sophisticated analytical methods.  Despite the
provocative experiments reported, up to this point little has
been said about the organ that we are studying, the human brain,
an organ that occupies scarcely one and one-half liters, weighs
little more than three pounds and is composed of 10,000 million
neurons or nerve cells, each with thousands of connections.  It
is the most complexly organized matter in the universe--without
question--without qualification.  Possibly it defies serious
comprehensive analysis, whatever mathematical model we apply.
Consider the fact that neurons in the brain make thousands of
connections with each other but the innumerable extra connections
that the larger human cortex, with its millions of apical dendrites,
multiplies virtually to infinity the brain's capacity for receiving, processing, and analyzing data.  And it is this sheer massive
power for handling data that challenges each of us to describe
its methods of function, electrical or otherwise.

Approaching the problem from the molecular point of view,
the capacity of each one of the neurons is staggering.  Biochemists
and cytologists point out that in a mature human brain each neuron
or nerve cell may have upwards of 20 million RNA molecules, thought
by some to serve as a "filing system" for memory.  It would appear
that the normal brain is a system capable of handling any load of

learning, memory, or data processing that one is likely to put upon
it. Considering the complexity of the brain, it is amazing that we
have reached the point that our computerized squiggles show credible
correlations with certain "mental activities."

As the processes by which the brain produces mind are inher-
ently covert and obstinately illusive, man through history has
been given full scale to his imaginative speculation, indeed poetic
inventiveness in explaining his experiential being and behavior,
normal or otherwise. From this state of ignorance has stemmed
much of the contrived and speculative explanations that has constituted the basis of psychological and psychiatric diagnosis
and treatment of man's behavioral difficulties and still clutter
the textbooks.

The fact that the brain is the organ of perception and cognition, that it is the essence of our thinking, our feeling, our
consciousness--and the consequence of this fact has barely begun
to penetrate the vast contrivances of psychological speculation.
It is to this point of view that this conference and conferences
similar to it, such as the NASA conference in San Francisco,
the Belgium conference in Brussels were directed and have contributed
so significantly.

Techniques other than the evoked potential technique have
emerged concomitantly with our methods in the last decade. Presently we have three notable approaches directed towards a better
understanding of the brain. One of course is refined chemical
analysis of the brain, e.g., catecholamine's metabolism and the
breakthrough demonstrating that certain amine-containing neurons
are not uniformly distributed in the brain. Another powerful
technique is computerized x-ray tomography, or the CAT scan,
making it possible to see inside the brain as never before, and
finally, of course, is our own computerized analysis of the brain's
electrical patterns and rhythms. One possible advantage of our
technique is that it is more dynamic than the others. That is,
we can observe electrical changes in the brain during cerebral
activity, or if you like, mental processes.

We are presently riding on a wave of optimism, optimism
that we have earned with the avalanche of experiments and studies
that have emerged in the generation since the technique was first
described by Dawson in the mid-fifties. We are recording certain
wave form patterns and configurations that correlate very highly
with mental states, information processing and the like. However,
I would like to sound a caveat in the midst of this enthusiasm.
This pertains to a return to the organ that we are studying, to
the brain. Since the late 1960s we have come to be rather cava-
lier about the neurogenesis or the underlying neuroanatomy of the
various components of the evoked potential. The all abiding concern

regarding detailed knowledge of the intracranial sources and
neural pathways that determine the wave form of the averaged
evoked potential (AEP) appears to be no longer a source of serious
concern.  I regret this for two reasons.  The first, of course,
is that the underlying neuroanatomy of the AEP has direct bearing
upon any interpretation of the changes we observe in the evoked
potential with disease, ingestion of drugs, aging, or those changes
that occur or are affected by psychological processes such as
information processing, cognition, and the like.

The second reason for my regret is the waning of excitement
and challenge that prevailed in the pursuit of the neurogenesis
of the various components of the evoked potential.  The speculations, arguments, theorizing; the "how," the "where" and the
"why" seemed to have gone.  This is, of course, still present
among some investigators, e.g., those studying and evaluating
far-field potentials or Jewett bumps and to a certain degree
those concerned with AEP components up to and during the time
of the vertex potential or roughly around 200-250 msec.  However,
any serious effort to pursue the source of long-latency components,
to my knowledge, is almost completely lacking.  It is generally
shrugged off with the notion that it must be cortical.  To me
this is tantamount to the German generality to a question without
answer, "Es liegt an der Luft" (it lies in the air).

Consequently, much as I admired the sophisticated mathematical
models that we have developed, the elaborate electronics and
computerized devices, I feel there is a need for serious neurophysiological investigation of the source of long-latency responses.
These waves relate critically to "biological psychiatry," and
to the problems that constitute the majority of papers presented
at this conference.  Despite this concern, I feel we have come
a long way, but missing is the skepticism and challenge that
often characterize new scientific observations or discoveries.

While there is no doubt about the reliability of these
phenomena, still disturbing questions remain unanswered.  Do
cerebral vascular changes in the brain contribute to the development of these late responses?  Following the resolution or expectancy of a particular stimulus is there some slight autonomic
or vascular change that produces a late slow positive shift?
Have experiments been tried to note the effects of cardiovascular
drugs, such as the nitrites on long-latency responses?  Are they
affected by hyperventilation?  What is the role of the autonomic
nervous system?  Does it take 300, 400 and often several hundred
milliseconds to "process" information, especially when the response
to such information processing often occurs before that period
of time?  What species differences exist?  Is it manifested in
those species such as the rat that are lissencephalic?  Will
long-latency components be differentially determined by a number

of conditions--physiological, pharmacological, and developmental?
These questions are pertinent in view of such information as
provided by the paper of Galbraith, Squires and Gliddeon who
demonstrated that one of the clearest P300s generated in their
Down's syndrome children was that of a child with an IQ of 8.

Let us turn now to the papers of this session. The three
papers that I am to discuss, parenthetically each very interesting
and well presented, have one thing in common. They each address
themselves to complex problems. The data they provide are descriptive. Explanations or analysis of the results are elusive.

The first paper for discussion is "Evoked Potential Correlates
of Central Information Processing in Mentally Retarded Individuals." Drs. Galbraith, Squires and Glidden are well known
for their work with sensory evoked responses in mentally retarded
children, especially those afflicted with Down's syndrome. Their
present paper departs from the usual approach of those studying
the evoked potential of retarded individuals and includes a comparison of the early far-field potentials or "Jewett bumps" with
retarded and normals. They also record the long-latency or P3
responses of these individuals. Their results show that from
the first synapse to cortex, the mentally retarded child differs
from the normal.

More specifically, the question was asked, what would be
the effects of increasing repetitive rate of the stimuli on the
amplitude and latency of components of far-field potentials?
The answer was surprising. While the largest overall amplitude
was found in the nonretarded children, and the lowest was seen
in the Down's syndrome children, surprisingly, mean latency of
wave components for the Down's syndrome group were consistently
shorter than the normal group. This infers faster conduction
and more rapid recovery time in the smaller brain stem of the
Down's syndrome child.

The results with the P3 component were equally unexpected.
While the Down's children ranged in IQ from 8 to 45, there was
no relationship between the amplitude of the P300 and the mental
abilities of the child. In point of fact, one of the most obvious
P3 waves was seen in a child with an IQ of 8.

These results are quite clear and convincing but difficult
to explain. Far-field auditory brain stem responses normally
consist of seven components in the initial 10 msec following
the click stimuli. As the interruption of auditory pathways at
the junction of the VIII nerve with the brainstem causes a loss
of response components following the first wave, it is generally
accepted that the origin of the first wave is the acoustic nerve.

Waves II and III are believed to reflect activity of the cochlear
nucleus, trapezoid body and possibly the superior olive.  The
lateral lemniscus and inferior colliculus are thought to generate
waves IV and V respectively.  Waves VI and VII, to my knowledge,
are not as yet defined.  While waves VI and VII are prominent
components in the auditory brain stem response of human subjects,
they are absent or almost impossible to define in experimental
animals such as the rat and the cat.  Consequently, all we can
say regarding the far-field experiments of Galbraith et al. is
that these brain stem structures differ in Down's syndrome youngsters.  This may be due to the smaller brain stem, hence fewer
number of snyapses or other factors that we as yet do not understand.

Interestingly, this is in contrast to the later components
which in the Down's individual arrive much later and are greater
in amplitude than those of matched normals.

I have only one minor criticism of this paper and that is
the inclusion of mental retardates of "uncertain" etiology.  I
find the study of Down's syndrome children an extremely worthwhile
endeavor in view of the homogeneity of these subjects, both in
the anatomical abnormalities of their brains as well as their
psychological makeup.  I believe that the study of subjects with
disorders of "uncertain etiology" may possibly yield "uncertain
results."

Dr. Roy John's paper, "A Neurometric Approach to Learning
Disabilities," was presented by Dr. Bernard Karmel.  Considerable
credit, I learn, should also be given Dr. Leslie Prichep, whose
interest in developmental psychopathology  has been a moving
force in the effort of this team to validate and apply the technology of "neurometrics," a quantitative electrophysiological
analysis of cognitively impaired populations.  She is particularly
interested in learning disabled children.  Dr. Karmel provides
much of the expertise of the complex methods employed in the
brain and behavior measures of this complex endeavor.

This presentation is based on two assumptions.  The first
is that the EEG and the evoked potential contain diagnostically
valuable information as yet not extracted.  The second is that
by a variety of mathematical and analytical techniques, a numerical taxonomy of certain diagnostic features will reveal clusters
of subjects with similar electrophysiological profiles of cerebral
malfunction.  Each of these clusters can be culled from the heterogeneous populations who display behavioral or perceptual difficulties.  Such a maneuver will shed more light on such situations
as learning disability in children as well as certain mental
problems that afflict the aged.

The host of measures employed demand some reasonable method of data reduction. Factor loading, abnormality vectors, distance matrix, and finally cluster analysis are all proposed to extract subgroups within the large sample which may share a set of abnormal features that constitute a cluster or diagnostic entity.

In the role of a discussant, I must confess I don't have the mathematical expertise to critically evaluate some of the methods of this paper. I gather from the comments from the audience, there is some disagreement, if not critical, at least vociferous.

I believe I could safely summarize by stating that Roy John et al. have launched into an interesting, worthwhile but complex endeavor with their "neurometrics." There is evidence of considerable effort and productivity. But at this point in time they still have a bit of a "sticky wicket."

The final paper in our section is that of Malcolm Preston from Johns Hopkins. Dr. Preston and his colleagues have done some interesting experiments using the evoked potential as a procedure in studying reading disability.

This group was particularly intrigued by a study by Conners in 1970 which was unique in that he studied a family wherein five of six members were affected with reading disability. Other data were gathered, but the family data yielded probably the most interesting findings. The index case, a teen-age boy, produced a noticeably attenuated evoked potential from the P3 electrode. There were similar findings in three other siblings, but not in the normal-reading mother.

P3 to some extent overlies the left angular and supramarginal gyri which have been presumed for years to be involved in reading ability. These structures are unique to humans and according to some are larger in the left hemisphere. It is questionable whether they exist in other primates. Conner's data was also in accord with the notion that heredity plays a role in some forms of developmental dyslexia, the number of affected children suggested an autosomal dominant mode of inheritance. As the Connor's experiment has never been successfully replicated, Preston et al. set out to investigate these findings.

In the three experiments they describe they repeatedly implicate P3 as being affected whenever words are used as stimuli. However, as they are in the midst of gathering control data to be compared with subjects afflicted with reading disability, some critical suggestions are offered.

The first is the change in amplitude that occurs with age, particularly in late components. These may be seen in this volume, Dustman et al., "The evoked response as a measure of cerebral dysfunction."  Major amplitude changes occur between ages seven and fifteen, ages involved in Preston's study.

In support of that point of view that evoked potentials may reveal genetic differences in brain function, I would like to briefly describe one of our efforts.  We had reason to believe that certain forms of centrencephalic epilepsy could have a genetic etiology.

The study had two goals.  The first was to note the nature of the visual evoked potential of patients with centrencephalic epilepsy.  The second was to compare evoked responses of close relatives of epileptics with matched controls and epileptic patients.  Would such responses be more like those of normal subjects or epileptic patients?

Results indicated that epileptic patients had significantly larger visual evoked potential amplitude than did matched control subjects.  The differences were most obvious in recordings from central areas and with late components.  Close relatives of the probands also possessed many of these same large amplitude characteristics.  They too differed from controls, occupying an intermediate rank in evoked potential amplitude between the patients and matched controls.  From such results a genetic basis for this disease might be argued.

I would suggest two additional procedures to Dr. Preston's proposed study.  The first is to include all siblings in addition to the reading disabled youngsters.  I also would suggest an array of electrodes, 4 or 5, in the general area of P3 to increase the possibility of recording subtle differences that may derive or be reflected from the angular or supramarginal gyri.

# VISUAL EVOKED POTENTIALS AND BRAIN DYSFUNCTION IN CHRONIC ALCOHOLICS

Bernice Porjesz and Henri Begleiter

Dept. of Psychiatry, Downstate Medical Center
State University of New York,
Brooklyn, New York, U.S.A.*

Chronic alcohol abuse is known to lead to brain dysfunction (Begleiter and Platz, 1972; Rankin, 1975). In an effort to ascertain some parallel between acute and chronic alcohol intake, the effect of single doses of alcohol on normal brain functioning is being studied. Extensive research has been conducted in order to investigate the effects of acute doses of alcohol on the normal human evoked potential. This has been examined with the auditory evoked response (AER) (Gross et al., 1966), the somatosensory evoked potential (SEP) (Lewis et al., 1970; Salamy and Williams, 1973; Porjesz and Begleiter, 1973), and the visual evoked potential (VEP) (Lewis et al., 1969, 1970; Porjesz and Begleiter, 1975; Rhodes et al., 1975), $P_3$ amplitude (Roth et al., 1977), the contingent negative variation (CNV) (Kopell et al., 1972; Roth et al., 1977), and the amplitude-intensity gradient (Spilker and Callaway, 1969).

Taken together, the results of these single dose alcohol studies with normal subjects concur that:
1) alcohol depresses the amplitude of the EP late components (Lewis et al., 1969; Salamy and Williams, 1973; Porjesz and Begleiter, 1975; Rhodes et al., 1975);
2) alcohol produces its maximal amplitude depression over association areas, as opposed to primary receiving areas (Salamy and Williams, 1973; Porjesz and Begleiter, 1975);
3) there is an inverse relationship between the dose of alcohol, the blood alcohol level, and the evoked potential amplitude (Salamy and Williams, 1973);
4) this EP amplitude depression represents decreases in single

* Supported by Grant No. AA02686

EP amplitudes, rather than increased latency variability (Salamy, 1973);

     5) alcohol depresses right hemisphere responses of visual evoked potentials to a greater degree than left (Lewis et al., 1969; Porjesz and Begleiter, 1975; Rhodes et al., 1975);

     6) alcohol dissipates hemispheric asymmetry, where present prior to alcohol ingestion (Lewis et al., 1969; Porjesz and Begleiter, 1975; Rhodes et al., 1975).

     The sites of action of single, acute doses of alcohol are important in that they may provide a clue as to the possible locus or loci of brain dysfunction resulting from prolonged, chronic alcohol abuse. However, there is a paucity of evoked potential experiments in alcoholics who are abstinent from alcohol for long periods of time, and are medication-free.

     A study in Beck's laboratory (Schenkenberg, Dustman and Beck, 1972) reported that while normal subjects manifested VEP amplitude asymmetry at central locations (with $C_4 > C_3$), alcoholic subjects did not. Furthermore, they also reported lower VEP amplitudes in their alcoholic samples at all electrode locations, namely frontal, central and occipital. In a recent dissertation from the same laboratory (Cannon, 1974), it was reported that late component occipital amplitudes of alcoholics were smaller than those of normal controls. Alcoholics also manifested delayed late component latencies for central and occipital locations.

     In our laboratory, we have studied the electrophysiological concomitants of withdrawal following cessation of chronic alcohol intake in animals (in rat: Porjesz et al., 1976; Begleiter and Porjesz, 1977; and monkey: Begleiter et al., 1978) as well as in humans (Begleiter et al., 1974). In one study (Begleiter et al., 1974) we examined the recovery function of somatosensory evoked potentials in alcoholics during intoxication and withdrawal and found increased CNS excitability during withdrawal. In all our studies, alcohol withdrawal was found to be accompanied by marked increases in the late component amplitude. This we postulate to be the result of brain hyperexcitability. Similar results were recently obtained by Coger et al. (1976), who examined the effects of alcohol withdrawal on the amplitude-intensity gradient.

     Taken together, the results of studies dealing with evoked potentials and chronic alcohol abuse suggest that:

     1) late component EP amplitudes are reduced in alcoholics;
     2) alcoholics manifest less EP hemispheric asymmetry than normal controls;
     3) alcohol withdrawal is accompanied by marked increases in late EP amplitude.

Consequently, it seems that the same EP components that are most sensitive to single doses of alcohol in the normal brain, are most susceptible to more permanent deficits in the chronic alcoholic. Specifically, alcoholics seem to manifest electrophysiological deficits in the late components of the EP, and show less hemispheric asymmetry than normals (right hemisphere more affected than left).

Alcohol seems to affect some intellectual abilities more than others; specifically, visual-spatial and visual-motor skills are impaired, while verbal skills remain intact. Results of neuropsychological tests have led to two major hypotheses regarding the sites of action of alcohol in the brain, namely: 1) that right-hemispheric functioning is affected (Parsons, 1975; Butters and Cermak, 1976) and 2) that there is frontal impairment (Jones and Parsons, 1971; Parsons, 1974; Tarter, 1975).

Evidence implicating the right hemisphere comes from neuropsychological tests, where alcoholics' scores on spatial tasks are more impaired than on verbal tasks, and their performance on spatial tasks is similar to performance of patients with right hemisphere lesions. In addition, they exhibit more impairment on manual tasks requiring the use of their left hand (Parsons, 1975).

Chronic alcohol abuse has also been shown to produce an impaired ability to process relevant dimensions of visual stimuli (Oscar-Berman, 1973). In a study of the ability of Korsakoff patients, alcoholics, and normals to adopt and modify problem solving strategies, Oscar-Berman found that once a Korsakoff or alcoholic patient adopts a particular response strategy, he perseverates this hypothesis despite the reinforcement contingencies. These results suggest that perhaps a general information processing deficit may account for many of the Korsakoff and alcoholic patient's cognitive difficulties.

Evidence is accumulating that demonstrates a deficit in cognitive performance in chronic alcoholics, resembling aberrations observed in frontal lobe brain damaged patients. Independent studies by Fitzhugh et al. (1960, 1965) and Parsons and his co-workers (Jones and Parsons, 1971) have found that alcoholics perform more similarly to brain damaged subjects than normal controls on the Halstead Category Test. The performance deficit of the alcoholics has been found to be related to the number of years of drinking, independent of age (Jones and Parsons, 1971).

In a more recent study, Tarter (1973) reported that alcoholic patients admitting to a history of alcoholism of greater than ten years were impaired in set persistence, set shifting, and error utilization compared to normal controls, while those subjects who describe themselves as alcoholics for a period of less than ten years, were deficient only in set persistence. In order to

ascertain whether the brain dysfunctions reported were a function
of socioeconomic class, Smith et al. (1973) studied alcoholics of
upper socioeconomic status. He demonstrated the same incidence of
impaired ability on the Halstead Category Test in these alcoholics
as exhibited by alcoholics of low socioeconomic status.

Thus, it seems from the foregoing brief literature review that
alcoholics have two general characteristics that interfere with
their conceptual performance: 1) they make numerous perseverative
errors, and 2) they show an inability to persist with correct cognitive sets.

These difficulties are typical of patients with frontal lobe
damage (Luria, 1973). Another typical characteristic of frontal
lobe patients and animals is their difficulty with inhibitory control. A study by Parsons et al. (1972) demonstrated that alcoholics
were impaired in their capacity to inhibit their own behavior.

There is also a growing body of evidence suggesting that alcohol has direct neurotoxic effects. Postmortem studies by Courville
(1955) indicated neuropathology of chronic alcoholics in the dorso-
lateral aspects of the frontal lobe, with atrophy as its main
characteristic. Similar results have been reported from other
laboratories using pneumoencephalography (Tumarkin et al., 1955;
Feuerlein, 1970; Brewer and Perrett, 1971). Most recently, CAT-Scan
techniques have demonstrated cortical atrophy in alcoholics compared
to normal controls (Carlen et al., 1976; Fox et al., 1976; Wilkinson
et al., 1976; Bergman et al., 1977; Tenner, Begleiter and Porjesz,
unpublished observations).

Thus, the evidence seems to implicate possible impaired right
hemisphere and frontal lobe functioning in alcoholics. In the present experiment, we investigated possible frontal lobe dysfunction
in alcoholics by testing their ability to change "sets". Most
evoked potential experiments with alcoholics use responses to blank
flashes that do not require the subject to be actively engaged in
any task (Sutton, 1968). The present design requires the subject
to shift attentional sets. Stimuli that are relevant in one run,
become irrelevant in another run.

The present study was designed to assess:
1) VEP differences between alcoholics and normal controls in
terms of brain loci that manifest the greatest aberrations in alcoholics;
2) dysfunction with regard to shifting attentional "sets" in
alcoholics;
3) the degree and type of evoked potential aberration.

## METHODS

### Subjects

The subjects were 14 right-handed adult male alcoholics with
a mean age of 35 and a minimum of eight years of heavy drinking
history.  They had a mean duration of heavy drinking of 13.4 years.
They had been abstinent from alcohol for a minimum of three weeks,
and were medication-free for at least 2.5 weeks.

Fourteen age and education matched right-handed males served as
normal controls (mean age 32).  The control subjects were occasional
"social" drinkers.  All subjects were tested for eye-dominance and,
in addition, a complete medical history was obtained.  The experimental and control subjects did not differ significantly with respect
to eye-dominance, age or education.

The same alcoholic subjects who participated in the present VEP
experiment were also tested on a battery of neuropsychological tests,
as well as sleep EEG patterns (in collaboration with B. Kissin and
A. Wagman).  The results of those scores and their relationship to
the VEP data, goes beyond the scope of the present paper and will be
published elsewhere.

### Electrodes

Gold-cup electrodes were placed bilaterally at frontal ($F_3$ and
$F_4$), central ($C_3$ and $C_4$), parietal ($P_3$ and $P_4$), and occipital ($O_1$
and $O_2$) scalp locations according to the 10-20 International System.
All recordings were monopolar, using the ears as references and
nasion as ground.  Resistances were maintained below 5000 ohms between brain loci and references.  Interaural resistances were kept
below .5 ohms.

### Procedure

Each subject was seated in a sound-attenuated IAC enclosure,
with his head resting on an adjustable chin rest, so that he was
looking directly into a viewing hood.  He was instructed to fixate
in the center of his visual field at all times.  A Grass PS-2 photostimulator, set at an intensity of 2, was mounted 50 cm from the
subject on the other side of a one-way mirror.  All subjects were
dark-adapted and then habituated to blank flashes (10 msec in duration and delivered at a regular rate of 1/2.5 sec, for a total of
64 flashes).

The experiment consisted of three types of runs, manipulating
the subject's attentional set, namely "no set" (NS), "flash-task-
relevant" (FTR), and "flash-task-irrelevant" (FTI), respectively.

<u>Stimuli</u>

The stimulus sequence consisted of a series of interspersed visual and auditory stimuli presented in random order at a random rate varying between one and five seconds apart. Interspersed among 64 single flashes were 10 double flashes, with an interstimulus interval (ISI) of 80 msec. The auditory stimuli consisted of 64 lower frequency tones and 10 tones of a higher frequency.

Each subject was presented with the identical stimulus sequence in all three of his runs, and this order of stimulus presentation was randomized across subjects. In addition, the order of presentation of the three experimental conditions (NS, FTR and FTI) was counter-balanced for both the alcoholic and normal control subjects. There was a five-minute break between runs throughout the experiment.

## EXPERIMENTAL CONDITIONS

<u>No Set (NS)</u>

During the NS condition, the subject was instructed to sit very still, look into the center of the viewer, and attend to all the stimuli. The randomized sequence of high and low tones, and single and double flashes, was then presented to the subject.

<u>Flash-Task-Relevant (FTR)</u>

During the FTR condition, the subject's task was to count the number of double flashes to himself and report his answer at the end of the run. The double flashes were fairly difficult to detect and, in order to ensure that the subject was able to discriminate between the single and double flashes, a training procedure preceded the actual run. Once the subject achieved the criterion of 5 correct consecutive discriminations, the run began. The subject was instructed to look into the center of the viewer and to sit as still as possible. The identical stimulus sequence as during the "no set" condition was then presented to the subject.

<u>Flash-Task-Irrelevant (FTI)</u>

During the FTI run, the subject was instructed to silently count the number of infrequent high tones while looking at the flashes. The subject reported his answer at the end of the run. A training procedure also preceded this run and after 5 correct discriminations, the run commenced. Again, the identical stimulus sequence was delivered.

<u>Visual Evoked Potentials (VEP's)</u>

Evoked potentials were obtained only to the 64 single flashes in all runs. They were amplified by means of a Grass model 78-B

Polygraph with a band width between .1 and 100 hz, and a gain setting of 5 $\mu$/V mm. The VEP's for each of the 8 electrodes were
sampled by 8 A/D converters in a PDP 11/40 computer for on-line
signal averaging of a 500 msec epoch (resolution 2 points/msec).

In order to minimize any possible differences between amplifiers
and A/D converters, halfway through each run, the amplifier and A/D
converters for each pair of bilateral brain locations were inter-
changed (such that the right-hemisphere and left-hemisphere recordings were switched).

The vertical electrooculogram (EOG) was recorded and averaged
in all subjects so that possible contamination from ocular artifacts
was ruled out.

## Measurements

Peak-to-peak amplitude and latency measures were obtained from
all leads by means of a display program developed in our laboratory.
Amplitude measures were taken as the perpendicular distance (in $\mu$/V)
between successive peaks, while latency measures were taken as their
time of occurrence (in msec). This paper will be limited to a discussion of the frontal and parietal results only. Occipital and
central results will be reported elsewhere.

### RESULTS

A two-way analysis of variance with repeated measures on one
factor was performed (Winer, 1962). The major amplitude difference
between the alcoholic and normal control samples is that the late
component of the VEP (110-190 msec) is significantly larger in the
normal controls, particularly under the FTR condition. This is true
for all four electrode placements (Figure 1). This effect is greatest over the right frontal area ($p < .01$). It is significant at
$p < .05$ for all other electrode placements.

In addition, the control group manifests hemispheric asymmetry
with regard to this component over the frontal area, with the right
hemisphere late wave being of a significantly larger amplitude than
that simultaneously recorded over the left hemisphere (Figure 2).
Dependent t-tests performed on differences between hemispheres revealed that this is highly significant for all tasks in the control
group ($p < .01$, $p < .025$, and $p < .005$ for FTR, FTI, and NS, respectively). The alcoholics, on the other hand, exhibit no hemispheric
asymmetry at all (not significant for any task).

Furthermore, the amplitude of this late component of the frontal
VEP bears a direct relationship to the degree of task-relevance only
in the normal controls (largest for FTR, next for FTI, and smallest

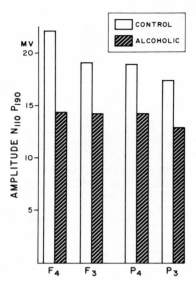

Figure 1.   Amplitude $N_{110}$-$P_{190}$ for all electrodes during the FTR
            task.   Amplitude values are based on group means
            (n=14/group) of peak-to-peak measurements.   Notice that
            the control group manifests a larger late component
            amplitude than the alcohol group.

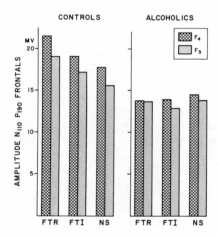

Figure 2.   Group mean amplitude $N_{110}$-$P_{190}$ for left and right frontal
            leads for all tasks separately.   Hemispheric asymmetry
            of amplitude ($F_4$>$F_3$) is displayed only by the control
            group, while the alcoholic group does not manifest any
            hemispheric asymmetry.

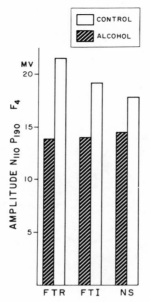

Figure 3.    Amplitude $N_{110}-P_{190}$ for the right frontal placement under
             the three experimental conditions:   FTR, FTI and NS.
             This amplitude is larger in the control group, and is
             directly related to the degree of task relevance
             (FTR>FTI>NS).   The amplitude remains the same across
             tasks in the alcoholic group.

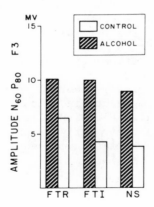

Figure 4.    Mean amplitude early component ($N_{60}-P_{80}$) recorded over
             left frontal scalp locations under the three experimental
             conditions (N=14/grp).   This early component amplitude is
             larger for the alcoholics than the normal controls for
             all tasks, particularly under the FTI condition.

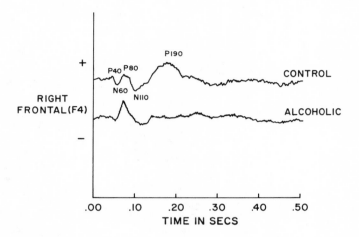

Figure 5. This illustration contains examples of VEP's recorded at
the right frontal electrode under an attention condition
(FTR), for one control subject (top trace) and one alcoholic subject (bottom trace). Notice the reduced late
component amplitude ($N_{110}$-$P_{190}$) in the alcoholic subject
as compared to the control, and the markedly enhanced
early components $N_{60}$-$P_{80}$ and $P_{80}$-$N_{110}$. As can be seen
in this illustration, the waveform is quite different in
the alcoholic and normal control subjects at frontal
locations. Typically, normal controls exhibit much
larger late components in comparison to their early
components, while the alcoholics manifest the reverse
waveform--with their early components being considerably
larger than their late components.

for no-set) (Figure 3). No relationship exists between degree of task relevance and late component amplitude in the alcoholics; in fact, this amplitude remains almost identical across tasks for them. This is true for both the right frontal electrode placement as well as the left. The slope of the amplitude measures taken across tasks indicates that the late component parallels the degree of task relevance only for normal control subjects. This relationship is significant not only for amplitude $N_{110}-P_{190}$ (Tukey test, p <.05) but also amplitude $P_{80}-N_{110}$ at frontal leads (Tukey test, p <.05, $F_4$; p <.01, $F_3$), only for the normal controls.

The early components, on the other hand, are of a larger amplitude in the alcoholics than the normal controls. This can be seen in amplitude $N_{60}-P_{80}$ over the frontal area, particularly for the FTI task (p <.01) (Figure 4). For the normal control group, it can be seen that there is a larger difference in amplitude between the FTR and FTI conditions, but not for the alcoholics.

The waveform of the frontal recordings are quite different for the alcoholic and control subjects (Figure 5). The alcoholic subjects manifest reduced late component amplitudes ($N_{110}-P_{190}$) and enhanced early component amplitudes ($N_{60}-P_{80}$ and $P_{80}-N_{110}$) when compared to the controls. The morphology of the frontal VEP for control subjects typically consists of a late component that is much larger than the early component. The alcoholics, on the other hand, typically exhibit the reverse waveform, where the early components are considerably larger than their late components.

The results obtained are illustrated in Figure 6, which is a schematic composite waveform, based on mean amplitude and response times of $F_4$, during the FTR task for both groups. Note the reduced late component amplitude in the alcoholic group ($N_{110}-P_{190}$) and the enhanced early components ($N_{60}-P_{80}$ and $P_{80}-N_{110}$).

The early component $P_{80}-N_{115}$ is also enhanced in the alcoholic group at parietal locations for all tasks. This is true for both the right and left parietal recordings, where it is significant at p <.05 for all tasks (Figure 7).

This component recorded at parietal leads shows hemispheric asymmetry of amplitude, where the right hemisphere has a larger amplitude than the left (Figure 8). This hemispheric asymmetry is highly significant for the control group at p <.005 for FTR, p <.05 for FTI, and p <.01 for NS. Hemispheric asymmetry is also present in the alcoholic group (at parietal) significant at p <.05 for all tasks. However, while this asymmetry is present in both groups, it is of a larger magnitude in the control group under the FTR and NS conditions.

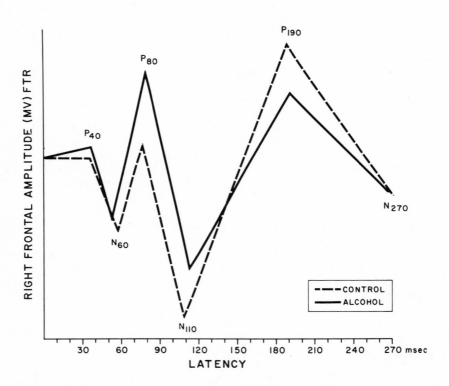

Figure 6.  This is a schematic composite right frontal waveform,
          based on the mean amplitudes and response times of all
          subjects combined for each group (N=14/grp).  The curves
          were obtained during the flash-task-relevant (FTR) task,
          where the subject is attending to the flash.  Note the
          decreased late component amplitude ($N_{110}$-$P_{190}$) in the
          alcoholic group, and the increased early component
          ($N_{60}$-$P_{80}$ and $P_{80}$-$N_{110}$).

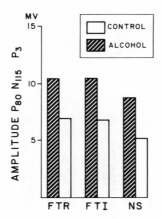

Figure 7. Mean amplitude early component ($P_{80}$-$N_{115}$) recorded at left parietal placements (N=14/grp). Note that this component is larger for all tasks in the alcoholic group.

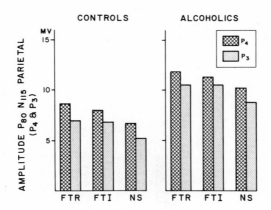

Figure 8. Bilateral recordings of $P_{80}$-$N_{115}$ over right and left parietal areas comparing each homologous pair for each group separately, under the three experimental conditions. Note the amplitude hemispheric asymmetry $P_4$>$P_3$) in the control group, and to a lesser degree in the alcoholic group for this amplitude.

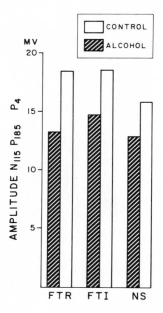

Figure 9.    Group means for right parietal amplitude $N_{115}$-$P_{185}$ for
             the alcoholic and control groups for the three experi-
             mental tasks.    Note the strikingly larger amplitude of
             this late component in the control group.

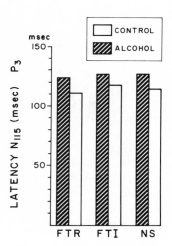

Figure 10.   Mean latencies ($N_{115}$) for each group for each of the
             three tasks.    Note that the alcoholics' latency occurs
             later than those of the normal subjects.

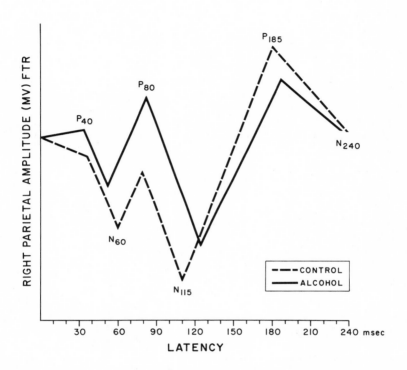

Figure 11.  This is a schematic illustration of the right parietal
            waveforms based on the mean amplitudes and latencies
            for the two groups, under the FTR task.  The late
            component ($N_{115}$-$P_{185}$) is reduced in the alcoholic
            group, while the early component amplitude ($P_{80}$-$N_{115}$)
            is enhanced.  Also note the latency shifts in the late
            components for the alcoholics ($N_{115}$ and $P_{185}$),
            occurring later in the alcoholic group.

As with the frontal leads, the late component of the parietal areas is also significantly larger for the control group than the alcoholic group, particularly under the FTR condition. This is true for both the left and right parietal recordings at $p < .05$, and is illustrated for the right parietal in Figure 9.

The time of occurrence of this late component, typically beginning around 115 msec occurs significantly later in the alcoholic group than in the controls. This significantly longer latency in the alcoholic group is most apparent during the FTR condition. This is true for both hemispheres (Figure 10).

Figure 11 is a schematic illustration of the right parietal results during the FTR task, based on the mean response amplitudes and latencies for the two groups. The late component ($N_{115}$-$P_{185}$) is reduced in the alcoholic group while the early component ($P_{80}$-$N_{115}$) amplitude is enhanced. Also note the latency shifts in the late components for the alcoholics ($N_{115}$ and $P_{185}$) occurring later in the alcoholic group.

## DISCUSSION

After many extensive attention experiments performed by Hillyard and his co-workers (Hillyard, 1977), Hillyard concludes that $N_1$ (approximately $N_{110}$ in the present paper) is indicative of the selection of target or non-target stimuli while later peaks ($P_3$) reflect memory-related cognitive or motor response selection.

In the present experiment, we found that the alcoholic subjects exhibited reduced late component amplitudes at all electrode sites. Furthermore, in the alcoholic sample, we found no difference in amplitude of the late component across different attentional tasks. Applying Hillyard's conclusions to the present experimental results, it can be hypothesized that the alcoholics are more impaired in the later stages of attentional processes. Information processing reaction-time experiments support this contention. Recent studies (Rundell et al., 1973; Tharp et al., 1974, 1975) have found that stimulus pre-processing and encoding are unaffected by alcohol, while alcohol affects the more central (output) stages of information processing, namely response selection and organization.

Similarly, support for this hypothesis comes from EP studies in many laboratories where acute doses of alcohol are administered to non-alcoholics (Lewis et al., 1970; Salamy and Williams, 1973; Porjesz and Begleiter, 1975; Rhodes et al., 1975). These studies report that alcohol primarily depresses the late components of the EP, while the early components are very resistant to its depressant effects. In addition, the maximal amplitude depression has been obtained over association areas of the brain.

The early components of the EP are generally taken to reflect sensory input. Hillyard maintains that in attentional processes they represent the selection of the target or non-target stimulus modalities or "sensory filtering." The human perceptual system is capable of rejecting or filtering irrelevant input at an early stage of processing.

In the present experiment, the high amplitude early component ($N_{60}-P_{80}$, $P_{80}-N_{110}$) manifested by the alcoholics in comparison to the controls, may be indicative of inappropriate filtering of sensory input (for example, for the $N_{60}-P_{80}$ component at frontal leads, the FTR and FTI responses had the same amplitude in the alcoholic). Perhaps this indicates a lack of selective-inattending to the irrelevant stimuli in alcoholics.

Nataanen (1975) postulates that an early amplitude enhancement of his $N_1$ peak (occurring at approximately 60-70 msec) indicates increased excitability or impulse activity related to preparation for a difficult discrimination (in his case pitch discrimination). According to Nataanen, the subjects must ask a series of questions in order to determine the relevance of a given stimulus, namely,
  1)  Is the stimulus task-relevant or not?
  2)  If task-relevant, is it a signal or not?

Using Natannen's approach to the present experiment, all stimuli are relevant in the attention and distraction runs in that they are necessary to make the decision. On the other hand, all our VEP's were obtained only to an irrelevant stimulus, namely, the single flash. However, its degree of relevance varied across the tasks. For the FTR task, the single flash was in the relevant stimulus modality; however, it was the non-signal (the signal being the double flash). In the FTI condition, not only was the flash the irrelevant signal, but it was also in the irrelevant stimulus modality.

Thus, the undifferentiated enhanced early component in the alcoholics is in response to irrelevant stimuli, and hence represents an inability to inhibit irrelevant input. This hypothesis is strengthened by the additional result that alcoholics differ most from normal controls for this component with regard to the flash-task-irrelevant condition. The control subjects' responses for the FTI condition are appropriately attenuated, as predicted by Hillyard's model.

The greatest late component difference between alcoholics and normal controls was found over the rightfrontal electrode placement. In addition, we found that while normal controls display hemispheric asymmetry with regard to this late component over the frontal area, alcoholics do not, and also manifested some loss of lateralization over parietal leads. This finding is in agreement with studies from Beck's laboratory (Schenkenberg et al., 1972; Dustman et al., this volume), indicating that hemispheric asymmetry typically manifested by normal subjects is not present in alcoholics. Similarly, studies with acute doses of alcohol administered to college students, in both his laboratory and ours, indicate that single doses of alcohol abolish hemispheric asymmetry when present and maximally depress responses from right central areas (Lewis et al., 1970; Porjesz and Begleiter, 1975; Rhodes et al., 1975). Taken together, these findings implicate possible impairment of right hemispheric functioning in chronic alcoholics.

Thus, it seems that the results of the present study with chronic alcohol ingestion, parallel results obtained with acute intake--suggesting that brain functioning that is impaired by acute alcohol doses is also more permanently impaired in the chronic alcoholic.

The results of the present experiment, that alcoholics exhibit an increased early component and decreased late component and delayed latencies, parallel the results obtained with samples of elderly people in Beck's laboratory (Cannon, 1974; Dustman et al., this volume).

It has been hypothesized that alcohol accelerates the aging process of the brain. Evoked potential studies of the aging process have demonstrated that the early components remain fairly stable until senescence, at which time amplitude increases occur. With aging, the amplitudes of the late components of the visual evoked response increase until adolescence, and progressively decrease thereafter. Furthermore, evoked potential latencies (VEP, SEP) decrease until adolescence and increase through old age. The VEP characteristics of the alcoholic patients in the present experiment resemble those obtained with elderly patients; namely, they have larger early components, smaller late components, and delayed late component latencies.

Similarities between alcoholics and elderly normal individuals have been independently found in neuropsychological (Fitzhugh et al., 1960; 1965) and neuroanatomical studies (Courville, 1955). Autopsy examinations between these two groups have revealed similarities in cortical atrophy and diffuse cell loss (Courville, 1955). It is interesting to note that at autopsy, chronic alcoholics exhibit progressive atrophy of the frontal lobes, particularly the dorso-lateral convolutions. With senescence, cell loss has been found mainly in the superior temporal gyrus and the frontal cortex, with the smallest loss at the post-central gyrus (Brody, 1970).

A recent experiment by Loveless and Sanford (1974) examined changes in preparatory set in elderly patients and contingent negative variation (CNV). They found that elderly subjects exhibited poor performance at long predictable foreperiods, accompanied by a

substantial difference in the form of the CNV.  This is less suggestive of the impaired ability to maintain a state of preparation than
of difficulty in controlling a sequence of psychological processes
so as to initiate preparation at an appropriate time.  Luria (1966)
suggests that a breakdown in the ability to follow through a series
of previously specific actions is a good indication of diffuse
frontal lobe damage.

The hypothesis that chronic alcoholism promotes the aging process of the brain has been proposed by a number of sleep researchers.
Extreme sleep disturbances in chronic alcoholics were first recognized by Gross and his co-workers (1966).  More recently, Johnson
et al. (1970) examined sleep (EEG patterns) in a group of alcoholic
patients withdrawn from alcohol for several days, who had been ex-
cessively drinking for 17 years.  They found that alcoholics had
fragmented sleep manifested by frequent awakenings, frequent changes
of EEG stage and, most importantly, found no slow wave sleep.  The
records revealed that the frequency of sigma spindles was low and
the frequency of well-formed K-complexes was considerably below
that found in normal subjects.  Generally, the sleep patterns of
alcoholic patients in Johnson's study resembled those of elderly
subjects.  Confirmation of these results has been reported by Lester
et al. (1973), who also found that alcoholics did not manifest any
stage 4 sleep.  They concluded that chronic alcoholism may impair
the cortical mechanisms necessary for spontaneous generation of high
voltage, slow-wave activity, and in that sense be associated with
premature aging of the brain.

At present, there is some reason to suppose that the generators
for such EEG phenomena are located in the frontal cortex.  In 1961,
Jouvet found that in the decorticate cat, only REM sleep occurred,
and the absence of SWS was quite striking.  Clemente and Sterman
(1967) reported that low frequency stimulation in certain basal and
cortical forebrain regions produced immediate sustained and diffuse
cortical synchronization.  Bilateral low frequency stimulation of
forebrain sites resulted in drowsiness and sleep within an average
of 30 seconds.  They conclude that the more frontal regions, together
with certain limbic and thalamic sites may constitute a critical
system capable of responding to conditions favoring behavioral inhibition and acting to bring the nervous system in line with the
physiological requirements at any instant.

The degree of reversibility (or lack of it) of electrophysiological changes produced by alcoholism is still an unresolved issue.
It is not clear whether the EEG aberrations reported in alcoholics
are withdrawal concomitants (which would be expected to dissipate
once the withdrawal symptomatology disappears) or whether they represent more long-lasting brain damage.  EEG abnormalities have been
reported to show their greatest improvements following the disappear-
ance of delirium and withdrawal symptomatology (Raffauf, 1974;

Mildovanska and Kukladziev, 1975); however, Bennett et al. (1956) have reported some improvements in abnormal EEG records as late as two months post-withdrawal. In our own laboratory (Porjesz, Begleiter, and Hurowitz, 1976; Begleiter and Porjesz, 1977) we have found that visual evoked responses of rats who had been chronically intubated with alcohol were no different from those obtained from naive rats following an abstinence period of two weeks. However, the two groups of rats responded very differently to a challenge dose of alcohol administered at that time.

Similarly, there are conflicting reports on the question of whether neuropsychological impairment in chronic alcoholics is permanent or reversible. Goodwin (Goodwin and Hill, 1975) claims that there is little or no evidence for permanent brain damage in alcoholics, unless coupled with nutritional deficits. Indeed, improvements have been reported in short-term memory (Jonsson et al., 1962; Weingartner et al., 1971), abstract thinking (Smith et al., 1971; Page and Linden, 1974), verbal understanding (Smith et al., 1971; Page and Linden, 1974), and perceptual-motor and psychomotor coordination (Long and McLachlan, 1974; Tarter and Jones, 1971; Templer, 1975).

However, major improvements in neuropsychological test scores have been reported to occur during the first 2-3 weeks of testing, with no further recovery over an 8-month abstinence period thereafter (Page and Linden, 1974; Page and Schaub, 1977). Despite these improvements in neuropsychological tests, abstract reasoning scores and visual-spatial skills remain below average (Jonsson et al., 1962; Smith et al., 1971; Page and Linden, 1974; Page and Schaub, 1977).

Thus, the issue of whether CNS aberrations observed in alcoholics are reversible or not, is still an unresolved issue and remains to be tested.

## ACKNOWLEDGMENTS

We would like to thank Robert Garozzo for his dedicated support and technical assistance and Dr. Wen-Huey Su for her invaluable statistical advice. We would also like to thank Laurence Pandolfo for his most helpful recruiting and screening of patients.

REFERENCES

Begleiter, H., DeNoble, V., and Porjesz, B.  Protracted brain
    hyperexcitability following ethanol withdrawal in monkeys
    (macacca Nemistrina).  In Alcohol Intoxication and Withdrawal,
    H. Begleiter (ed.), Vol. 4, Plenum Press, New York, 1978
    (in press).

Begleiter, H. and Platz, A.  The effects of alcohol on the central
    nervous system in humans.  In The Biology of Alcoholism,
    B. Kissin and H. Begleiter (eds.), Vol. 2, Plenum Press,
    New York, 1972, pp. 293-343.

Begleiter, H. and Porjesz, B.  Persistence of brain hyperexcitability
    following chronic alcohol exposure in rats.  Adv. Exp. Med. Biol.,
    1977, 85b: 209-222.

Begleiter, H., Porjesz, B., and Yerre-Grubstein, C.  Excitability
    cycle of somatosensory evoked potentials during experimental
    alcoholization and withdrawal.  Psychopharmacologia, 1974,
    37: 15-21.

Bennett, A. E., Doi, L. T., and Mowery, G. L.  The value of electro-
    encephalography in alcoholism.  J. Nerv. Ment. Dis., 1956,
    124(1): 27-32.

Bergman, H., Borg, S., Hindmars, T., Idestrom, C. M., and Myrhed, M.
    Computed-tomography of the brain and psychometric assessment
    of alcoholic patients: Some preliminary results.  Presented at
    World Congress of Psychiatry, Hawaii, 1977.

Brewer, C. and Perrett, L.  Brain damage due to alcohol consumption:
    An air-electroencephalographic, psychometric and electro-
    encephalographic study.  Brit. J. Addict., 1971, 66: 170-182.

Brody, H.  Structural changes in the aging nervous system.  Interdisc.
    Top. Geron., 1970, 7: 9-21.

Butters, N. and Cermak, L. S.  Neuropsychological studies of alco-
    holic Korsakoff patients.  In Empirical Studies of Alcoholism,
    Goldstein and Neuringer (eds.), Ballinger, Cambridge, 1976,
    pp. 153-193.

Cannon, W. G.  Cortical evoked responses of young normal, young
    alcoholic, and elderly normal individuals.  Unpublished doctoral
    dissertation, University of Utah, 1974.

Carlen, P. L., Wilkinson, A., and Kiraly, L.  Dementia in alcoholics:
    A longitudinal study including some reversible aspects.
    Neurology, 1976, 26: 355.

Clemente, C. D. and Sterman, M. B.  Limbic and other forebrain
    mechanisms in sleep induction and behavioral inhibition.  In
    Progress in Brain Research, R. Adey and T. Tokizone (eds.),
    Vol. 27, Elsevier, Amsterdam, 1967, pp. 34-47.

Coger, R. W., Dymond, A. M., Serafetinides, E. A., Lowenstein, I.,
    and Pearson, D.  Alcoholism:  Averaged visual evoked response
    amplitude - intensity slope and symmetry in withdrawal.  Biolog.
    Psychiat., 1976, 11(4): 435-443.

Courville, C. B.  Effects of Alcohol on the Nervous System of Man.
    Los Angeles, San Lucas Press, 1955.

Dustman, R. E., Snyder, E. W., Callner, D. A., and Beck, E. C.  The
    evoked response as a measure of cerebral dysfunction.  In
    Evoked Brain Potentials and Behavior, H. Begleiter (ed.), 1978,
    (this volume).

Feuerlein, W. and Heyse, H.  Die Weite der 3-Hirn Kammer bei Alko-
    holkern.  Ergebnisse echoenzephalographischer Messungen.
    Arch. Psychiat. Nervenkv., 1970, 213: 78-85.

Fitzhugh, L. C., Fitzhugh, K. B., and Reitan, R. M.  Adaptive abili-
    ties and intellectual functioning of hospitalized alcoholics.
    Quart. J. Stud. Alc., 1960, 21: 414-443.

Fitzhugh, L. C., Fitzhugh, K. B., and Reitan, R. M.  Adaptive abili-
    ties and intellectual functioning of hospitalized alcoholics:
    Further considerations.  Quart. J. Stud. Alc., 1965, 26: 402-411.

Fox, J., Ramsey, R., Huckman, M., and Proske, A.  Cerebral ventricular
    enlargement: Chronic alcoholics examined by computerized tomog-
    raphy.  J. Amer. Med. Assoc., 1976, 236: 365-368.

Goodwin, D. W. and Hill, S. Y.  Chronic effects of alcohol and other
    psychoactive drugs on intellect, learning and memory.  In Alcohol,
    Drugs and Brain Damage, G. Rankin (ed.), A.R.F., Ontario, 1975,
    pp. 55-70.

Gross, M. M., Begleiter, H., Tobin, M., and Kissin, B.  Changes in
    auditory evoked response induced by alcohol.  J. Nerv. Ment.
    Dis., 1966, 143: 152-156.

Hillyard, S. A.  Electrophysiological assessment of attentional
    processes in man.  Presented at NIMH Conference on Event Related
    Potentials.  Airlie, Virginia, April, 1977.

Johnson, L. C., Burdick, J. A., and Smith, J.  Sleep during alcohol
    intake and withdrawal in the chronic alcoholic.  Arch. Gen.
    Psychiat., 1970, 22: 406-418.

Jones, B. M. and Parsons, O. A.  Impaired abstracting ability in
    chronic alcoholics.  Arch. Gen. Psychiat., 1971, 24: 71-75.

Jonsson, C. O., Cronholm, B., and Izikowitz, S.  Intellectual changes
    in alcoholics.  Psychometric studies on mental sequels of pro-
    longed intensive abuse of alcohol.  Quart. J. Stud. Alc., 1962,
    23: 221-242.

Jouvet, M.  Telencephalic and rhombencephalic sleep in the cat.
    In The Nature of Sleep.  G. E. Wolstenholme and M. O'Connor
    (eds.)  Little Brown and Co., Boston, 1961.

Kopell, B. S., Tinklenberg, J. R., and Hollister, L. E.  Contingent
    negative variation amplitudes:  Marijuana and alcohol.
    Arch. Gen. Psychiat., 1972, 27: 809-811.

Lester, B. K., Rundell, O. H., Cowden, L. C., and Williams, H. L.
    Alcoholism, alcohol and sleep.  Adv. Exp. Med. Biol., 1973,
    35: 261-280.

Lewis, E. G., Dustman, R. E., and Beck, E. C.  The effect of alcohol
    on sensory phenomena and cognitive motor tasks.  Quart. J. Stud.
    Alc., 1969, 30: 618-633.

Lewis, E. G., Dustman, R. C., and Beck, E. C.  The effects of alcohol
    on visual and somatosensory evoked responses.  Electroenceph.
    clin. Neurophysiol., 1970, 28: 202-205.

Long, A. and McLachlan, J.  Abstract reasoning and perceptual-motor
    efficiency in alcoholics.  Quart. J. Stud. Alc., 1974, 35(4):
    1120-1129.

Loveless, N. E. and Sanford, A. J.  Effects of age on the contingent
    negative variation and preparatory set in a reaction-time task.
    J. Gerontol., 1974, 29: 52-63.

Luria, A. R.  Higher Cortical Functions in Man.  Translated by Basil
    Haigh, Basic Books, Inc., New York, 1966.

Luria, A. R.  The Working Brain.  Penguin, Great Britain, 1973.

Mildovanska, P. and Kukladziev, B.  EEG study of patients with alco-
    holic delirium.  Electroenceph. clin. Neurophysiol., 1975,
    39: 672.

Nataanen, R.  Selective attention and evoked potentials in humans –
    a critical review.  Biolog. Psychol., 1975, 2: 237–307.

Oscar-Berman, M.  Hypothesis testing and focusing behavior during
    concept formation by amnesic Korsakoff patients.
    Neuropsychologia, 1973, 11: 191–198.

Page, R. D. and Linden, J. D.  "Reversible," organic brain syndrome
    in alcoholics: A psychometric evaluation.  Quart. J. Stud. Alc.,
    1974, 35: 98–107.

Page, R. D. and Schaub, L. H.  Intellectual functioning in alcoholics
    during six months abstinence.  J. Stud. Alc., 1977, 38: 1240–1246.

Parsons, O. A.  Brain damage in alcoholics: Altered states of uncon-
    sciousness.  Alc. Tech. Rep., 1974, 2: 93–105.

Parsons, O. A.  Brain damage in alcoholics: Altered states of con-
    sciousness.  Adv. Exp. Med. Biol., 1975, 59: 569–584.

Parsons, O. A., Tarter, R. E., and Edelberg, R.  Altered motor con-
    trol in chronic alcoholics.  J. Abn. Psychol., 1972, 80: 308–
    314.

Porjesz, B. and Begleiter, H.  The effects of alcohol on the somato-
    sensory evoked potential in man.  Adv. Exp. Med. Biol., 1973,
    35: 345–350.

Porjesz, B. and Begleiter, H.  Alcohol and bilateral evoked brain
    potentials.  Adv. Exp. Med. Biol., 1975, 59: 553–567.

Porjesz, B., Begleiter, H., and Hurowitz, S.  Brain excitability
    subsequent to alcohol withdrawal in rats.  In Tissue Responses
    to Addictive Substances, D. H. Ford and D. H. Clouet (eds.),
    Spectrum, New York, 1976, pp. 461–469.

Raffauf, H. J.  Convulsive attacks and EEG in connection with alco-
    holism.  Electroenceph. clin. Neurophysiol., 1974, 36: 90.

Rankin, J. G.  Alcohol, drugs and brain damage.  Proceedings of a
    symposium:  Effects of chronic use of alcohol and other psycho-
    active drugs on cerebral functioning.  Addict. Research Founda-
    tion of Ontario, Toronto, 1975.

Rhodes, L. E., Obitz, F. W., and Creel, D.  Effect of alcohol and
    task on hemispheric asymmetry of visually evoked potentials in
    man.  Electroenceph. clin. Neurophysiol., 1975, 38: 561–568.

Roth, W. T., Tinklenberg, J. R., and Kopell, B. S. Ethanol and marihuana effects on event-related potentials in a memory retrieval paradigm. Electroenceph. clin. Neurophysiol., 1977, 42: 381-388.

Rundell, O. H., Tharp, V., Lester, B. K., and Williams, H. L. Some effects of acute intoxication on information processing stages. Alc. Tech. Rep., 1973, 1: 25-32.

Salamy, A. The effects of alcohol on the variability of the human evoked potential. Neuropharmacology, 1973, 12: 1103-1107.

Salamy, A. and Williams, H. L. The effects of alcohol on sensory evoked and spontaneous cerebral potentials in man. Electroenceph. clin. Neurophysiol., 1973, 35: 3-11.

Schenkenberg, T., Dustman, R. E., and Beck, E. C. Cortical evoked responses of hospitalized geriatrics in three diagnostic categories. Proceedings of the 80th Annual Convention, American Psychological Association, 1972, pp. 671-672.

Smith, J. W., Burt, D. W., and Chapman, R. F. Intelligence and brain damage in alcoholics: A study in patients in middle and upper social class. Quart. J. Stud. Alc., 1973, 34: 414-422.

Smith, J. W., Johnson, L. C., and Burdick, J. A. Sleep, psychological and clinical changes during alcohol withdrawal in NAD-treated alcoholics. Quart. J. Stud. Alc., 1971, 32: 982-994.

Spilker, B. and Callaway, E. Effects of drugs on "augmenting/reducing" in averaged visual evoked response in man. Psychopharmacologia, 1969, 15: 116-124.

Sutton, S. The specification of psychological variables in an average evoked potential experiment. In Average Evoked Potentials: Methods, Results, and Evaluation. NASA SP-191, Washington, D.C., 1968, pp. 237-297.

Tarter, R. An analysis of cognitive deficits in chronic alcoholics. J. Nerv. Ment. Dis., 1973, 157: 138-147.

Tarter, R. E. Psychological deficit in chronic alcoholics: A review. Intn'l. J. Addict., 1975, 10(2): 327-368.

Tarter, R. and Jones, B. Motor impairment in chronic alcoholics. Dis. Nerv. Sys., 1971, 32: 632-636.

Templer, D. I. Trail Making Test performance of alcoholics abstinent at least a year. Intn'l. J. Addict., 1975, 10(4): 609-612.

Tenner, M., Begleiter, H., and Porjesz, B.   CAT-scan and evoked
    potentials in chronic alcoholics.  (Unpublished observations,
    1978.)

Tharp, V. K., Rundell, O. H., Williams, H. L., and Lester, B. K.
    Alcohol and information processing.  Psychopharmacologia, 1974,
    40: 33-52.

Tharp, V. K., Rundell, O. H., Jr., Lester, B. K., and Williams, H. L.
    Alcohol and secobarbital: Effects on information processing.
    Adv. Exp. Med. Biol., 1975, 59: 537-552.

Tumarkin, B., Wilson, J. D., and Snyder, G.  Cerebral atrophy due
    to alcoholism in young adults.  U.S. Arm. Forc. Med. J., 1955,
    6: 67-74.

Weingartner, H., Faillace, L. A., and Markley, H. G.  Verbal informa-
    tion retention in alcoholics.  Quart. J. Stud. Alc., 1971,
    32: 293-303.

Wilkinson, A., Rankin, J. G., and Kiraly, L.  Organic brain syndrome
    in chronic alcoholism: A reversible encephalophathy?  Presented
    at:  11th Annual Conference, Canadian Foundation on Alcohol and
    Drug Dependencies, Toronto, Canada, June, 1976.

Winer, B. J.  Statistical Principles in Experimental Design.  McGraw-
    Hill, New York, 1962.

# RELATIONSHIPS BETWEEN BEHAVIORAL AND ELECTROCORTICAL RESPONSES OF

# APHASIC AND NON-APHASIC BRAIN-DAMAGED ADULTS TO SEMANTIC MATERIALS

Sue A. Pace, Dennis L. Molfese, A. L. Schmidt,
W. Mikula, C. Ciano

Southern Illinois University at Carbondale
Carbondale, Illinois

## INTRODUCTION

Disorders of semantic processing are well recognized components of the syndrome of aphasia. Specific disabilities described in the literature include the following:

1. failure of naming on confrontation (Geschwind, 1967)
2. paraphasia (Beyn and Vlasenko, 1974; Goodglass, 1976)
3. paralexia (Marshall and Newcombe, 1966)
4. reduced verbal productivity (Milner, 1964) and/or reduction in vocabulary (Pizzamiglio and Appicciafuocco, 1971)
5. dependency upon neologisms and circumlocutions (DeRenzi et al, 1966)
6. inability to match a stimulus to its spoken name (Geschwind, 1967). This symptom is also referred to by Luria (1966) as extinction of word meaning characterized by disintegration of audio-visual synthesis and a disconnection between visual images and their spoken word names.
7. reduced fluency or notable delay in evoking contentive words, particularly nouns, verbs and adjectives (Schuell and Jenkins, 1961)
8. disturbance of ability to generate divergent semantic operations as described by Guilford and Hoepfner (1971). This is, aphasics display an inability to generate a number and a variety of logical semantic alternatives to given information. (Chapey et al, 1976.)

Researchers studying these semantic disabilities have concluded that confusion of words which are associated by category are common

(Rinnert and Whitaker, 1973; Weinstein and Keller, 1963). Gardner
(1974) demonstated convincingly that the naming errors of aphasics
are intercategorical, and as well retain the same paradigmatic
relationship of the preferred word. Apparently even the most global
aphasics retain some categorical associations.

Errors can most often be explained in terms of categorical
association based on: (a) similarities in function; e.g. "cigarette" for ash tray, "telescope" for compass, (b) similarities in
sound; e.g. "love" for glove, "fashing pen" for fountain pen, and
(c) spatial and temporal contiguity; e.g. interchange of part for
a whole, "seat" for chair and, for example, the aphasic substitutes
the name of an object located in the proximity of a desired one.

Goodglass et al (1966) also identified frequent substitution
of a secondary lexical entry rather than the most commonly elicited
word, e.g. "plant" for the target word bush. He found that the
category of words most frequently subject to misnaming is objects.
Aphasic patients who misname objects frequently use the same words
that normals use when asked to respond to a word with the first
word they think of, i.e., high word association (Schuell and
Jenkins, 1961).

Apparently ease of word-finding is related not only to category
but also to input-output modalities. Errors appear regardless of
whether patients are asked to name objects, match words to pictures,
match spoken to printed words or write words to dictation. However, the difficulty experienced does not remain the same for both
comprehension and production. While objects are usually the most
difficult category for aphasics to name, it is an easy category
for aphasics to comprehend (Goodglass et al, 1966).

These findings suggest that semantic storage and retrieval are
maintained by complex neural mechanisms which code the distinctive
features of words, as well as the learned associations between
specific words and other semantic entries in the storage system.
Certain aspects of the code may be retained and other aspects lost
following cerebral damage. The neural mechanisms associated with
this clinical phenomenon are worthy of exploration.

This study was designed to investigate the behavioral and
electrocortical responses of a group of brain damaged subjects
some of whom demonstrated disorders of semantic processing. The
researchers proposed to investigate the relationships between the
semantic abilities of the subjects and the electrocortical responses to semantic stimuli as measured by Auditory Evoked Potentials.

METHODOLOGY

Subjects

Two groups of subjects participated in this study.  The groups
selected for study were:  three left hemisphere brain-damaged adults
and three right hemisphere brain-damaged adults.  The two groups
of subjects were selected from the population of patients under-
going treatment at the University Clinics.  The subject characteristics are presented in Table I.

Table I

Subject Characteristics

| Left Damaged Subjects | Sex | Age | Months Post Stroke |
|---|---|---|---|
| 1 | M | 57 | 66 |
| 2 | F | 59 | 43 |
| 3 | F | 62 | 13 |
| Right Damaged Subjects | Sex | Age | Months Post Stroke |
| 1 | F | 27 | 6 |
| 2 | M | 65 | 24 |
| 3 | F | 65 | 36 |

All subjects in both groups of subjects had experienced a
single incident of cerebral vascular accident.  Symptomology was
of sudden onset.  The outstanding symptomology for the left-damaged patients was right hemiparesis accompanied by loss of functional speech.  The right-damaged patients experienced left hemiparesis with no reported speech loss at onset or henceforth.  All
patients in both of the clinical groups retained motor dysfunction
and were continuing in physical therapy.  The left-damaged patients
were also continuing in speech therapy.

The ages of the left-damaged group ranged from 57 to 62 years,
mean group age of 59.3 years.  For this group, months post stroke
ranged from 13 to 66 months.  All of these patients began therapy
no less than six months following onset of symptoms.  All of these
subjects had been employed previous to illness in professional or
business positions.  None had regained language functioning to permit their return to previous or other employment.

The ages of the right-damaged group ranged from 27 to 65 years,
mean group age of 52.3 years.  For this group months post stroke
ranged from 6 to 36 months.

The right-damaged patients were reported by self, family, and physician to have retained normal speech and language functions. The attending physical therapist reported no receptive or expressive language problems. These observations were confirmed by the researchers. The subjects were oriented for place and time. They experienced no difficulty in reporting accurately remote and current events. They had complete and correct recall of the circumstances surrounding their illness. Verbal performance of these subjects in conversation could not be distinguished from normal.

The left-damaged patients were fluent aphasics as defined by the Goodglass and Kaplan categories (1972). Their speech retained melody and contained a variety of grammatical constructions. There was, however, notable presence of paraphasia and/or circumlocutions in discourse and frequent word-finding difficulties as evidenced by delay in selection/recall of contentive words, that is, words belonging to the grammatical classes nouns, verbs, and adjectives. Language was functional for all left-damaged patients but communication was hampered by a less-than-efficient production system. Utilizing Jakobson categories (1961), these patients should be classified as similarity aphasics. This group of aphasics demonstrated both semantic and formal paraphasias as have been observed by Lecours and Rouillon (1976). That is, there are both conceptual relationships between substituted and target words, e.g. "book" for magazine and morphological relationships, e.g. "beauty" substituted for beautiful.

The topography of the brain lesions for the subjects under study was not obtainable. The medical records of all of the three left-damaged patients contained diagnoses of "infarction associated with occlusion of the middle cerebral artery." None of the subjects were on antidepressants or anticonvulsant drugs and none were reported to have experienced seizures at the time of testing. One subject in the right damaged group reported use of a tranquilizing medication. None of the subjects had histories of alcohol or drug abuse or had received treatment for psychotic disabilities.

Handedness data are insufficient to document manual laterality; however, all subjects in the study were reported by self, family, and physician to have relied upon the right hand in habitual manual tasks pre-onset of the cerebral vascular accident.

Behavioral Measurements

The principal behavioral tool of this study, used to measure language performance of the left-damaged subjects, was the Porch Index of Communicative Ability (Porch, 1973). This test is at present widely used in aphasia centers. It permits the clinician to describe response behaviors of patients in numerical terms on a sixteen-step scale in a way which is very meaningful to all clinicians who are familiar with the test. The test is a composite of eighteen subtests which are designed to measure verbal, gestural, and graphic skills. It allows one to evaluate specific levels of the output modalities and to make inferences about input and integrative abilities. A total of 180 responses is obtained, and each response is scored according to a sixteen-point binary choice system based on the dimensions of accuracy, responsiveness, completeness, promptness, and efficiency. The test yields an overall communicative ability mean score, as well as mean scores of the subject's performance within the verbal, gestural and graphic modalities.

The PICA test does not tax the language system and does not require the subject to produce a complex linguistic string. The most difficult subtest requires only that the patient describe the function of a familiar object in a semantically and syntactically correct sentence. It is, however, very sensitive to semantic disorders, permitting a reduction of scores for delayed or incomplete responses.

The typical aphasia pattern with left hemisphere insult across modalities is gestural performance equal to or slightly better than verbal performance which in turn is better than graphic performance. The graphic subtests are the most sensitive of the modalities to minimal damage even though allowances are made for the inefficiency of the left hand in writing for those patients who habitually write with the right hand.

The PICA was used in this study to assess the functional capabilities of the aphasic subjects and to confirm the presence of semantic disorders as the outstanding symptom of the aphasia syndrome.

## Electrocortical Measurements

Sixteen word pairs produced by a native English speaker with a general American dialect were used as stimuli in the present study. These included words from the two categories which are furniture and animals. Two of the words in each category were high frequency members and two were low frequency members as defined by the Battig and Montague norms (1969). The stimuli presented are shown in Table II.

Eight replications of each word were recorded in random order on one channel of a Sony stereo Tape Recorder (Model TC-560). A 80 Hz square wave (1/4 volt in amplitude) was recorded on the second channel of the tape recorder 40 msecs prior to the onset of the speech stimuli.  This 80 Hz pulse served as a marker to identify the beginning of each stimulus presentation and the subsequent auditory evoked potential.

Table II

Stimuli

|      | Furniture | Animals |
|------|-----------|---------|
| High | Bed       | Dog     |
|      | Lamp      | Rat     |
|      |           |         |
| Low  | Rug       | Bull    |
|      | Bench     | Wolf    |

The stimuli were presented in pairs such that the subject heard a category name, i.e., furniture or animal, followed by a second word that is a high or low member from that category or from the second category.

The interstimulus interval between pair members varied randomly from 4 up to 6 seconds while the interval between pairs varied from 7 up to 12 seconds.

The stimuli were presented to each S in a sound dampened, air conditioned and electrically shielded room through a speaker suspended approximately 1 meter above the subject's head.  The stimulus intensity at the subject's ears was 80 dB SPL.

Grass silver scalp electrodes were placed on the scalp over the superior temporal regions of the left and right hemispheres at $T_3$ and $T_4$ and over the parietal region $P_3$.  (Ten-Twenty Electrode System of the International Federation, Jasper 1958.)  The temporal region sites were selected in order to record neural activity in the secondary auditory zones in response to verbal stimuli presented through the auditory channel.  The $P_3$ site was chosen to record activity from the angular gyrus, a region of the neocortex which participates in the semantic/syntactic component of the Central Language System (Whitaker, 1971).  The electrodes were referred to linked ear lobes.  Resistances of the electrodes for each side of the head were monitored before and after the test session and maintained under 5 K Ohms and within 1 K Ohm of each other. The recording electrodes were connected to four Analogue Devices Isolation Amplifiers (Model 273 J) powered by two Analogue Devices Power Supplies (Model 940).  This system served as a safeguard unit

in the event of a worse case failure to protect the subject from
the risk of shock.

The output of each amplifier was connected to a modified Tek-
tronic AM502 differential amplifier with the bandpass flat between
0.1 Hz and 30 Hz.  The amplifier gain controls were set at 20K.
The amplified auditory evoked potentials and the stimulus trigger
were recorded on a Vetter modified cassette FM tape recorder for
later off-line analysis on a PDP-12 computer and an IBM-370.

Two telegraph keys were positioned three inches apart directly
in front of the subjects who were instructed to place one hand over
the two keys.  Subjects were then instructed that they would hear
pairs of words and that they should press one key if the words were
related, and the other if they were not.  Several extra-list examples were then given the subjects in order to verify that they
understood the task.  The correctness of the categorical identification of the word pairs was recorded by the researchers during
the course of the experiment.  The position of the keys in relation
to the match/mismatch conditions was varied randomly across subjects.

Subjects were also instructed to remain as motionless as
possible during the testing session.

## RESULTS

### Verbal Abilities of Left-Damaged Group

The PICA mean scores are presented in Table III.

### Table III

### PICA Mean Scores

| Modalities Subjects | Overall | Gestural | Verbal | Graphic |
|---|---|---|---|---|
| 1 | 11.42 | 13.06 | 13.77 | 7.68 |
| 2 | 12.42 | 12.55 | 13.55 | 11.50 |
| 3 | 13.12 | 12.70 | 14.15 | 12.90 |

With respect to verbal abilities this particular group of
aphasics can be described as moderate to mild in deficit ratings.
Table IV presents the PICA percentiles and deficit ratings for
the three left-damaged subjects.  No subject's verbal abilities
fell below the 50th percentile as compared with the PICA standardization group of left-hemisphere-damaged patients.  The subjects

functioned satisfactorily and handled most basic communication
tasks fairly well, requiring little assistance.

On the verbal subtests, no subjects produced error or poorer
responses.  The poorest responses produced by any subject were related responses, e.g. "smoke" for cigarette, "light" for match, or
"pen" for pencil.  For all three subjects delayed responses were
common; that is, the subject needed additional processing time to
respond.  In general, the patients filled the time with inter-
jections, gestures and/or incomplete responses that were then improved; e.g. (item, knife) "Uh....I cut meat with it," or (item,
match) "light....I light a fire."  Functions were usually described
in terms of the person, using the first person pronoun: e.g. "I
eat," "I write," "I smoke," etc.  Incomplete responses were also
frequent in this group of subjects.  Examples of incomplete
responses are as follows:
    Number violations:  "cigarettes" for cigarette or "match"
                           for matches.
    Subject-predicate disagreement:  I eats with a fork,"
                           "Cigarette are for smoking."
    Syntax incomplete:  "for a fire" rather than for lighting
                           a fire.

Table IV

PICA Percentiles and Ratings

| Modalities | Overall | Deficit | Gestural | Deficit | Verbal | Deficit | Graphic | Deficit |
|---|---|---|---|---|---|---|---|---|
| Subjects | % | Rating* | % | Rating* | % | Rating* | % | Rating* |
| 1 | 59 | Mod | 58 | Mild | 76 | Mild | 53 | Mkd |
| 2 | 73 | Mod | 48 | Mod | 73 | Mild | 83 | Mod |
| 3 | 93 | Mild | 68 | Mod | 89 | Mild | 96 | Mod |

*1 -  7  Severe
 7 - 10  Marked
10 - 13  Moderate
12 - 15  Mild

As can be seen by inspection of Table V, all subjects improved
performance as task difficulty decreased.  All subjects experienced
difficulty in describing function and in naming objects.  One of
the three subjects continued to produce delayed, distorted or incomplete responses on sentence completion tasks.  None of the subjects experienced difficulty in imitative naming.

Table V

PICA Verbal Subtest Scores*

| Subtests | I | IV | IX | XII |
|---|---|---|---|---|
| Subjects | Describe Function | Name Object | Sentence Completion | Imitative Naming |
| 1 | 12.2 | 12.9 | 15 | 15 |
| 2 | 10.6 | 13.6 | 15 | 15 |
| 3 | 13.8 | 14.1 | 14.7 | 15 |

*Mean Scores

All of the subjects demonstrated some residual disability in graphic output although discrepancy between subject performance was greatest in this modality with subject #1 demonstrating a marked deficit (53rd percentile) and subject #3 retaining a moderate deficit (96th percentile). All subjects reported an inability to write and initially rejected writing tasks. This reluctance to write may however be related to awkwardness with the left hand.

During the recording of electrocortical data, the subjects were asked to identify words as related or not related. The researchers recorded errors of subjects, finding that the mean percent errors for the left-damaged subjects was 2.08 (128 responses per subject). Mean percent of errors for the right-damaged group was 3.12. One subject in this group made 10 errors. More than half of these errors were on the words bull and wolf.

## Electrocortical Data

The AEPs from each subject were digitized and averaged on a PDP-12 computer using a modified version of "Averager" (Decus No. 12-84). Averages were based on amplitude measures at 6 msec intervals over a 510 msec period following stimulus onset for a total of 85 points. These averages were based on 16 samples obtained independently for the high and low members of each category so that an average was obtained based on four repetitions of the members of the high and low groups of each category. In this manner, averages were obtained for the following:
1.  2 categories (furniture/animals)
2.  2 category membership frequencies (high/low)
3.  2 conditions of match (match/mismatch)
4.  3 recording sites ($T_3$, $P_3$, $T_4$)
Twenty-four averaged evoked potentials were obtained for each subject and 144 averages were obtained for the two brain-damaged groups.

Following the procedures outlined by Molfese et al (1976), Molfese (in press) and Chapman, McCrary, Bragdon and Chapman (in press), an 85 (time point variables) x 144 (averaged evoked potential cases) input data matrix was obtained for the two brain-damaged groups. Intercorrelations among the 85 variables were subjected to a principal components factor analysis with the varimax rotation of factors with an Eigen = 1.0 criterion (BMD08M).

Twelve factors accounting for 94.64% of the total variance were selected with the Eigen = 1.0 criterion and then rotated using the varimax method (Mulaik, 1972) with the BMD08M computer program (Dixon, 1972). The centroid (the average evoked potential for the entire data set) and the twelve factors are presented in Figure 1.

The factor scores for each factor were treated separately as the dependent variables in a series of twelve independent analyses of variance (Myers, 1972) using the BMD08V computer program (Dixon, 1972). The groups (2) x electrode sites (3) x categories (2) x frequency (2) x match (2) analyses of variance were performed in order to identify possible relationships existing between the factors and specific levels of the independent variables. The Scheffé procedure (Winer, 1962) for making a posteriori comparisons was implemented to examine the interactions between subject and stimulus variables which relate to the simple main effects identified.

These analyses determined that the AEP responses of the left-damaged subjects differed from those of the right-damaged subjects. Significant main effects for groups were found for three of the twelve factors: Factor 1 ($F = 9.61$, df = 1, 4, $p < .05$), Factor 6 ($F = 12.79$, df = 2, 4, $p < .05$), and Factor 9 ($F = 15.71$, df = 1, 4, $p < .05$). The waveforms for the three factors which reflected group differences were characterized by major amplitude changes occurring late in the waveforms. The latencies of the portions of the waveforms in which the major activity occurred are listed in Table VI. In Factor 1 and in Factor 6 late positive responses occurred. In Factor 9 the major components were negative in polarity. Differences between the left damaged and the right damaged groups are found in the waveforms which are displayed in Figure 2.

In addition to the main effects for electrode placement sites which reflected hemisphere differences for Factor 6, interaction between subject groups, electrode placement sites and stimulus frequency was found to contribute to the variability of the AEP responses. This interaction is shown in Figure 3. The waveforms for Factor 6 are displayed in Figure 4. The left damaged group differed significantly from the right damaged group in the following:

1. AEP responses recorded from $T_4$ for the low frequency stimuli ($F = 14.98$, df = 2, 8, $p < .025$)

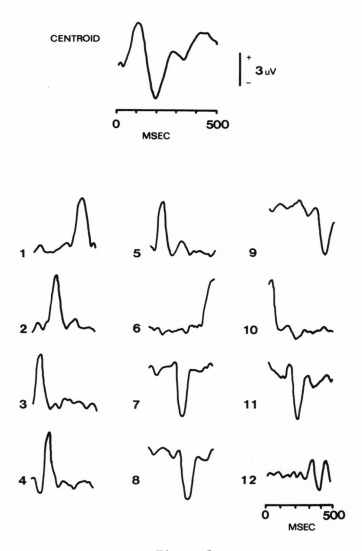

Figure 1
Centroid and Factor Waveforms

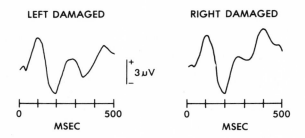

Figure 2

Waveforms for Left and Right Damaged Subject Groups

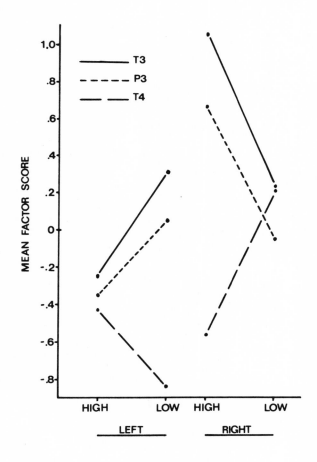

**5**

Figure 3
Factor 6 Interaction

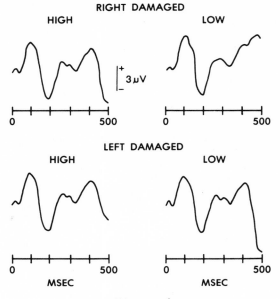

Figure 4
Factor 6 Waveforms

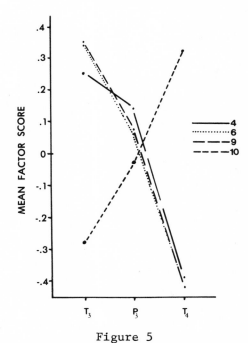

Figure 5
Main Effects for Electrode Placement Site

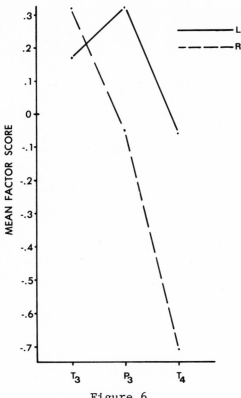

Figure 6
Factor 4 Interaction


Table VI

Factor Latencies

| Factor | Latency (msec) |
|--------|----------------|
| 1      | 336 – 438      |
| 2      | 156 – 234      |
| 3      | 30 –  96       |
| 4      | 120 – 186      |
| 5      | 72 – 138       |
| 6      | 456 – 510      |
| 7      | 252 – 312      |
| 8      | 288 – 366      |
| 9      | 408 – 492      |
| 10     | 6 –  54        |
| 11     | 210 – 270      |
| 12     | 354 – 414      |

2.  AEP responses recorded from $T_3$ for the high frequency stimuli (F = 18.32, df = 2, 8, p < .001)
3.  AEP responses recorded from $P_3$ for the high frequency stimuli (F = 14.4, df = 2, 8, p < .025)

For the high frequency stimuli differences were found in the responses recorded for the left damaged subjects from electrode placement sites $T_3$ and $P_3$ (F = 16.23, df 2, 8, p< .025). With these stimuli differences between $T_3$ and $T_4$ were also found for this group of subjects (F = 11.25, df = 2, 8, p< .05).

For the right damaged group the responses recorded from $T_3$ and $P_3$ differed when the stimuli were of high frequency (F = 22.7, df = 2, 8, p < .001).  There were also significant differences between the high and low frequency stimuli for the right damaged group in the AEP responses recorded from $T_3$ (F = 11.44, df = 2, 8, p < .05); from $P_3$ (F = 10.08, df = 2, 8, p <.05); and from $T_4$ (F = 11.08, df = 2, 8, p < .05).

Significant main effects for electrode placement site were found in four factors:  Factor 4 (F = 30.00, df = 2, 8, p < .001), Factor 6 (F = 4.95, df = 2, 8, p < .05), Factor 9 (F = 5.81, df = 2, 8, p < .05), and Factor 10 (F = 5.90, df = 2, 8, p < .05).  The effects are plotted in Figure 5.  The effects were due to differences in the AEP responses of the left and right temporal areas. The two hemispheres were responding differentially to the verbal stimuli.

The differences between the evoked responses of the two hemispheres occurred early and throughout the waveforms.  The major activity for Factor 10 occurred at 6 - 54 msec.  A major change in amplitude occurred for Factor 4 at 12 - 186 msec.  Late amplitude changes characterized Factors 6 and 9.  For Factors 1, 6, and 10 the major components were positive in polarity while a negative peak characterized Factor 9.

A Groups x Sites interaction (F = 16.49, df = 2, 8 p < .025) was found for Factor 4.  The AEP responses obtained from $T_3$ and $T_4$ differed for the right-damaged subjects but did not differ significantly for the left-damaged subjects.  This interaction is presented in Figure 6.

These data support previous research which has indicated that the electrocortical activity of the two hemispheres differs when the activity is elicited by the presentation of verbal stimuli through the auditory channel.  The differences which occur are however related to the neurological status of the two hemispheres and to stimulus variables.  The AEP responses from the two hemispheres were different for left-brain damaged subjects as compared to those from right-brain damaged subjects.

DISCUSSION

The findings of this study support previous research which identified hemisphere differences as measured by auditory evoked responses to linguistic stimuli. The findings also indicate that two groups of brain damaged subjects can be distinguished on the basis of the AEP responses as well as by their language performances.

The group of aphasic subjects in this study demonstrated mild to moderate word finding problems. They experienced very little difficulty in sentence completion tasks but their naming on confrontation was delayed or incomplete. The right-brain damaged subjects evidenced no language disabilities. The waveforms evoked by the auditory presentation of linguistic stimuli differed for these two groups of subjects; however, the differences noted were related to placement of recording electrode and to linguistic stimulus characteristics.

It appears that hemisphere differences are less prominent for the left-damaged subjects than for the right-damaged subjects. Differences between the right and left temporal areas did, however, emerge in the left-damaged subjects related to the stimulus frequency variable. These differences were observed for Factor 6. Damage to the left cerebral hemisphere may result in increased participation of the right hemisphere in the processing of verbal material. Alternatively, the presence of right hemisphere damage may result in greater activity in the left temporal areas in response to verbal material presented to the auditory system. This relationship between the loci of cerebral damage and the electrocortical responses of the temporal areas can not be interpreted in the absence of a control group of neurologically normal subjects.

The latencies of the factors reflecting group differences are interesting. Hemisphere differences occurred early in the waveforms. This finding would appear to indicate laterality within subcortical systems in response to verbal stimuli. Hemisphere differences occurring later in the waveforms indicated that the left and right auditory association areas of the neocortex are also responding to the stimuli in different ways.

Differences between the left and the right brain-damaged groups appeared late in the waveforms. This finding was expected since cortical damage differentiated the two groups. The two brain-damaged groups could not, however, be differentiated on the basis of the functioning of the subcortical systems. The language systems of the aphasics in this study were mildly impaired. Extension of this research to include severe aphasics may reveal that the subcortical systems which serve the Central Language System may also be impaired by cerebral vascular accident.

Certain methodological limitations restrict the interpretation
of the results of this study.  The sample size was small and the
left-damaged subjects represented a single type of aphasia.  Further, data from neurologically intact subjects of comparable age
are not available for comparison at this time.  The specific loci
and extent of the neurological damage of the subjects were not
determined. Several stimulus and task characteristics were manipulated and the sample of stimulus characteristics was restricted.
The number of factors emerging was very likely related to the number of variables under study.

This preliminary study does indicate that AEP data may be useful in the examination of clinical populations with language disabilities.  The study of the neuroelectrical responses of aphasics
may provide insight into the neural mechanisms associated with
semantic confusions.  Individual subject and group analyses of responses to specific stimulus characteristics should receive further
attention.

## BIBLIOGRAPHY

Battig, W. and Montague, W.  1969.  Category norms for verbal items
    in 56 categories: an application and extension of the Connec-
    ticut category norms. Journal of Experimental Psychology
    Monograph.  80 (3).  1-47.

Beyn, E. S. and Vlasenko, I. T.  1974.  Verbal paraphasias of
    aphasic patients in the course of naming actions.  British
    Journal of Disorders of Communication.  9.  24-34.

Chapey, R., Rigrodsky, S. and Morrison, E. B.  1976.  Divergent
    semantic behavior in aphasia.  Journal of Speech and Hearing
    Research.  19.  664-677.

Chapman, R. M., McCrary, J. W., Bragdon, H. R., and Chapman, J. A.
    (in press)  Latent components of evoked potentials functionally
    related to information processing.  In Cerebral Evoked Poten-
    tials In Man.  J. E. Desmedt, Ed. London: Oxford University
    Press.

DeRenzi, E., Pieczuro, A., and Vignolo, L. A.  1966.  Oral aprexia
    and aphasia.  Cortex.  2.  50-73.

Dixon, W. J.  Ed.  1972.  BMD Biomedical Computer Program: X-series
    Supplement.  Berkeley: University of California Press.

Gardner, H.  1974.  The naming and recognition of written symbols
    in aphasic and alexic patients.  Journal of Communication
    Disorders.  7.  141-153.

Geschwind, N.  1967.  The variety of naming errors.  Cortex.  3.
    97-112.

Goodglass, H., Klein, B., Carey, P. W., Jones, K. J.  1966.
    Specific semantic word categories in aphasia.  Cortex.  2.
    74-89.

Goodglass, H., and Kaplan, E.  1972.  The Assessment of Aphasia
    and Related Disorders.  Philadelphia: Lea and Febiger.

Goodglass, H. 1976. Agrammatism. In Studies in Neurolinguistics: Volume 1. H. Whitaker and H. A. Whitaker, Eds. New York: Academic Press.

Guilford, J. P., and Hoepfner, R. 1971. The Analysis of Intelligence. New York: McGraw Hill.

Jakobson, R. 1961. Aphasia as a linguistic problem. In Psycholinguistics: A Book of Readings. New York: Holt.

Jasper, H. L. 1958. The ten-twenty electrode system of the international federation of societies for electroencephalography: Appendix to report of the committee on methods of clinical examination in electroencephalography. The Journal of Electroencephalography and Clinical Neurophysiology. 10. 371.

Lecours, A. R., and Rouillon, F. 1976. Neurolinguistic analysis of jargonaphasia and jargonagraphia. In Studies in Neurolinguistics: Volume 2. H. Whitaker and H. A. Whitaker, Eds. New York: Academic Press.

Luria, A. 1966. Higher Cortical Functions in Man. New York: Basic Books.

Marshall, J. C., and Newcombe, F. 1966. Syntactic and semantic errors in paralexia. J. Neuropsychologia. 4. 169–176.

Milner, B. 1964. Some aspects of frontal lobectomey in man. In The Frontal Granular Cortex and Behavior. J. Warren and K. Akert, Eds. New York: McGraw-Hill.

Molfese, D. L., Nunez, V., Seibert, S. M., and Raminaiah, N. V. 1976. Cerebral Asymmetry: changes in factors affecting its development. Annals of the New York Academy of Sciences, Vol. 280. New York: New York Academy of Sciences, 821–833.

Molfese, D. L. (in press) Neuroelectrical correlates of speech perception in adults. Brain and Language.

Mulaik, S. A. 1972. The Foundation of Factor Analysis. New York: McGraw-Hill.

Myers, J. L. 1972. Fundamentals of Experimental Design: Second Edition. Boston: Allyn and Bacon.

Pizzamiglio, L. and Appicciafuocco, A. 1971. Semantic comprehension in aphasia. Journal of Communication Disorders. 3. 280–288.

Porch, B. E. 1973. Porch Index of Communicative Ability: Administration, scoring and interpretation. Vol. 2. Palo Alto: Consulting Psychologists Press.

Rinnert, C. and Whitaker, H. A. 1973. Semantic confusions by aphasic patients. Cortex. 9 (1). 56–81.

Schuell, H. and Jenkins, J. 1961. Reduction of vocabulary in aphasia. Brain. 84. 243–261.

Weinstein, E. A. and Keller, N. J. 1963. Linguistic patterns of misnaming in brain injury. J. Neuropsychologia. 1. 79–90.

Whitaker, H. A. 1971. On the Representation of Language in the Human Brain. Edmonton: Linguistic Research, Inc.

Winer, B. J. 1962. Statistical Principles in Experimental Design. New York: McGraw-Hill.

# THE EVOKED RESPONSE AS A MEASURE OF CEREBRAL DYSFUNCTION

R. E. Dustman, E. W. Snyder, D. A. Callner, E. C. Beck

Veterans Administration Hospital and University of Utah

Salt Lake City, Utah  84148

It has been scarcely a generation since Dawson (1947,1954) described and developed the technique for summing and averaging the brain's electrical response to repeated stimuli.  Since then, there has been an avalanche of research including many aspects of behavior in species ranging from worms to man.  What was first thought to be a fairly simple response has come to be seen as a complex pattern of as many as 15 identifiable wave components or reproducible patterns of polarity, amplitude and duration that lasts for hundreds of milliseconds.  Recently great strides have been made in understanding the neurogenesis of these components, thereby strengthening both the clinical and research applications of the technique.

Contributing to the volumes of research that have emerged have been the technological advances and the development of small relatively inexpensive computers allowing researchers to average or sum the brain's electrical responses efficiently and rapidly.  But probably the most critical factor in the momentum of research has been the repeatedly reinforced finding that the evoked response technique is more useful in assessing brain function than the conventional EEG (Beck, 1975; Beck, Dustman & Lewis, 1975).

Clinical application of the evoked response has been successfully attempted in many branches of medicine, even dentistry.  For example, in ophthalmology the evoked response is of special value in the areas of refraction, infant visual acuity, diseases of the optic nerve, color blindness, amblyopia and field defects (Sokol, 1976).

In neurology, neurosurgery and audiology the technique has found widespread acceptance.  The somatosensory evoked response has

321

been applied in an effort to localize peripheral and spinal cord lesions as well as to define the locus and extent of cerebral lesions (Alajouanine et al., 1958; Giblin, 1964; Larson, Sances, & Christenson, 1966; Bergamini & Bergamasco, 1967; Gossman et al., 1968; Williamson, Goff, & Allison, 1970; Croft, Brodkey, & Nulsen, 1972; Perot, 1973; Nakanishi et al., 1974; Cracco, 1975). The auditory evoked response has been found useful in evaluating hearing loss, particularly with prespeech and mentally defective children (Rapin, 1964; Cody & Bickford, 1965; Barnet & Lodge, 1966; Davis, 1966; Davis et al., 1967; Rapin & Graziani, 1967). Lately the visual evoked potential has been successfully used in the early detection of multiple sclerosis (Namerow, 1970; Namerow & Enns, 1972; Halliday, McDonald, & Mushkin, 1973; Asselman et al., 1975). The technique appears to be superior to the conventional EEG in determining cerebral death (Behrens, Beck, & Dustman, 1973; Trojaborg & Jørgensen, 1973; Beck, Dustman, & Lewis, 1975; Starr, 1976).

In psychiatry, despite the complexity of the problem, you will learn from this conference that tremendous strides have been made with the application of the technique to psychopathology and in providing new insights and inroads into the relationships between psychological phenomena and its underlying physiological determinants (Begleiter, Porjesz, & Garozzo, 1977; Buchsbaum, 1977; Callaway, 1977; Roth, 1977; Shagass, 1977).

Over the past decade our efforts have been mainly in the direction of clinical application of the technique. We have not had the temerity for an excursion into the mind, mental states, information processing and the like, but have been content to study differences that emerge among different clinical categories with the brain alert but without any imposed task or performance. The data that have accumulated indicate that this is a rich vein of knowledge that, despite the exciting findings of other approaches, is yielding interesting and important answers and bringing into focus additional questions regarding cerebral function.

We report on several experiments that involve both humans and experimental animals. These range from an analysis of the evoked potentials of a large group of Down's syndrome subjects, aged 5 to 62, through experiments with alcohol and methadone, analysis of the somatosensory evoked response in patients afflicted with amyotrophic lateral sclerosis and ending, with a sense of finality, in describing the use of the evoked potential for assessing "brain death."

## Procedures and Equipment

Evoked responses were recorded from human subjects while they were seated in an electrically shielded, sound deadened, darkened

room.  Although electrode placements varied slightly from one study
to another, electrodes were usually placed at $F_3$, $F_4$, $C_3$, $C_4$, $O_1$
and $O_2$ according to the International Ten-Twenty System (Jasper,
1958), and on the forehead above the nasion.  The last was used to
record eyeblinks when they occurred.  All recordings were unipolar,
both ear lobes combined serving as reference.  Brain waves were
amplified by an eight-channel Grass EEG polygraph and, together with
pulses accompanying stimuli, were stored on magnetic tape.  The
stored EEG was digitized at a rate of 500/sec by a PDP-9 computer
which also summed and averaged evoked responses.  Individual responses which were contaminated by muscle, eyeblink, or other artifact were excluded from the averaging process.

Visual stimuli of 10 µsec duration were generated by a Grass
photic stimulator which projected flashes into a reflecting hemisphere 70 cm in diameter.  The hemisphere, partially surrounding the
field of view, insured a relatively constant level of retinal illumination regardless of the position of the subject's head.  At a
stimulator setting of PS2 the measured luminance at the subject's
eyes, 40 cm from the center of the hemisphere, was 12 lux.  Subjects
were asked to fixate on a black dot attached to the center of the
hemisphere.

Somatosensory potentials were evoked by 0.25 msec electrical
pulses.  Stimulus intensity was determined by the method of ascending and descending limits and was calculated from subjective
thresholds.  Stimuli were delivered to the index finger of the
dominant hand through two silver clip electrodes.  A copper cuff
was placed on the forearm to ground the spread of shock artifact.

In two studies to be reported we investigated the relationship
of single trial response (STR) amplitude and variability to averaged
evoked response amplitude.  An STR is an evoked response elicited
by the presentation of a single stimulus.  A mean STR amplitude
and variability measure was obtained for each of several sets of
10 consecutive STRs.

For each set of 10 STRs a mean amplitude reflecting the voltage
fluctuations occurring within a specified time interval was calculated.  This measure is analogous to measuring the total length of
line comprising a segment of a response tracing.

Variability measures were calculated for the same time intervals by means of Pearson product-moment coefficients of correlation.
The digital values comprising each STR in a set were correlated with
those of each of the nine remaining STRs.  The correlations were
converted to Fisher Z-scores which have a normal sampling distribution, and a mean of the Z-scores was used as an estimate of variability.

## AGE RELATED CHANGES IN THE EVOKED RESPONSES OF
## DOWN'S SYNDROME AND NORMAL SUBJECTS

A substantial part of our research has been directed towards a description of evoked response characteristics in normal subjects spanning a wide age range.  Since we have found that age is a critical variable when evoked responses are interpreted (Dustman & Beck, 1966; Dustman & Beck, 1969; Schenkenberg & Dustman, 1970; Dustman, Schenkenberg, & Beck, 1976), these normative data are used for comparison purposes when disease entities are investigated.

Before we discuss age-related changes in Down's syndrome subjects, a review of our normative data is necessary.  Figure 1 illustrates age-related changes in VERs, AERs, and SERs.  Both VERs and SERs show a gradual reduction in late wave amplitude with increasing age.  This trend is most apparent in the VERs recorded from occipital scalp.  A negative wave peaking at about 220 msec is large in the youngest group and diminishes in amplitude, becoming very small or absent, in the responses of the oldest subjects.  An earlier negative wave, N150, behaves differently.  It is small in the VERs of the youngest subjects and gradually grows in size, to become a prominent landmark in the responses of the older people.  Also of interest are early VER waves, i.e., those occurring prior to 90 msec.  These are larger and occur later in the VERs of older subjects and are readily identified in the group VERs of subjects whose mean age was 41 years or older (see Fig. 1).

Another portrayal of age-related changes in the VERs of normal subjects is shown in Figure 2.  The evoked responses are from occipital and central scalp of 425 normal subjects aged 4-86 years. Figure 3 clearly shows that VERs recorded from central scalp do not exhibit the large age-related amplitude changes seen in occipitally derived VERs.  The pattern of amplitude changes associated with increasing age, which was discussed with reference to the occipital VERs portrayed in Figure 1, can also be seen in Figure 2.

While we had previously studied the evoked responses of Down's syndrome children (Bigum, Dustman, & Beck, 1970), we conducted a second investigation of Down's syndrome to evaluate age-related changes in evoked responses associated with this disorder.  There have been repeated observations that Down's syndrome individuals show signs of premature and accelerated aging.  During adulthood, many of the neurological and psychological signs of senility such as cortical atrophy, premature graying, loss of skin turgor, and changes in personality occur at an earlier age in DS than in normals (Penrose, 1966; Benda, 1969).  Neurohistological abnormalities occur in the brains of DS people which appear to be similar to those found in the brains of patients with Alzheimer's and Pick's diseases (Jervis, 1948-49, 1970; Solitaire & Lemarche, 1966; Neuman, 1967; Olson & Shaw, 1969; Roizan et al.,1972; Burger & Vogel, 1973). The average weight of the DS brain is consistently less than that

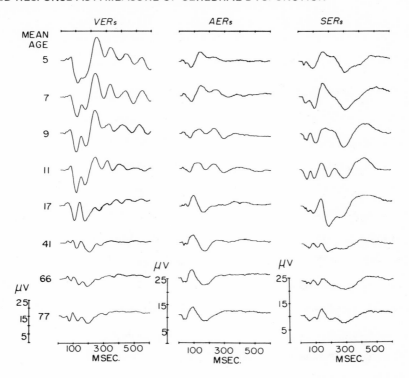

Figure 1.  A comparison of group VERs, AERs, and SERs during maturation and aging.  Each trace was obtained by averaging the evoked
responses of the 20 subjects, 10 males and 10 females, in each
group.  VERs are from $O_1$; AERs and SERs are from $C_3$.  The mean age
of each group is shown at the left of the figure.  (From Dustman,
Schenkenberg, and Beck, in R. Karrer (Ed.), Developmental psychophysiology in mental retardation and learning disability, C. C.
Thomas, 1976)

of age-matched normal controls (Yakovlev, 1962; Benda, 1969) and
shows a slower rate of growth from infancy to adulthood (Benda,
1969).  In addition, Solitaire and Lemarche (1967) report that
the brain weight of DS adults reduces faster with increasing age
than the brain weight of normals.  Many areas of the DS brain show
evidence of delayed and incomplete myelin development (Benda, 1969).

    The following study (Callner, 1975; Callner et al., 1977) was
designed to determine whether the premature aging seen in DS individuals is reflected in the evoked response, and if aging trends
were observed, whether they would parallel trends reported above
for normal subjects.  For example, do late waves of VERs recorded
from occipital scalp of Down's subjects show a decrement in amplitude at an earlier age than was found for normals?

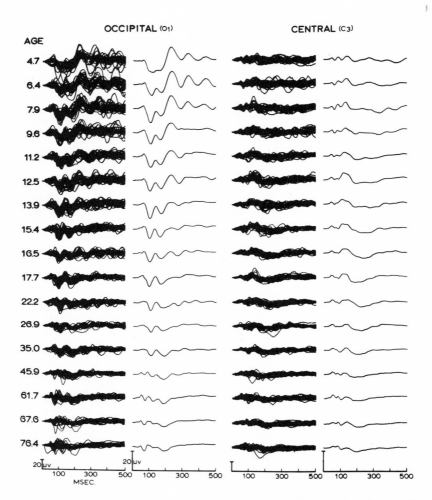

Figure 2.   Changes in the VER during maturation and aging.   Portrayed are VERs of 425 individuals ranging in age from 4 to 86.
Each of the 17 age groups, designated by mean age at the left of
the figure, is composed of 25 subjects (rather equally divided,
male and female).   It may be seen that the configuration of the
VER changes with age and that the trend of these changes is
obvious both in the individual and the group. (From Beck and Dustman,
in N. Burch and H. L. Altshuler (Eds.), Behavior and brain electrical activity, Plenum, 1975).

VERs, AERs and SERs were recorded from 66 DS subjects ranging in age from 5 to 62 years and compared with similar data previously recorded from age and sex matched normal controls (Schenkenberg & Dustman, 1970). The subjects were divided into six age groups of 11 individuals. Table I gives the mean age and IQ for the six groups. Each DS subject was examined by a pediatric neurologist who excluded those found to have moderate to severe sensory deficits or medical, neurological or ophthalmological disorders other than those typically associated with Down's syndrome. None of the DS subjects had a history of seizures during the preceding three years, and none was taking psychoactive medication. All were cooperative, capable of focusing their attention and able to follow simple verbal instructions.

Figure 3 illustrates group VERs recorded from occipital, central and frontal scalp of the normal and DS subjects. The wave patterns of the occipital VERs of the two groups are reasonably similar in appearance. As can be seen, however, VERs recorded from central and frontal areas of the DS individuals are much larger than those of the normal controls.

Age related changes in VERs and SERs are portrayed in Figure 4, in which each tracing was obtained by averaging the responses of the 11 subjects in each age group. Data for frontally derived VERs are not shown as the results closely paralleled those from central scalp. Age-related changes in amplitude were more evident in responses of normal subjects than in those of the DS individuals. With respect to VERs recorded from occipital scalp of the normals, amplitudes of most waves decreased significantly with advancing age (see also Figs 1 & 2). For the Down's subjects, only wave P100 became reliably smaller as age increased, while amplitudes of other waves did not change significantly.

Table I. Summary of age and IQ data for six age groups of normal and Down's subjects. Each group includes eleven subjects.

| | Normal | | | | Down's Syndrome | | | |
| | Age (Yrs) | | I.Q. | | Age (Yrs) | | I.Q. | |
| | Mean | S.D. | Mean | S.D. | Mean | S.D. | Mean | S.D. |
|---|---|---|---|---|---|---|---|---|
| 1 | 8.2 | 2.4 | 118.3 | 8.2 | 8.4 | 2.4 | 32.7 | 3.1 |
| 2 | 14.4 | 2.2 | 111.2 | 10.3 | 15.1 | 2.1 | 32.4 | 4.0 |
| 3 | 21.0 | 3.4 | 115.3 | 8.4 | 21.2 | 2.8 | 31.1 | 5.8 |
| 4 | 29.5 | 1.8 | 116.1 | 5.8 | 29.6 | 1.2 | 31.3 | 4.7 |
| 5 | 35.5 | 4.1 | 113.2 | 6.3 | 36.0 | 2.9 | 30.5 | 4.3 |
| 6 | 51.2 | 5.8 | 119.1 | 8.2 | 50.7 | 4.8 | 30.6 | 5.7 |

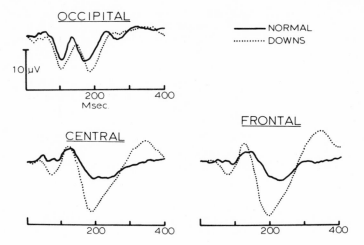

Figure 3.   A comparison of VERs recorded from three scalp areas of normal and Down's syndrome individuals.   Each response was averaged from the VERs of 66 subjects ranging in age from 5-62 years.   Note that the responses of the Down's patients recorded from central and frontal areas, are much larger than those of the normals.

 

 

        For VERs and SERs recorded from central scalp, the responses of the DS subjects were noticeably larger than those of the normal controls at each age level.   The amplitude difference tended to be accentuated in the older age groups for central and frontal VERs.

        We investigated the relationship of single trial response (STR) amplitude and variability to averaged evoked response amplitude for two reasons.   First, we were curious to find out whether the larger averaged evoked responses found for DS subjects might be related to reduced variability among their STRs.   That is, if STR wave forms are more similar from one response to another there would be less cancellation during the averaging process and the resulting averaged response would be larger.   Second, others have reported that the averaged evoked responses of infants (Barnet, Ohlrich & Shanks, 1971) and of normal children (Lichy, Veselý, Adler & Zizka, 1975) show a habituation effect, i.e., the responses become progressively smaller with repeated stimulation, while those of DS children of similar age do not.   Analyses of STRs would suggest whether the habituation found for normals was the result of decreasing amplitude or increasing variability of STRs with continued stimulation, or to a combination of the two factors.

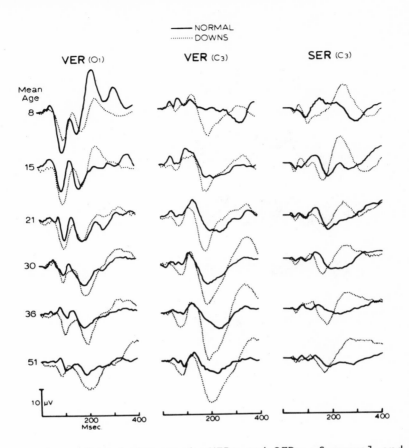

Figure 4.  Age related changes in VERs and SERs of normal and
Down's syndrome individuals.  Each tracing was averaged from the
VERs of 11 subjects within an age group.  The mean age for each
group is shown at the left.


Only data related to visual stimulation will be reported.

The 100 STRs from which each VER was averaged were divided
into ten successive blocks of 10 STRs each. Only odd numbered
blocks were analyzed to reduce computation time.  A mean amplitude
and variability measure encompassing the 80-220 msec interval of
each STR was obtained for each set.  In addition, a VER was
averaged from the 10 STRs in each set and the amplitude of the
VER was calculated using the procedure for obtaining the amplitude
of an STR.  The STRs and VERs of one subject are portrayed in
Figure 6.

SINGLE TRIAL
RESPONSES                          AVERAGED VER

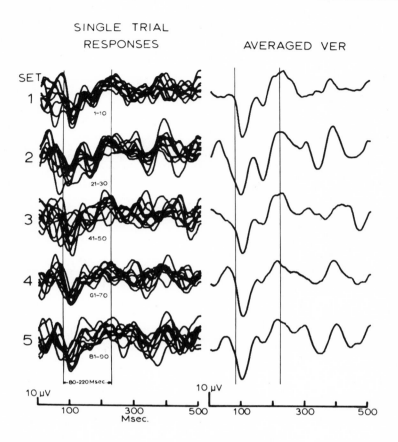

Figure 5.  Five sets of 10 superimposed single trial responses (STRs)
are shown in the left column, while the VER averaged from each set
of 10 STRs is traced in the right column.  The vertical lines delineate the 80-220 msec interval from which variability and amplitude
measures were obtained (see text).  The numbers beneath each set of
STRs, e.g., 1-10, indicate the STRs selected for analysis from a
total of 100 obtained from each subject for a particular electrode
site.  Note that the voltage calibrations for the two columns are
different.


        Figure 6 summarizes the VER and STR results for occipital
and central areas.  VER amplitudes of normal subjects changed
significantly across sets.  For responses from occipital scalp,
the mean amplitude of set 1 was reliably larger than that of sets
3, 4, and 5 (p <.02) while for central VERs the amplitudes of both

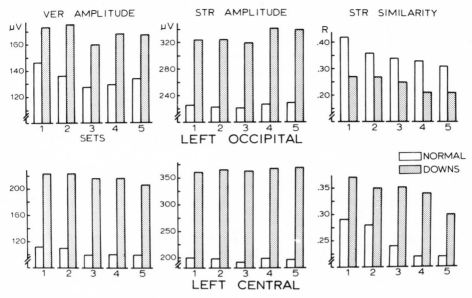

Figure 6.   Results of VER amplitude and STR amplitude and similarity
analyses for 66 normals and 66 Down's syndrome subjects.   VER
amplitude and STR similarity for the normal group showed reliable
habituation effects across sets.   Occipital STRs of the normal subjects were more similar (less variable) than those of the Down's
subjects while the opposite was true for STRs from central scalp.
Measures were from an 80-220 msec interval of VERs and STRs.


sets 1 and 2 were reliably larger than those of the remaining
sets (p <.02).   VER amplitudes of the DS subjects did not change
significantly across sets.   Thus, the 10 flash VERs of normals
demonstrated an habituation effect across time while those of
the DS people did not.

     The mean STR amplitudes did not change reliably across sets
for either group, although the mean amplitude of the Down's STRs
were much larger than those of the normals (p <.001).   Measures
of STR variability, however, paralleled the results reported above
for VER amplitude.   For normal subjects, STRs became less similar
(more variable) with repeated stimulation (p <.001, occipital;
p <.01 central).   Mean correlations did not differ across sets
for the Down's subjects.

     It is interesting to note the pattern of STR correlations
between the two groups of subjects.   Occipital STRs of normal subjects were more similar than those of the DS subjects (p <.005)
while the reverse was true for central STRs; intercorrelations
were larger for the Down's group (p <.01).   This may help to

explain the averaged evoked response results portrayed in Figures
3 and 4, in which there are minimal VER amplitude differences between the occipital responses of the two groups, while the central
VERs of the DS subjects are much larger than those of the normals.
A combination of larger STR amplitudes and a higher degree of similarity among the central responses of the Down's group would produce the enhanced averaged VER amplitudes.  The increased variability of the Down's occipital STRs apparently counteracted their
larger STR amplitudes, such that their averaged occipital VERs
were reasonably similar in amplitude to those of the normals.

The larger STR amplitudes found for the Down's subjects
paralleled power spectral analysis (PSA) results obtained from the
EEGs of the two groups.  To obtain a relative estimate of EEG
amplitude of the normals and Down's, PSA was computed on 100 one-
second epochs of EEG recorded during the VER run of each subject.
Each one-second epoch immediately preceded a flash.  Since flashes
were presented at 2-3 second intervals, each epoch, with the exception of the first, followed a flash by 1-2 seconds.  Power was computed over a frequency band of 3-14 Hz.  The EEGs of the DS subjects
generated about two and a half times as much power as did the EEGs
of the normals thus indicating that their background brain waves
were larger.

We found that Down's syndrome individuals have larger evoked
responses than do normals, which is consistent with earlier reports
for VERs (Bigum et al., 1970; Galbraith, Glidden, & Busk, 1970;
Glidden, Galbraith, & Busk, 1975), AERs (Barnet & Lodge, 1967;
Barnet, Ohlrich, & Shanks, 1971; Straumanis, Shagass, & Overton,
1973a) and SERs (Bigum et al., 1970; Straumanis et al., 1973b). We
did not, however, observe age-related changes in the evoked responses of DS subjects similar to those found for normals.  Rather
than late component amplitudes becoming smaller with increasing age,
wave components of the DS subjects, in some instances, become larger.

The enhanced amplitudes of the DS subjects likely reflects
deficits in the central inhibition of afferent stimuli.  Others
have also suggested that the brains of DS individuals are characterized by inhibitory deficits (Barnet & Lodge, 1967; Bigum et al.,
1970; Marcus, 1970; Glidden et al., 1975; Crapper et al., 1975).

The absence of age-related trends among the DS group may be
related to both defective central inhibition and the levels of
stimulus intensity employed in our experiments.  Glidden, Busk,
and Galbraith (1975) found that when DS and normal subjects were
exposed to progressively brighter stimuli, the amplitude of VERs
recorded from the DS subjects increased at a faster rate than that
for normals.  Thus, had we used less intense stimuli, the responses
of the DS group may have shown more definite age-related changes.
That is, deficits in the central inhibition of afferent stimulation

may result in enhanced averaged evoked responses to visual intensities typically used with normal subjects which mask possible age-
related changes in VER amplitude.  This "overstimulation" hypothesis
may best be tested by employing stimuli which are closer to a threshold level.

Two additional comments should be made regarding these data.
This study replicates the findings of Barnet et al. (1971) and
of Lichý et al. (1975) showing that the evoked responses of normals
habituate (show a response decrement) across time, while those of
DS subjects do not.  From our data it appears that the phenomenon
of habituation may be related more to increased variability of
STR wave form than to a reduction in single trial response amplitude.
The next study reports data which support this idea.

### THE CONTRIBUTION OF SINGLE TRIAL RESPONSE AMPLITUDE AND VARIABILITY TO AVERAGED VISUALLY EVOKED RESPONSE AMPLITUDE OF CHILDREN AND ADULTS

In an effort to determine whether the larger VER amplitudes
found in children (see Figs 1 & 2) might be related to STR variability, we studied the STRs of 20 eight and nine year old children
and of 20 adults ranging in age from 36-52 years.  VERs to 100
flashes had been recorded from four scalp areas ($C_3$, $C_4$, $O_1$, $O_2$)
of each subject.  The first 60 STRs of each VER were divided into
six successive sets of 10 STRs.  Amplitude and variability measures
were computed for three time intervals for each set:  0-100,
100-200, and 200-300 msec.

Age differences can be quickly summarized.  STR amplitudes,
similar to averaged VER amplitudes, were much larger in the
responses of the youngsters while STR variability was not different.
Thus, STR variability did not contribute to the VER amplitude differences between the children and adults.

Inspection of the STR data for the two groups combined (N=40)
suggests an habituation effect similar to that discussed in the
previous study.  Figure 7 shows the mean correlations across the
six sets of 10 STRs for the four scalp areas.  These data are for
the 100-200 msec interval.  For the four electrode sites combined,
STR intercorrelations decreased significantly across sets (p <.001),
the largest decrease occurring during the first two sets.  STR
amplitudes did not change reliably across sets.  Again, VER habituation appears to be related to increased STR variability rather than
to a decrease in STR amplitude.  A consistent, but nonsignificant,
hemispheric trend can be seen in Figure 7 with STRs from the
right side being less variable than those from the left.

How strong is the relationship between STR variability and
averaged evoked response amplitude?  We had 2880 measures of STR

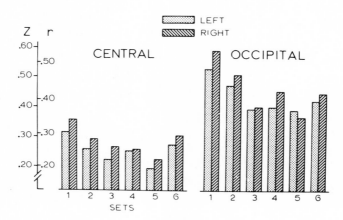

Figure 7. Results of STR similarity analyses for responses recorded from $C_3$, $C_4$, $O_1$, and $O_2$ electrode sites of 40 subjects (20 children and 20 adults). Note that the STRs in the first set were more similar (higher correlation) than those in the remaining sets. For each subject each set was composed of 10 successive single trial responses.

variability and amplitude and a similar number of VER amplitude measures (40 subjects, 4 scalp areas, 6 sets, 3 time intervals). Figure 8 is a scatter plot of the 2880 measures in which the abscissa shows the degree of similarity, or the converse, variability, for each set of 10 STR wave forms for a particular time interval. To eliminate individual differences in response size, amplitude was expressed as a percent: VER amplitude/STR amplitude x 100. If each of the 10 STRs in a set was identical to the others, the mean of the intercorrelations would be unity and one would expect that the mean amplitude of the 10 STRs would be equal to the amplitude of the VER averaged from these STRs. In this instance, VER amplitude would be 100 percent of the respective mean STR amplitude. As variability among STR wave forms increases, VER amplitude, because of the averaging process, should decrease and concomitantly percent amplitude would become smaller. The Y-coordinate of the scatter plot is percent amplitude. As can be seen in Figure 8, the relationship between the two variables was exceptionally strong. The correlation between STR similarity and the amplitude measure was 0.932.

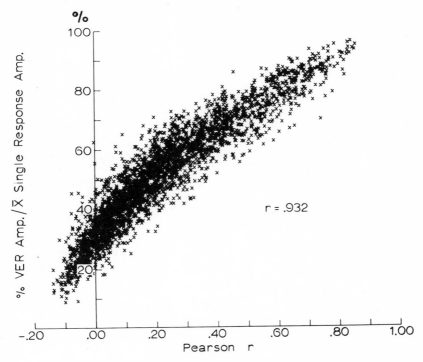

Figure 8.  The relationship of STR similarity to VER amplitude.  VER amplitude (Y-axis) is expressed as a percent of mean STR amplitude: VER amplitude/STR amplitude.  The X-axis represents the mean inter-correlation of the 10 STRs within a set from which the corresponding VER and STR amplitudes were derived.  A total of 2880 data points are plotted (40 subjects, 4 electrode sites, 6 sets, 3 time inter-vals).  The time intervals were 0-100, 100-200, and 200-300 msec. The correlation between similarity and VER amplitude measures was 0.932.

## THE RELATIONSHIP OF ALCOHOLISM TO AGING

There is some evidence which suggests that alcoholism may be conducive to premature aging.  For example, Courville (1955) reported striking similarities in cortical atrophy and diffuse cell loss in alcoholics and normal oldsters.  Patterns of psychometric test scores have also shown parallels between alcoholism and aging (Fitzhugh, Fitzhugh & Reitan, 1965; Williams, Ray & Overall; 1973).

Two studies were conducted in our laboratory to investigate

the possibility that alcoholism leads to early aging.  In the first,
the evoked responses of alcoholics and normals were investigated,
while in the second, dependent measures were scores on a battery
of neuropsychological tests and the Wechsler Adult Intelligence
Test.  The same subjects were included in each study.

Three groups of 20 right handed male subjects were studied
(Cannon, 1974; Blusewicz, Schenkenberg, Dustman & Beck, 1977).
The first group, young normals, consisted of non-drinkers and
social drinkers with a mean age of 31 years.  The second group,
young alcoholics, consisted of problem drinkers whose mean age was
33 years.  The alcoholics had a mean duration of problem drinking
of 13.3 years and a mean period of abstinence from alcohol of
approximately 40 days at the time they were studied.  To be included in the study each must have experienced drinking related
problems in four of the six following areas:  1) at least a 10 year
history of drinking; 2) severe withdrawal symptoms such as delirium
tremens and seizures; 3) loss of job; 4) divorce or separation;
5) legal problems such as bankruptcy; 6) medical and/or psychiatric
hospitalization.

The third group, elderly normals, consisted of non-drinkers
and social drinkers whose mean age was 71 years.  The mean educa-
tional levels of the three groups were comparable.

### Evoked Responses, Alcholism and Aging

Visual evoked responses were recorded from each subject.
Figure 9 is a graphic portrayal of VERs recorded from occipital
and central scalp of the three groups.

Two trends were observed in the visual evoked response data
which 1) differentiated the oldsters from the two younger groups,
and 2) highlighted similarities between the oldsters and young
alcoholics.  With respect to the first, the latencies of most
wave components were reliably longer in the VERs of the elderly
as compared to the two younger groups.  In addition, the amplitudes
of two earlier occipital waves, P60 and N80, and two earlier central
waves, N45 and P60, were significantly larger in the responses of
the oldsters.

Parallels between the alcoholics and oldsters was reflected
primarily in VERs from occipital scalp.  The amplitudes and
latencies of two later waves, P100 and N140, of the young alcoholics
and elderly normals were equivalent and significantly different from
those of the young normals (p <.01).  These waves were smaller and
occurred later in the responses of the alcoholics and oldsters
(see Fig. 9).  With one exception, centrally derived VERs of the
alcoholics and elderly normals were different.  A late VER wave

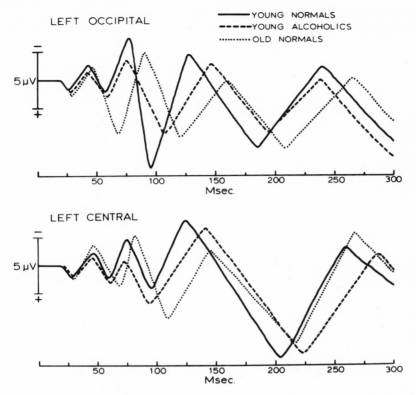

Figure 9.  Visual evoked responses from occipital and central
scalp of 20 young normals, 20 young alcoholics and 20 elderly
normal subjects.  The tracings were constructed by plotting the
mean latency and amplitude values of the various VER waves and
drawing interconnecting lines between the mean values.

from central scalp, N140, occurred reliably later in their responses than in those of the young controls (p <.01).

## Psychometric Test Scores, Alcoholism and Aging

        Eight tests drawn from a battery developed in our laboratory,
the Reitan Indiana Neuropsychological Test Battery, and the
Wechsler Adult Intelligence Scale (WAIS) were administered to each
subject.  Detailed descriptions of the Neuropsychology Tests and
scoring procedures can be found in Reitan (1955); Graham and
Kendall (1960); Grundvig, Needham, Ajax and Beck (1970); Blusewicz
(1975).  A brief description of each test follows.
        1)  Spiral Aftereffect.  A rotating spiral wheel is viewed
and the duration of an aftereffect (an illusion that the wheel
reverses direction after it is stopped) is measured.

2) Complex Reaction Time. The subject presses a response switch as quickly as possible following the illumination of two of four differently colored lights.

3) Graham-Kendall Memory for Designs. The subject draws from memory each of 15 designs which are individually flashed on a screen for one-half second.

4) Category Test. This test has seven parts. For each a series of geometric figures and designs is viewed and the subject abstracts and reports a principle which runs through the series.

5) Tactual Performance. The subject while blindfolded is requested to place blocks of varying shapes and sizes into corresponding spaces on a form board.

6) Trails-B. A measure is made of the time required for a subject to connect circled numbers and letters in correct sequence. The correct sequence is 1 to A, A to 2, 2 to B., etc.

7) Tapping. A measure is made of the number of times a subject can tap a telegraph key with his index finger during an interval of 10 seconds.

8) Rhythm. The subject is required to make a judgement of same or different with regard to 30 pairs of tape-recorded rhythmical patterns.

A comparison of the three groups on each of the tests can be seen in Figure 10. Striking age effects were observed. The young normals performed significantly better than the oldsters on every test. Means for the young alcoholics, with the exception of Spiral Aftereffect, fell between those of the young and elderly controls. On all but two tests, Category and Tactual Performance, they too performed reliably better than the oldest group. Their scores on four tests, Memory for Designs, Category, Tactual Performance, and Trails-B, were significantly lower than those of their age-matched controls.

An impairment index was calculated for each subject from his scores on selected tests of the Reitan Battery (Category, Tactual Performance, Trails-B, Tapping, and Rhythm) according to the procedures outlined in Reitan's Manual for Administration of Neuropsychological Test Batteries for Adults and Children (undated). The impairment index provides a global measure of neuropsychological functioning (Reitan, 1955) and, in comparison to young normals, an indication of neurological damage.

Similar to the profile resulting from the neuropsychological test scores, the Impairment Index scores of the young alcoholics fell between those of the young and elderly normal groups (see Fig. 10). The mean for each group was significantly different from those of the other two groups (p <.01).

Figure 11 portrays mean WAIS verbal and performance scaled subtest scores for each of the three groups of subjects. A pattern

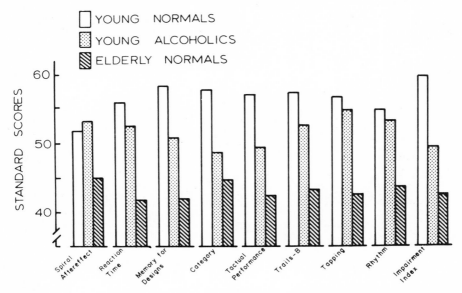

Figure 10. A summary of neuropsychology test scores for 20 young normals, 20 young alcoholics and 20 elderly normals. Scores were converted to standard scores having a mean of 50 and a standard deviation of 10. For each test a higher score indicates better performance.

of results similar to that reported for the neuropsychology tests (see Fig. 10) was found, with the scores of the young alcoholics being better than those of the oldsters but poorer than those of their age-matched controls. In general, the young alcoholics resembled the oldsters more with respect to verbal than to the performance subtests. For example, only one verbal subtest, Similarities, significantly differentiated the two groups, while the scores of the alcoholics on all performance subtests, except Block Design, were significantly higher than those of the elderly normals. Again, the effects of age alone are evident. The young normals' scores on all subtests but Arithmetic and Digit Span were reliably larger than those of the oldsters.

The results of these studies were similar. Each clearly showed marked differences between the young and elderly normal groups. VER early waves were larger in the responses of the oldsters, while late waves were smaller and most of the waves had delayed latencies. In addition, the oldsters' performance on both the Neuropsychological and WAIS tests were decidely inferior to the performance of the young normal group.

Despite the nearly 40 year age difference between the young

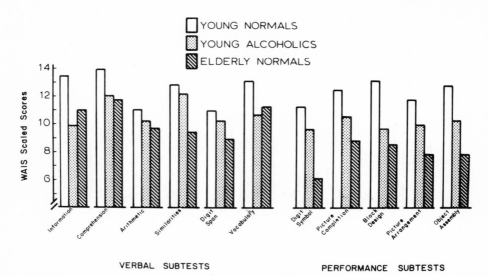

Figure 11. Wechsler Adult Intelligence Test scores for three groups of 20 subjects: young normal, young alcoholic and elderly normal.

alcoholics and normal oldsters, the evoked responses and test performances of the two groups exhibited a surprising number of similarities. It is interesting to note that the WAIS scores of the alcoholics and elderly normals were more alike on verbal than performance subtests and that the two groups achieved scores which were more similar on those neuropsychology tests which measured reasoning and short term memory, i.e., Category and Tactual Performance, than on those which measured more fundamental sensory-motor functions. In accord with the above are the evoked response findings. Later VER wave components, presumed to be associated with central processing and cognitive functioning, did not differentiate the alcoholics from the oldsters while the two groups were clearly different with respect to earlier waves which are believed to reflect the reception of sensory stimuli.

EVOKED RESPONSES OF PATIENTS WITH AMYOTROPHIC LATERAL SCLEROSIS (ALS)

This uncommon and fatal disease is probably best known as the disease that killed Lou Gehrig, famous first baseman for the New York Yankees, and Ezzard Charles, world champion boxer.

Little is known about the etiology and pathophysiology of ALS but the clinical course of the disease has been well described. The disease is highly selective for the moto-neuron and soma as with poliomyelitis. Thus by definition ALS is a chronic, progressive degenerative disease involving both the upper motor systems, the corticospinal and corticobulbar tracts and the lower motor neurons or ventral horn cells in the final common pathway of the spinal cord. The duration of the disease is one to five years, death generally resulting from involvement of bulbar motor cells. Thus the majority of these patients die of respiratory failure, dysphagia, or aspiration pneumonia.

Our interest in the disease, beyond our hope to contribute information contributing to earlier and possibly more reliable diagnoses, lies in the fact that moto-neuron involvement is so precise, e.g., upper motor neuron involvement is limited primarily to the somatic efferent motor cells of area 4. There is no involvement of visceral efferents such as urinary sphincter or certain abdominal reflexes. As a disease that selectively destroys the Betz cells in area 4 of the motor cortex, the lateral and ventral corticospinal tracts and the anterior horn cells in the spinal cord, it provides an experimental model that the most skilled surgeon could not provide. Motor systems from cortex through the pyramidal tracts to anterior horn cells are selectively destroyed with no disturbance of any of the sensory input or afferent systems. Bereft of motor input or modification, the somatosensory system may function quite differently. We may learn what components of the somatosensory evoked response are affected, or possibly even derived, from motor involvement. A number of answers regarding the reciprocal relationship of afferent-efferent systems may be answered. For example, there is evidence (Lawrence & Kuypers, 1968a,b; Nyberg-Hansen, 1966) that pyramidal tract collaterals enter the substantia gelatinosa of the dorsal horn of the spinal cord, thereby providing a neuroanatomical substrate for influence on or control of afferent impulses which may mediate tactile or proprioceptive sensation. Furthermore, when sensory nerves and the pyramidal tract are simultaneously stimulated (electrically), the evoked potentials from the sensory nerve stimulation, recorded both at the spinal cord level and at the cortex, change markedly (Nyberg-Hansen, 1966).

There are other reasons to believe that there may be motor or pyramidal feedback acting directly on the somatosensory system. Lesions which release reflexes like the grasping or groping reflex are often regarded as cortical, implying a direct link between somatosensory and pyramidal neurons. Some of the abnormal reflexes noted in patients with ALS may result from altered proprioceptive and tactile input at the spinal cord level. That is, some of the spinal release mechanisms producing hyperflexia, often seen in the disease, may result from modification of tactile input at the cord level because of the reduction of pyramidal output, i.e., reduced inhibition of afferent input at the spinal cord level. Thus, there may be an interruption of inhibitory collaterals that go through internuncial neurons acting on dorsal horn cells.

Finally, psychologists make much of what they call S-R or stimulus-response relationships. Does the response have the significance they argue or is it just an addendum to the real course of events that are occurring between sensory systems? Thus there are those who maintain that behavior, learning and the like, are mainly determined by repeated association of stimulus and response, that is, S-R theorists. If this is so, there should be reciprocal relationships of sensory and motor systems throughout the motor system. Evoked responses should reflect such relationships. That is, afferent input in the somatosensory evoked response of patients with amyotrophic lateral sclerosis should be different than that of normal individuals. These differences, if indeed there are such differences, should shed some light on the functional relationships between sensory and motor systems in the human nervous system.

We are currently studying 20 patients, ranging in age from 35 to 60 years. Thirteen of these are confirmed ALS patients, all having supporting findings from muscle biopsy and EMGs. Seven show serious anterior horn cell degeneration and most probably have ALS. We are recording somatosensory evoked potentials of approximately 50 control subjects in this age range so that each patient will have an age and sex matched control. Our methods for recording, data analysis, etc., have been previously described. Somatosensory stimuli are presented at five different intensities, 1-1/2, 2, 2-1/2, and 3 times threshold, and at 80 volts. VERs are being recorded to diffuse and patterned light. Additionally each subject is given a series of sensory tests such as the Critical Flicker Fusion, Auditory Flutter Fusion, and Stroop Color Test as a check on other sensory systems.

At this time the somatosensory evoked potentials of the patients appear to differ from those of the matched controls. Further, there is a difference between the confirmed ALS patients and the anterior horn cell disease patients. Figure 12 illustrates a comparison of the SERs and VERs of nine patients and nine controls. It should be noted that the somatosensory evoked potentials of the patients differ in amplitude from those of the normals, while the visual evoked potentials appear not to discriminate the two groups. Data at this time are not sufficient for statistical analysis, but trends appear to be emerging as may be seen in the figure.

Because ALS involves three distinct but related phenomena, degeneration of ventral horn cells, bilateral involvement of long motor tracts with progressive muscular atrophy, and progressive bulbar-palsy, it was described for many years as three different diseases. This is understandable as the initial manifestations may be spasticity, or atrophy with flaccidity, or both depending upon the degree or involvement of the upper and lower moto-neurons. In 1883 Dejerine integrated the symptoms into one complex as

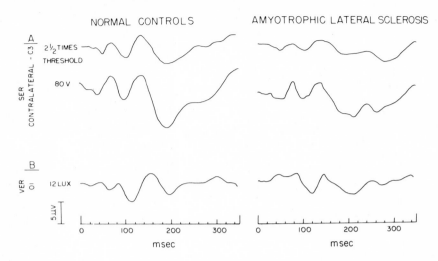

Figure 12.  A comparison of composite somatosensory and visual
evoked potentials of nine matched normal controls and nine
amyotrophic lateral sclerotic patients.  In A of the figure
differences in amplitudes and wave form configuration between
patients and controls may be seen.  In B, where visually evoked
potentials are compared, differences are not so evident.

essentially one disease, and it has been accepted since as one
disease which presents differently at different stages.  Consequently, the differences that we have noted between patients
presenting with confirmed ALS symptoms and those with anterior
horn disease may be a consequence of which part of the somatosensory system is most affected at the time of testing.

     A number of patients have been tested as many as four times
and there appears to be a gradual attenuation in the amplitude
of three components over time,  a positive wave at about 40 msec,
a negative wave at about 70 msec, followed by a positive wave
at about 110 msec.  There also is a trend in the direction of
increased latency with increasing severity of the disease.
Consequently, from the data we have acquired, despite the fact
that ALS is considered to be a purely motor disease, selectively
destroying only motor neurons, it appears that certain components
of the evoked somatosensory response are affected in some way by
motor or pyramidal feedback acting on the somatosensory system.
It is also possible that there are unobserved lesions of some
sensory systems.

EVOKED RESPONSES AND SLEEP CYCLES DURING SUSTAINED
INGESTION OF METHADONE IN MONKEYS

The characteristics of narcotic tolerance and dependence have
been extensively studied in recent years (for review, see Clouet
& Iwatsubo, 1975). It is apparent that a multitude of variables
determine the degree of dependence and the severity of the withdrawal syndrome. Unfortunately, relatively little attention has
been directed toward those effects, physiological or psychological,
which may accrue following prolonged ingestion of a narcotic.
Indeed, many "chronic" studies are limited to several hours, most
encompass a few days and a few are extended over several weeks.
Many of these studies have demonstrated that "chronic" exposure
to a narcotic causes biochemical, physiological and behavioral
changes which do not occur following acute or subacute administration of the drug (Domino & Wilson, 1975). Such changes may persist
despite the development of tolerance to other effects of the drug
(Esposito & Kornetsky, 1977). Thus, Eibergen and Carlson (1975)
provide convincing evidence that sustained methadone ingestion leads
to dopamine receptor supersensitivity which persists even after
many months in a drug-free environment. Similarly, Crowley et al.
(1975) determined that 10 weeks of methadone maintenance effected
obvious motor stimulation and altered social behavior in monkeys.
There was no evidence that the animals became tolerant to these
drug effects.

With tens of thousands of patients in methadone maintenance
programs, studies such as these provide useful and needed information. Perhaps the information that the drug is relatively safe
with generally nondebilitating side effects (Dobbs, 1971; Dole,
1970) is sufficient to warrant its use in prolonged maintenance
programs. However, except for the reliable information that the
EEGs of methadone patients show a decrease in alpha frequency
(Gritz et al., 1975; Isbell et al., 1947, 1948, 1949; Martin
et al., 1973; Roubicek et al., 1969), little is known regarding
the effects on the brain of long-term (e.g., one year) methadone
ingestion. Therefore we have repeatedly examined the visual
evoked responses (VERs) and sleep cycles of a group of monkeys
prior to and throughout a year of methadone maintenance, and for
over five months of withdrawal. In addition, plasma methadone
concentrations were determined for each animal throughout the
period of investigation.

## VER Studies

Twelve young adult, stump-tailed macaques (Macaca arctoides)
were stereotaxically implanted with stainless steel screw electrodes
contacting dura and with depth electrodes positioned according to
an atlas (Snider & Lee, 1961) in mesoreticular formation and hippocampus. However, only VERs recorded from striate cortex will be

described herein as histological confirmation of depth electrode
placement is not yet complete.  Electrodes were connected to
a small pedestal which was anchored to the skull (Shearer et al.,
1976).  Animals were allowed at least three weeks to recover from
surgery before recording began.

All animals were confined to plastic restraining chairs for
many months prior to and throughout the maintenance period except
for regular exercise periods.  During VER recording the restrained
animal was positioned with its eyes near the center of a reflecting
hemisphere into which 10 μsec flashes of light were delivered.
VERs were summed from blocks of 50 flashes which were presented
at about two second intervals during artifact free periods of EEG.

Following baseline recording, six monkeys began sustained
ingestion of methadone while six control animals received placebo
on the same schedule.  Methadone HCl dissolved in water was administered orally at 8:00 A.M., 4:00 P.M., and 9:30 P.M. daily in an
effort to keep the animals continually exposed to safe levels of
the drug.

During the initiation of methadone treatment the total daily
dose was increased rapidly to 15 mg/kg/day over a two-week period
and VERs were recorded at least four days per week between 12:00
Noon and 1:30 P.M.  Maintenance on 15 mg/kg/day began after the
second week.  Blood samples were drawn immediately after a recording session and plasma was extracted for radioimmunoassay of methadone content (Snyder et al., 1977).

During the initiation of methadone treatment neither the
animals' behavior nor their VERs changed appreciably from baseline.
However, occasionally throughout the first half year of maintenance,
at doses typically causing no depression, four of the animals occasionally evidenced moderate to severe drug intoxication while no
control animal ever evidenced a similar reaction (Snyder et al.,
1977).  Toxic reactions were sudden, unpredictable, and occurred
with no obvious precipitating factors such as illness, trauma or
decrease in body weight.  The reactions always occurred within
three hours of the morning dose and whenever nalorphine HCl was
administered respiratory depression was reversed within three
or four minutes.  Evoked responses during intoxication were characterized by a marked decrease in the amplitudes of all components,
early and late, and an increase in latencies (Fig. 13).  In each
instance intoxication was accompanied by marked increases in plasma
methadone concentration.  In one case the reaction was so severe
that, although nalorphine restored breathing the animal had suffered severe brain damage and died soon thereafter.

Other than the occasional behavioral and electrophysiological
depression of sudden intoxication, overall changes in the VER during

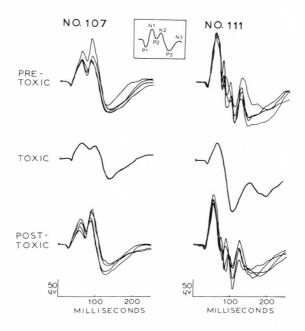

Figure 13.   VERs recorded from two monkeys prior to, during and following sudden toxic reactions.

the 12-month maintenance period were relatively minor, exhibiting a nonsignificant decrease in amplitude of most components (see Fig. 15 below).  However, the effects of the drug on sleep cycles were obvious, highly significant and persistent.

## Sleep Studies

While all opioids apparently disrupt normal sleep, the time course and extent of disruption during sustained drug ingestion have received scant attention.  Most narcotic analgesics produce a decrease in the proportion of REM and Stage 3-4 sleep after the first few doses (Echols & Jewett, 1972; Henderson, et al., 1970; Lewis et al., 1970, 1972) with a gradual return to approximate predrug levels after a week to 10 days.  Then, upon withdrawal a marked increase in REM and Stage 3-4 sleep typically occurs. Unfortunately, these studies provide little information regarding the long-term effects of narcotic analgesics on sleep. Attempts have been made to extend the period of study. Thus, six ex-heroin addicts, after six weeks of abstinence from opioids, were studied over a three-month "control phase" during which single doses of methadone and morphine were ingested (Kay, 1975). The subjects were then administered daily doses of methadone for approximately three months during which their sleep was recorded twice. Withdrawal extended for 22 weeks and it was demonstrated that Stage 3-4 and REM sleep remained well above control values for the six subjects (see also Martin et al., 1973). However, when compared to the mean value of 37 ex-heroin addicts studied separately, the REM sleep during withdrawal was only marginally elevated. In short, the pattern of sleep disruption during the initiation of methadone treatment, the quality of sleep during maintenance, and the nature of tolerance to the sleep-disruptive effects of the drug remain obscure. Similarly, the evidence for a REM "rebound" following long-term methadone ingestion is tentative. The importance of resolving these issues is apparent given the evidence that the effects of this widely prescribed drug may be cumulative (Goodman & Gilman, 1970). Therefore, we have studied over 50 nights of sleep in each of four stump-tailed macaques throughout a year of methadone maintenance and for five months following withdrawal.

Implanted animals were allowed at least five months to adapt to the restraining chairs and EEG recording procedure before baseline sleep recording began. Sleep records were then obtained for 14 consecutive nights during baseline and the initiation of drug treatment. Thereafter, during a year of drug maintenance and for many months of withdrawal, sleep was recorded at the intervals described below. Each recording session was preceded by three nights of adaptation to the procedure. At 4:30 P.M. on an adaptation or recording night EMG and EOG electrodes were applied and the EEG connector lead was attached to the animal's pedestal. At 9:30 P.M. the drug (or placebo during baseline and withdrawal) was administered, the animals were enclosed in separate, sound attenuating and vented isolation booths, lights were extinguished and white noise was turned on. At 6:00 A.M. the animals were removed from the booths. Sleep records were scored according to the Rechtschaffen and Kales (1968) technique and the following measures were derived: percent REM and non-REM (NREM) and percent awake based upon the total eight-hour recording session. In addition, the average interval length, total frequency and onset latency for each measure were obtained.

During the six night baseline period there were no consistent changes in the monkeys' sleep patterns. That is, none of the measures showed significant differences across nights as determined

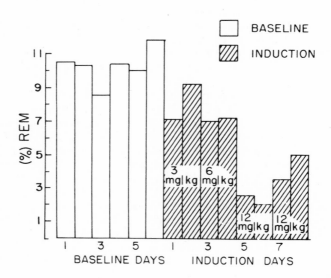

Figure 14.   Percent REM sleep during baseline and for eight days
of methadone induction during which time the dose was increased
rapidly.   Single factor analysis of variance indicates a significant
drug effect (p <.01).

by a single factor analysis of variance.   Our hopes that the
institution of the pre-recording adaptation period would eliminate
the uneconomical "first night effect" (Agnew et al., 1966) were
fulfilled.

Obvious changes in the monkeys' sleep occurred with the initiation of drug treatment.   As is apparent in Figure 14, percent REM
decreased significantly to reach its lowest level on the sixth
night of treatment.   Both percent NREM and percent awake were
slightly though nonsignificantly larger during induction as compared
to baseline.

Since the frequency of REM episodes did not decrease significantly during the initiation of drug treatment, it would appear
that the decrease in percent REM was due to a decrease in the

average length of a REM episode.

Percent REM sleep during the 12 months of methadone maintenance is portrayed in Figure 15.  As is evident, percent REM remained markedly below baseline values for the first eight months.  Single factor analyses of variance with tests for nonadditivity and appropriate transformations (Meyers, 1969) indicated that during the maintenance period percent REM was significantly below predrug and withdrawal values.  As was the case during the initiation of drug treatment, percent NREM and percent awake were both somewhat elevated but the differences were not significant.

By the eleventh month of maintenance the percent REM was within two standard deviations of the predrug baseline mean and remained there throughout withdrawal.  Similarly, the other sleep measures were not significantly different from baseline during the withdrawal period.

In short, percent REM was the most sensitive indicator of drug effect and remained suppressed for at least eight months of maintenance.  Upon withdrawal percent REM was slightly greater than predrug values.  However, the mean value across monkeys evidenced no statistically significant "rebound."

It has long been recognized that drug effects may evidence tolerance differentially (Clouet & Iwatsubo, 1975).  That is, a rat may develop tolerance to the analgesic effects of morphine but not to its convulsive properties.

The results of our studies suggest that sustained methadone ingestion may have markedly different effects depending upon which "system" is examined.  Generally stable evoked responses were interspersed with periods of sudden methadone intoxication with gross electrophysiological depression, while REM sleep remained uniformly suppressed until the seventh or eighth month of maintenance (Fig. 15) despite progressively smaller maintenance doses.

These results restate the apparent insensitivity of nonnociceptive sensory pathways to opioids (Borison, 1971) while confirming and expanding the evidence for opioid induced REM sleep suppression.  Any evidence of protracted drug effects on sleep is of obvious significance especially when the drug under study is currently being administered to many thousands of patients across the country.  Whether our results are species-specific is not known.  However, the REM suppression was of sufficient duration and magnitude to warrant further testing with similar techniques in human subjects.  The absence of a clearly defined REM rebound following drug withdrawal is of particular interest, given the evidence that such a rebound occurs in humans (Kay, 1975).  It is possible that extended periods (e.g., two months) of stable, relatively normal REM sleep

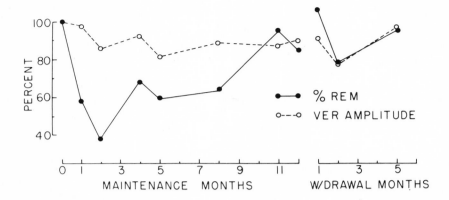

Figure 15.   Percent REM sleep and total VER amplitude over the period of extended drug ingestion and withdrawal.

prior to withdrawal preclude a rebound despite earlier REM deficits.

### THE EVOKED POTENTIAL AS A TECHNIQUE FOR ASSESSING CEREBRAL DEATH

During the past several years modern resuscitative procedures have made it difficult to define death in terms of the traditional signs alone, and have brought about an increased awareness of the problems of defining "brain death."  This in turn has led physicians to evaluate levels of unconsciousness when attempting to determine when an individual is dead.  Thus, with modern advances in medical technology and the increasing demand for organ transplantation, all techniques available should be applied for a reliable evaluation of cerebral death.  Presently, the "isoelectric" or "flat" EEG has been an indicator of cerebral death when confirmed at two examinations within 24 hours.  The pronouncement of brain death necessitates recording at high gain or sensitivity which may invalidate the interpretation of the EEG due to pickup of the electrocardiogram, ballistocardiogram and any mechanical vibration that may occur.

To rely on the EEG alone in diagnosing brain death also poses other problems.  Conditions such as barbiturate intoxication, anoxia and ischemia often result in prolonged isoelectric EEG, which occasionally is not conclusive evidence of cerebral death (Wulff, 1959; Meyer & Gastaut, 1961; Bird & Plum, 1968; Hossman & Sato, 1970).  In fact patients with isoelectric EEG have survived  (see Figure 16).  With barbiturate intoxication there have been reports of survival after hours and even days of flat EEG.  A similar situation has been seen in patients in hypothermia.

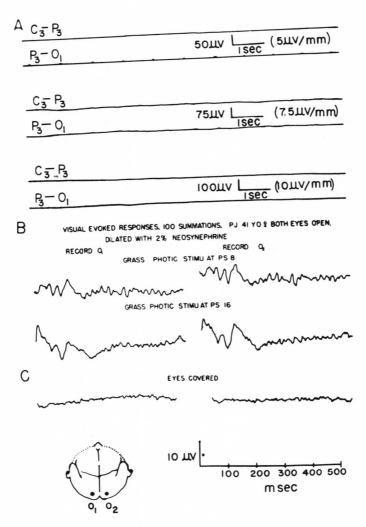

Figure 16.   The visually evoked potential during EEG silence.
A.   An isoelectric EEG at three different gain settings in a 41
year old vegetative female with extensive cerebral injury.
B.   Visual evoked potentials may be elicited and, although
distorted, they change with light intensity and disappear when the
eyes are closed.   (From Beck, Dustman, & Lewis, 1975, by courtesy
of the Editor of International Journal of Neurology)

This study was a comparison of the EEG and the evoked potential during epochs of serious cerebral embarrassment induced by various means and characterized by isoelectric cortical activity. Three different situations were experimentally produced: cerebral ischemia, barbiturate intoxication, and anoxia.

Twelve cats, four for each condition, permanently implanted stereotaxically with an array of cortical and subcortical electrodes were studied. Electrodes were on marginal and middle Sylvian gyri, in the center median, mesencephalic reticular formation, and hippocampus. Visually evoked responses were recorded throughout the experiment. Critical measures were: (1) changes in EKG and blood pressure until the lower limits of each of these functions were reached, (2) EEG from onset until the occurrence of continuous isoelectric activity, (3) the averaged peak-to-peak amplitude of the positive/negative sequence of primary evoked responses and that of the succeeding positive/negative secondary sequence, and (4) latencies of these same potentials.

The animals were deeply anesthetized, tracheotomized, curarized, and placed under artificial ventilation with room air while body temperature was kept constant at 35-37° C with heating pads. Several evoked response control records were obtained from each animal prior to the induction of the experimental condition. Asphyxia was induced by turning off the mechanical respirator and the anoxic state was allowed to continue for one minute following the cessation of all spontaneous electrical activity. Cerebral ischemia was produced by clamping the innominate artery anterior to the point of bifurcation from the aortic arch. Arterial blood supply to the brain was interrupted for one minute following the cessation of all spontaneous electrical activity. Barbiturate intoxication was produced by sodium pentobarbital in small successive doses of 10 to 20 mg every fifteen minutes until an isoelectric EEG resulted. Cats were later sacrificed, brains were perfused with saline and formaldehyde and electrode placements were confirmed.

After asphyxic anoxia was induced, the EEG activity was characterized by slowing, attenuation, and finally becoming isoelectric. By three minutes these transitions were complete. The ischemic condition produced a much more rapid isoelectric EEG than did the anoxic; the EEG became flat in less than one minute after clamping. Following the cessation of the anoxic and ischemic episodes, the spontaneous cerebral activity was seen to reappear in approximately one minute. The small amplitude returning activity gradually increased so that "normal EEG" had fully returned in two to five minutes.

During the anoxic and ischemic episodes the primary or early component of the response survived well beyond the time the EEG had become isoelectric. In the anoxic state the primary component eventually disappeared, even though seemingly normal EEG ultimately

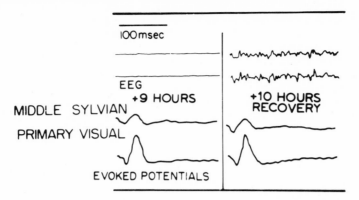

Figure 17.  EEG activity, top of figure, and visually evoked potentials from middle Sylvian and primary visual cortex recorded during
intense barbiturate intoxication and following recovery of EEG.
EEG was isoelectric for 9 hours, however, primary components of the
evoked potential never disappeared during that period.

returned.  EEG and evoked potential changes during barbiturate
intoxication were of great interest in that, in this condition,
the evoked response endured with little change in amplitude throughout all the experiments despite 9-12 hours of isoelectric EEG (see
Fig. 17).  The EEG changes during baribiturate intoxication were
similar to the anoxic and ischemic changes, although the progres-
sion was, of course, slower and recovery took much longer.

These results suggest that the evoked response technique
provides valuable information in the presence of ambiguous EEG
activity, particularly with suspected deaths due to overdose
of barbiturate or other depressants.  Interference from extracerebral potential sources and artifacts in the EEG may be minimized or eliminated when the cortical evoked response to sensory
stimuli is examined concomitantly with the EEG.  The characteristic
wave form of the response, visual, auditory, etc., minimizes confusion with artifact.  Trojaborg & Jørgensen (1973) tried such
a procedure with 50 patients and found that the absence of the
evoked response was a reliable evidence of brain death in unconscious, unresponsive patients.  The technique is particularly
indicated when death is a result of suspected suicide attempts
with barbiturates and other depressants.  Figure 17 is an illustration of the usefulness of the technique, indicating that even
though the EEG has been isoelectric for several hours, the evoked
potential continues.  Starr (1976) reports a similar useful

application of the auditory evoked response, relying on far-field potentials which are believed to be generated from the brain stem.

In summary we feel that our studies show that the cerebral evoked response can provide useful insights and information regarding brain dysfunction in a variety of disorders and situations even when efforts are not made to impose cognitive tasks on the subjects. Indeed, in some instances, as for example with Down's syndrome and cortically damaged patients, procedures need to be relatively simple and straightforward.

## ACKNOWLEDGEMENTS

Supported by the Medical Research Service of the Veterans Administration, research projects 1973-06, 1973-08, 0864-02, 0864-05, and by the National Institutes of Health research grants, DA00388 and AG00568.

We wish to acknowledge Drs. M. J. Blusewicz and W. G. Cannon, principal investigators of the experiments which investigated the relationship of alcohol to aging; Dr. E. M. Behrens, principal investigator of the experiments of techniques for assessing cerebral death, and Dr. T. Schenkenberg for his contributions to the study of changes in evoked responses during aging.

## REFERENCES

Agnew, H. W., Wilse, W. B. and Williams, R. L. The first night effect: An EEG study of sleep. Psychophysiology 2:263-266, 1966.

Alajouanine, T., Scherrer, J., Barbizet, J., Calvet, J. and Verley, R. Potentiels evoques corticaux chez des sujects atteints de troubles somesthetiques. Rev. Neurol. (Paris) 98:757-761, 1958.

Asselman, P., Chadwick, D. W. and Marsden, C. D. Visual evoked responses in the diagnosis and management of patients suspected of multiple sclerosis. Brain 98:261-282, 1975.

Barnet, A. B. and Lodge, A. Diagnosis of deafness in infants with the use of computer-averaged electroencephalographic responses to sound. J. Pediat. 69:753-758, 1966.

Barnet, A. B. and Lodge, A. Click evoked EEG responses in normal and developmentally retarded infants. Nature, 214:252-255, 1967.

Barnet, A. B., Ohlrich, E. S. and Shanks, B. L.  EEG evoked re-
    sponses to repetitive auditory stimulation in normal and
    Down's syndrome infants. Dev. Med. Child Neurol. 13:321-329,
    1971.

Beck, E. C.  Electrophysiology and Behavior.  In M. R. Rosenzweig
    and L. W. Porter (Eds.), Annual Review of Psychology 26:
    233-262, 1975.

Beck, E. C. and Dustman, R. E.  Changes in the evoked response in
    maturation and aging in man and macaque.  In N. R. Burch (Ed.),
    Behavior and brain electrical activity.  New York:  Plenum
    Press, Pp. 431-472, 1975.

Beck, E. C., Dustman, R. E. and Lewis, E. G.  The use of the
    averaged evoked potential in the evaluation of central
    nervous system disorders.  Int. J. Neurol. 9:211-232, 1975.

Begleiter, H., Porjesz, B. and Garozzo, R.  Affect and evoked
    potentials.  In H. Begleiter (Ed.), Evoked brain potentials.
    New York: Plenum, 1979, in press.

Behrens, E. M., Beck, E. C. and Dustman, R. E.  The averaged visual
    evoked potential as a technique for assessing cerebral death.
    Society for Neuroscience, 3:326, 1973.

Benda, C. E.  The child with mongolism.  New York:  Grune &
    Stratton, Inc., 1960.

Benda, C. E.  Down's syndrome.  New York:  Grune & Stratton, 1969.

Bergamini, L. and Bergamasco, B.  Cortical evoked potentials in
    man.  C. C. Thomas, Springfield, Ill., 1967.

Bigum, H. B., Dustman, R. E. and Beck, E. C.  Visual and somato-
    sensory evoked responses from mongoloid and normal children.
    Electroencephalogr. Clin. Neurophysiol. 28:202-205, 1970.

Bird, T. D. and Plum, F.  Recovery from barbiturate overdose coma
    with a prolonged isoelectric EEG.  Neurology 18:456-460,
    1968.

Blusewicz, M. J.  Neuropsychological correlates of chronic
    alcoholism and aging.  Unpublished doctoral dissertation.
    Pennsylvania State University, 1975.

Blusewicz, M. J., Schenkenberg, T., Dustman, R. E. and Beck, E. C.
    WAIS performance in young normal, young alcoholic, and
    elderly normal groups:  An evaluation of organicity and mental
    aging indices.  J. Clin. Psychol., in press, 1977.

Borison, H. L. Sites of action of narcotic analgesic drugs. The nervous system. In D. H. Clouet (Ed.). Narcotic drugs, biochemical pharmacology. New York: Plenum, pp. 342-365, 1971.

Buchsbaum, M. S. Signal to noise ratio and response variability in affective disorders and schizophrenia. In H. Begleiter (Ed.), Evoked brain potentials. New York: Plenum, 1977, in press.

Burger, P. C. and Vogel, F. S. The development of the pathologic changes of Alzheimer's disease and senile dementia in patients with Down's syndrome. Am. J. Pathol. 74:457, 1973.

Callaway, E. In H. Begleiter (Ed.), Evoked brain potentials. New York: Plenum, 1977, in press.

Callner, D. A. Developmental trends in the visual, auditory, and somatosensory evoked responses of normal and Down's syndrome individuals. Unpublished doctoral dissertation, University of Utah, 1975.

Callner, D. A., Dustman, R. E., Madsen, J. A., Schenkenberg, T. and Beck, E. C. Life span changes in the averaged evoked responses of Down's syndrome and normal subjects. Am. J. Ment. Defic., 1977, in press.

Cannon, W. G. Cortical evoked responses of young normal, young alcoholic and elderly normal individuals. Unpublished doctoral dissertation, Brigham Young University, 1974.

Clouet, D. H. and Iwatsubo, K. Mechanisms of tolerance to and dependence on narcotic analgesic drugs. Annu. Rev. Pharmacol. 15:49-71, 1975.

Cody, E. T. R. and Bickford, R. G. Cortical audiometry: An objective method of evaluating auditory acuity in man. Proc. Mayo Clinic, 40:273-277, 1965.

Courville, C. B. Effects of alcohol on the nervous system of man. San Lucas, Los Angeles, 1955.

Cracco, R. O. Clinical application of averaged evoked responses to somatic stimulation. Int. J. Neurol., 9:233-246, 1975.

Crapper, D. R., Dalton, A. J., Skopitz, M., Scott, J. W., and Hachinski, V. C. Alzheimer degeneration in Down's syndrome. Arch. Neurol. 32:618-623, 1975.

Croft, T. J., Brodkey, J. S. and Nulsen, F. E.  Reversible spinal
    cord trauma:  A model for electrical monitoring of spinal cord
    function.  J. Neurosurg., 36:402-406, 1972.

Crome, L.  Some morbid-anatomical aspects of mental deficiency.
    J. Ment. Sci. 100: 894-902, 1954.

Crome, L., Cowie, V., and Slater, E.  A statistical note on cere-
    bellar and brain-stem weight in mongolism.  J. Ment. Defic.
    Res., 10:69-72, 1966.

Crowley, T. J., Hydinger, M., Stynes, A. J. and Feiger, A.  Monkey
    motor stimulation and altered social behavior during chronic
    methadone administration.  Psychopharmacologia 43:135-144,
    1975.

Davis, H.  Validation of evoked-response audiometry (ERA) in deaf
    children.  Int. Audiol. 8:77-81, 1966.

Davis, H., Hisch, S. K., Shelnutt, J. and Bowers, C.  Further
    validation of evoked response audiometry (ERA).  J. Speech
    Hear. Res. 10:717-732, 1967.

Dawson, G. D.  Cerebral responses to electrical stimulation of
    peripheral nerve in man.  J. Neurol. Neurosurg. Psychiatry
    10:134-140, 1947.

Dawson, G. D.  A miltiple scalp electrode for plotting evoked
    potentials.  Electroencephalogr. Clin. Neurophysiol. 6:
    153-154, 1954.

Dejerine, J.  Arch. Physiol. Norm. Path. (Fr.) 2:180-226, 1883.

Dobbs, W. H.  Methadone treatment of heroin addicts.  J. Am. Med.
    Assoc. 218:1536-1541, 1971.

Dole, V. P.  Biochemistry of addiction.  In Annual review of bio-
    chemistry, 39:821, 1970.

Domino, E. F. and Wilson, A. E.  Brain acetylcholine in morphine
    implanted rats given naloxone.  Psychopharmacologia 41:19-
    22, 1975.

Dustman, R. E. and Beck E. C.  Visually evoked potentials:  Ampli-
    tude changes with age.  Science 151:1013-1015, 1966.

Dustman, R. E. and Beck, E. C.  The effects of maturation and
    aging on the wave form of visually evoked potentials.  Electro-
    encephalogr. Clin. Neurophysiol. 26:2-11, 1969.

Dustman, R. E., Schenkenberg, T. and Beck, E. C.  The development of the evoked response as a diagnostic and evaluative procedure.  In R. Karrer (Ed.), Developmental psychophysiology of mental retardation.  Springfield, IL: C. C. Thomas, 247-310, 1976.

Dustman, R. E., Schenkenberg, T., Lewis, E. G., and Beck, E. C.  The cerebral evoked potential:  Life-span changes and twin studies.  In J. E. Desmedt (Ed.), Visual evoked potentials in man: New developments.  Oxford:  Clarendon Press, pp. 363-377, 1977.

Echols, S. D. and Jewett, R. E.  Effects of morphine on sleep in the cat.  Psychopharmacologia 24:435-448, 1972.

Eibergen, R. D. and Carlson, K. R.  Dyskinesias elicited by Methamphetamine:  Susceptibility of former methadone-consuming monkeys.  Science 190:588-589, 1975.

Esposito, R. and Kornetsky, C.  Morphine lowering of self stimulation thresholds:  Lack of tolerance with long term administration.  Science 195:189-190, 1977.

Fitzhugh, L. C., Fitzhugh, K. B. and Reitan, R. M.  Adaptive abilities and intellectual functioning of hospitalized alcoholics:  Further considerations.  Q. J. Stud. Alcohol 26:402-411, 1965.

Galbraith, G. C., Gliddon, J. B. and Busk, J.  Visual evoked responses in mentally retarded and nonretarded subjects.  Am. J. Ment. Defic. 75:341-348, 1970.

Giblin, D. R.  Somatosensory evoked potentials in healthy subjects and in patients with lesions of the nervous system.  Ann. N. Y. Acad. Sci. 112:93-142, 1964.

Glidden, J. B., Galbraith, G. C., and Busk, J.  Effect of preconditioning visual stimulus duration on visual evoked responses to a subsequent test flash in Down's syndrome and nonretarded individuals.  Am. J. Ment. Defic. 80:186-190, 1975.

Glidden, J. B., Busk, J. and Galbraith, G. C.  Visual evoked responses as a function of light intensity in Down's syndrome and nonretarded subjects.  Psychophysiology 12:416-422, 1975.

Goodman, L. S. and Gilman, (Eds.)  The pharmacological basis of therapeutics.  New York: MacMillan, p. 243, 1970.

Gossman, M., White, R. J., Taslitz, N. and Albin, M. S.  Electro-
    physiological responses immediately after experimental injury
    to the spinal cord.  Anat. Rec. 160:473, 1968.

Graham, F. K. and Kendall B. S.  Memory-for-designs test:  revised
    manual.  Percept. Mot. Skills 11:147-188, 1960.

Gritz, E. R., Sheffman, S. M., Jarvik, M. E., Haber, J., Dymond,
    A. M., Coger, R., Charuvastra, V. and Schlesinger, J.  Physio-
    logical and psychological effects of methadone in man.  Arch.
    Gen. Psychiatry 32:237-242, 1975.

Grundvig, J. L., Needham, W. E., Ajax, E. T.,and Beck, E. C.  The
    use of the Sensory Perceptual Examination in the diagnosis of
    degree of impairment of higher cerebral functins.  J. Nerv.
    Ment. Dis. 151:114-119, 1970.

Halliday, A. M., McDonald, W. I. and Mushin, J.  Visual evoked
    response in diagnosis of multiple sclerosis.  Br. Med. J.,
    661-664, December 1973.

Henderson, A., Nemes, G., Gordon, N. B. and Roos, L.  Sleep and
    narcotic tolerance.  Psychophysiology 7:346-347, 1970.

Hossman, K. A. and Sato, K.  Recovery of neuronal function after
    prolonged cerebral ischemia.  Science 168:375-376, 1970.

Isbell, H., Wikler, A., Eddy, N. B., Wilson, J. L., Moran, C. F.
    Tolerance and addiction liability of 6-Dimethylamino-4-4
    Diphenylheptanone-3 (Methadon).  J. Am. Med. Assoc.,
    888-894, December 1947.

Isbell, H., Wikler, A., Eiseman, A., Daingerfield, M. and Frank, K.
    Liability of addiction to 6-dimethylamino-4-4-diphenyl-3-
    heptanone (methadone, "amidone", or "10820") in man.  Arch.
    Int. Med. 82:362-392, 1948.

Isbell, H. and Vogel, V. H.  The addiction liability of methadone
    (Amidone, Dolophin 10820) and its use in the treatment of the
    morphine abstinence syndrome.  Am. J. Psychiat. 105:909-914,
    1949.

Jasper, H. H.  The ten-twenty electrode system of the international
    federation.  Electroencephalogr. Clin. Neurophysiol. 10:
    371-375, 1958.

Jervis, G. A.  Early senile dementia in mongolian idiocy.  Am. J.
    Psychiat. 105:102-106, 1948.

Jervis, G. A. Premature senility in Down's syndrome. Ann. N. Y. Acad. Sci. 171:559-561, 1970.

Kay, D. C. Human sleep and EEG through af cycle of methadone dependence. Electroencephalogr. Clin. Neurophysiol. 38:35-43, 1975.

Larson, S. J., Sances, A., Jr., and Christenson, P. C. Evoked somatosensory potentials in man. Arch. Neurol. 15:88-93, 1966.

Lawrence, D. G. and Kuypers, H. G. The functional organization of the motor system in the monkey. I. The effects of bilateral pyramidal lesions. Brain 91:1-15, 1968a.

Lawrence, D. G. and Kuypers, H. G. The effects of lesions on the descending brain-stem. Brain 91:15-33, 1968b.

Lewis, J. F., Lewis, S. A. and Tinker, M. Chlormethazole, sleep and drug withdrawal. Psychol. Med. 2:239-247, 1972.

Lewis, S. A., Oswald, I., Evans, J. I., Arkindele, M. O. and Tomsett, S. L. Heroin and human sleep. Electroencephalogr. Clin. Neurophysiol. 28:374-381, 1970.

Lichy, J., Vesely, C., Adler, J. and Zizka, J. Auditory evoked cortical responses in Down's syndrome. Electroencephalogr. Clin. Neurophysiol. 38:440, 1975. (abstract)

Marcus, M. M. The evoked cortical response: A technique for assessing development. Calif. Ment. Health Res. Digest 8:59-72, 1970.

Martin, W. R., Jasinski, D. R., Haertzen, C. A., Kay, D. C., Jones, B. E., Mansky, P. A. and Carpenter, R. W. Methadone--a reevaluation. Arch. Gen. Psychiat. 28:286-289, 1973.

Meyer, A. and Jones, J. Histological changes in the brain in mongolism. J. Ment. Sci. 85:206-221, 1939.

Meyer, J. S. and Gastaut, H. Cerebral anoxia and the electroencephalogram. Springfield, IL: C. C. Thomas, 1961.

Myers, J. L. Fundamentals of experimental design. Boston: Allyn and Bacon, p. 166, 1969.

Nakanishi, T., Shimada, Y. and Toyokura, Y. Somatosensory evoked responses to mechanical stimulation in normal subjects and in patients with neurological disorders. J. Neurol. Sci. 21:289-298, 1974.

Namerow, N. S.  Somatosensory recovery function in multiple scle-
    rosis patients.  Neurology 20: 813-817, 1970.

Namerow, N. S. and Enns, N.  Visual evoked responses in patients
    with multiple sclerosis.  J. Neurol. Neurosurg. Psychiatry
    35:829-833, 1972.

Neumann, M. A.  Langdon Down syndrome and Alzheimer's disease.
    J. Neuropathol. Exp. Neurol. 26:149-150, 1967.

Nyberg-Hansen, R.  Functional organization of descending supraspinal
    fibre systems to the spinal cord:  Anatomical observations and
    physiological correlations.  Ergebn. Anat. Entwicki-gesch 39:
    1-48, 1966.

Olson, M. I. and Shaw, C.  Presenile dementia and Alzheimer's
    disease in mongolism.  Brain 92:147-156, 1969.

Penrose, L. S.  Down's anomaly.  Boston:  Little, Brown & Company,
    1966.

Perot, P. L., Jr.  The clinical use of somatosensory evoked poten-
    tials in spinal cord injury.  Clin. Neurosurg. 20:367-381,
    1973.

Rapin, I.  Evoked responses to clicks in a group of children with
    communication disorders.  Ann. N. Y. Acad. Sci. 112:182-203,
    1964.

Rapin, I. and Graziani, L. J.  Auditory evoked responses in normal,
    brain-damaged, and deaf infants.  Neurology 17:881, 1967.

Rechtschaffen, A. and Kales, A.  (Eds.).  A manual of standardized
    terminology, techniques and scoring system for sleep stages of
    human subjects.  Los Angeles, CA., BIS/BRI, UCLA, 1968.

Reitan, R. M.  Investigation of the validity of Halstead's measures
    of biological intelligence.  AMA Arch. Neurol. and Psychiatry
    73:28-35, 1955.

Roizon, L., Jervis, G., Kaufman, M. A., Popovich, I. and Hoshimoto,
    S.  Senile plaque pathogenesis in Down's, Alzheimer's, and
    senile diseases.  J. Neuropathol. 31:188, 1972.

Roth, W. T.  Late event-related potentials in schizophrenia.  In
    H. Begleiter (Ed.), Evoked brain potentials.  New York:
    Plenum, 1977, in press.

Roubicek, J., Zaks, A. and Freedman, A. M.  EEG changes produced by heroin and methadone. Electroencephalogr. Clin. Neurophysiol. 27:667, 1969.

Shagass, C.  Sensory evoked potentials in psychosis.  In H. Begleiter (Ed.), Evoked brain potentials. New York:  Plenum, 1977, in press.

Shearer, D. E., Snyder, E. W., Beck, E. C. and Dustman, R. E.  A miniature, readily available electrode pedestal for recording cerebral and other electrophysiological activity from several species. Lab. Anim. Sci. 26:630-632, 1976.

Schenkenberg, T. and Dustman, R. E.  Visual, auditory and somato-sensory evoked response changes related to age, hemisphere and sex. Proc. Am. Psychol. Assoc., 183-184, 1970.

Snider, R. S. and Lee, J. C.  A stereotaxic atlas of the monkey brain.  Chicago: University of Chicago Press, 1961.

Snyder, E. W., Dustman, R. E., Straight, R. C., Wayne, A. W. and Beck, E. C.  Sudden toxicity of methadone in monkeys:  Behavioral and electrophysiological evidence.  Pharmac., Biochem., Behav. 6:87-92, 1977.

Sokol, S.  Review:  Visually evoked potentials: Theory, techniques and clinical applications.  Survey of Ophthalmol. 21:18-44, 1976.

Solitare, G. B. and Lemarche, J. B.  Alzheimer's disease and senile dementia as seen in mongoloids:  Neuropathological observations. Am. J. Ment. Defic. 70:840-848, 1966.

Solitare, G. B. and Lemarche, J. B.  Brain weight in the adult mongol.  J. Ment. Defic. Res. 11:79-84, 1967.

Starr, A.  Auditory brain-stem responses in brain death.  Brain 99: 543-554, 1976.

Straumanis, J. J., Shagass, C. and Overton, D. A.  Auditory evoked responses in young adults with Down's syndrome and idiopathic mental retardation.  Biol. Psychiatry 6:75-79, 1973a.

Straumanis, J. J., Shagass, C. and Overton, D. A.  Somatosensory evoked responses in Down's syndrome.  Arch. Gen. Psychiatry 29:544-549, 1973b.

Trojaborg, W. and Jørgensen, E. O.  Evoked cortical potentials in patients with "isoelectric" EEGs. Electroencephalogr. Clin. Neurophysiol. 35:301-309, 1973.

Williams, J. D., Ray, C. G. and Overall, J. E.   Mental aging and
    organicity in an alcoholic population.   J. Consult. Clin.
    Psychol. 41:392-396, 1973.

Williamson, P. D., Goff, W. R. and Allison, R.   Somato-sensory
    evoked responses in patients with unilateral cerebral lesions.
    Electroencephalogr. Clin. Neurophysiol., 28:566-575, 1970.

Wulff, M. H.   The barbiturate withdrawal syndrome:  A clinical and
    EEG study. Electroencephalogr. Clin. Neurophysiol. Supplement
    14: 173, 1959.

Yakovlev, P. I.   Morphological criteria of growth and maturation of
    the nervous system in man.   In L. C. Kalb, R. L. Masland, &
    R. E. Cooke (Eds.), Mental retardation.   Baltimore:   Williams
    & Wilkins Company, pp. 3-46, 1962.

# EVOKED POTENTIALS IN PATIENTS WITH NEUROLOGICAL DISORDERS

Roger Q. Cracco, M.D.

S.U.N.Y. Downstate Medical Center

Brooklyn, N.Y.

Averaged evoked potentials have been investigated in the research laboratory for many years but it is only in the last few years that the clinical applications of these methods have received emphasis. In the preceding three chapters of this volume clinically oriented research is presented. These investigations and other related material are discussed in the first part of this chapter. The second part consists of a brief review of the applications of evoked potential methods in the clinical evaluation of patients with neurological disorders.

A number of clinical possibilities must cross the mind of the clinical neurologist when confronted with a patient who is a known alcoholic including peripheral neuropathy, myopathy, delirium tremens, cerebellar degeneration, Wernike-Korsakoff's syndrome, central pontine myelinolysis, the syndrome of degeneration of the corpus callosum and cerebral atrophy. Thus, alcoholism can effect the entire neuraxis from cerebral cortex to muscle. Some of these disorders are thought to be due to alcohol directly, others to nutritional factors including vitamin deficiencies and the cause of others is uncertain. Conditions such as hepatic encephalopathy, head trauma and post traumatic epilepsy are also associated with alcoholism. Lastly, since many alcoholics have severe personality disorders, it is likely that a significant proportion of them have underlying brain disease predisposing them to their habit. Therefore, disorders of neurological function in alcoholic patients have multiple possible causes. In any study of these patients, it would be important to try to determine the specific cause of a given abnormality.

In this context, the observation of Lewis et al (1970) and Porjesz and Begleiter (1975) that the hemispheric assymetry of certain late evoked potentials recorded in normal subjects over central head regions is abolished by a single dose of alcohol is important. This demonstrates that this is related to alcohol and is not the result of vitamin deficiency or other factors associated with alcoholism. It also indicates that this finding results from functional rather than structural changes. Whether this finding is a direct effect of alcohol or is secondary to differences in level of arousal or attention is, however, uncertain.

Porjesz and Begleiter's observation (1975) that certain late evoked potentials recorded over central head regions in normal subjects are depressed by a single dose of alcohol whereas potentials of similar latency recorded over occipital regions are relatively unaffected is of interest since it suggests that these potentials arise in multiple generators, some of which are more affected by alcohol than others. There is evidence in humans and in animals that many evoked potential components arise in multiple generators.

Porjesz and Begleiter's observation (this volume) that certain late evoked potentials recorded over the frontal lobes are lower in amplitude in alcoholic patients than in normals and that the evoked potential recorded over the right frontal lobe is maximally affected suggests that frontal lobe function, and particularly right frontal lobe function, is impaired in these patients. There is clinical and pathological evidence to support the presence of frontal lobe involvement in the alcoholic patient. Additionally, the frontal lobes contain numerous association areas and experimental work in the monkey suggests that evoked potentials arising in association areas are affected by alcohol to a much greater extent than those arising in primary sensory areas (Himwick and Callison 1972). However, maximum response amplitude in evoked potential studies is probably not sufficient proof for the location of the generator or generators of a potential and, depending on the location and orientation of the unknown generator sources, it is possible that an abnormality in generators located in areas other than the frontal lobes is responsible for the lower amplitude response recorded over this region. For example, subcortical or temporal lobe generators with certain orientations could conceivably produce evoked potentials recorded maximally over the frontal lobes. It would, therefore, be useful to determine whether evoked potentials are similarly affected in patients with known discrete frontal lobe lesions such as tumors. If this were so, then this would be convincing evidence that this finding in alcoholic patients results from dysfunction in frontal lobe generators.

Dustman et al and Porjesz and Begleiter (this volume) found
that the early evoked potentials are increased in amplitude in
alcoholic patients.  This is consistent with the hypothesis that
there is a lack of inhibition at the input level of sensory processing in these patients.  However, information concerning the role
of inhibitory or excitatory mechanisms in the genesis of evoked
potentials will remain uncertain until more is known about the
generator sources of the potentials.  Studies concerning the
generator sources of some of the earlier potentials is currently
under way.  Since late potentials can be easily recorded in an
animal model (Porjesz et al 1976; Begleiter and Porjesz 1977;
Begleiter et al 1978), it seems that it will also be possible to
learn more about the nature of their generator sources.

The hypothesis that alcoholism accelerates the aging process
is supported by Dustman et al and Porjesz and Begleiter (this volume).
Although alcoholism and aging must have certain things in common
which produce the similarities in evoked potential and results of
psychological testing in the two groups, this does not necessarily
indicate that the dysfunction has an identical pathophysiological
substrate or that one process accelerates the other.  While there
is experimental evidence that alcohol can produce neuronal loss
and gliosis, there is no general agreement that the pathological
picture which results is typical of the normal aging process.
More evidence will be required before this hypothesis can be accepted.

With respect to the value of electrophysiologic tests in
cerebral death discussed by Dustman et al (this volume), it should
be emphasized that, at the present time, the clinical examination
is of primary importance in making this diagnosis.  Electrophysiological tests including the EEG are of value only in confirming the
diagnosis.  There is some question as to whether an EEG should
always be required in confirming the diagnosis.  When the EEG is
used, the strict criteria recommended by the Federation of EEG
Societies should be followed.  It should be pointed out that these
criteria were not fulfilled in most of the patients reported to
have survived after an isoelectric EEG was recorded.

Two problems may lead to clinical and EEG signs of cerebral
death in patients whose coma may be reversible.  One is hypothermia.
This source of potential error can be excluded merely by assuring
that the body temperature is not less than $35^{\circ}C$ when the diagnostic
tests are carried out.  The other is depressant drug intoxication.
In this situation evoked potential measures may be of value as
Dustman et al and others suggest but even here a large experience
will be necessary with these procedures before their value can be
assessed.  In the meantime, a very conservative approach seems
justified in making  the diagnosis of cerebral death in patients who

may have depressant drug intoxication.  In the vast majority of
patients, evoked potential studies are unnecessary to confirm the
diagnosis of cerebral death.

    Dustman et al's finding (this volume) that certain components
of the somatosensory evoked response are altered in patients with
amyotrophic lateral sclerosis is interesting.  As they suggest,
this may be due to abnormal motor or pyramidal feedback acting on
the somatosensory system.  An alternate explanation is that the
sensory system itself is impaired in a sub-clinical fashion.  A
third possibility is that the evoked potential changes are secondary to a psychological disturbance possibly associated with depression.

    Dustman et al's study of patients with Downs Syndrome (this
volume) indicate that, like the clinical features, the appearance
of the evoked response may be sufficiently characteristic to
suggest the diagnosis in these patients.  It would be important if
similar results are obtained in patients with other chromosomal
abnormalities where the diagnosis is less evident on the clinical
examination.   It would also be important to correlate the evoked
potential changes with post mortem findings in these patients.

    Dustman et al's work on single trial responses (this volume)
is an important contribution.  They produced evidence which suggests that response habituation in these patients does not result
from a decrease in the amplitude of each single evoked potential
but results rather from variability in the amplitude of the individual evoked potentials.  This work emphasizes that the evoked
response is a statistical procedure.  Information concerning the
nature of the individual potentials which make up the averaged
evoked response is obviously important and should increase the
value of this method since the individual components may vary in
different ways in patients with different cerebral disorders.
It would be important, however, to exclude the possibility that
the variation in individual evoked potential amplitude is due to
fluctuations in background noise level (EEG activity etc) rather
than to changes in the amplitude of the individual evoked potentials.

    Pace has used natural stimuli-words-rather than unnatural
stimuli such as clicks in her evoked potential study of aphasic
patients (this volume).  This is obviously imperative in any
evoked potential study of aphasia.  The use of more natural stimuli
should be the aim of many future evoked potential studies.  Although
her results are preliminary, the research may suggest that certain
relationships exist between the site of the lesion, semantic disability and verbal stimulus characteristics.  Such relationships are
important to pursue.  It would be worthwhile in these patients to
record over other head regions besides the temporal parietal scalp.

Functional disturbances to verbal stimuli might be expected from
brain areas remote from the areas of known structural damage.  It
would be important to extend these studies to include non fluent
aphasics.  It would also be of great importance to clinical neuro-
logists and neurosurgeons if a non-invasive evoked potential technique could be developed which would reliably determine which
cerebral hemisphere is dominant for speech.  The only way this can
currently be accomplished is by the Wada test which involves the
injection of barbiturate into the carotid arteries.  This procedure
is not risk-free and can only be justified in a few patients.

In Pace's study the wave forms which are being analyzed are
themselves statistical derivations.  While it is true that the
averaging process itself is a statistical procedure, this is not
usually considered to be an advantage.  Averaging methods are
usually employed because the small signal to noise ratio of scalp
recorded cerebral evoked potentials prevents these potentials from
being reliably recorded without the use of these methods.  It seems
that making the procedure more statistical, and getting further
away from the actual waveforms, may lead to misinterpretation
unless the derived waveforms are used to clarify the experimental
effects obtained with original waveforms.

It seems that future clinical investigations involving the late
evoked potentials should place greater emphasis on asking questions
relating to the patients behavioral aberrations in addition to
observing differences in evoked potential waveform.  The neural
substrate generating these potentials should be challenged to a
greater degree by delivering more complex stimuli or requiring
multiple behavioral tasks.  In this way it may be possible to
determine whether a problem results from a functional disturbance
at the input or output stage of central processing. Such information
could ultimately lead to the definition of more specific diagnostic
categories in patients with mental retardation, dementia or psychiatric disturbances.  Additionally, it would be important to investigate the event related potentials that precede motor behavior in
patients with movement disorders.  These studies could provide a
more precise understanding of the nature of the wide variety of
movement disorders which are seen in the neurology clinic.

## REFERENCES

Begleiter, H. and Porjesz, B.  Persistance of brain hyperexcitability
following chronic alcohol exposure in rats.  Advances in Exptl.
Medicine and Biology, 1977.

Begleiter, H., DeNoble, V. and Porjesz, B.  The effects of alcohol
on cortical and subcortical evoked potentials in the monkey.
Psychopharmacology, 1978 (in press).

Himwich, H.E. and Callison, D.A.  The effects of alcohol on evoked potentials of various parts of the central nervous system of the cat.  The Biology of alcoholism, 2:67-84 (Plenum Press) 1972.

Lewis, E.G., Dustman, R.E. and Beck, E.C.  The effects of alcohol on visual and somatosensory evoked responses.  Electroenceph. clin. Neurophysiol., 28: 202-205, 1970.

Porjesz, B. and Begleiter, H. Alcohol and bilateral evoked potentials.  In: Adv. Exp. Med. Biol., 59, M.M. Gross (Ed), Plenum Press, N.Y., 553-567, 1975.

Porjesz, B., Begleiter, H. and Hurowitz, S.  Brain excitability subsequent to alcohol withdrawal in rats.  In:  Tissue responses to addictive drugs.  D.H. Ford and D.H. Clonet (Ed), Spectrum, N.Y., 461-469, 1976.


## CLINICAL APPLICATIONS OF AVERAGED EVOKED POTENTIALS

In order for a laboratory method to have widespread use in the clinic, it must be sensitive, reliable and provide relevant information which cannot be obtained from available safer, cheaper and simpler methods.  These are difficult criteria to meet and it is only in the last few years that evoked potentials have found some clinical application.  The method has the great advantage that it provides a non-invasive technique for assessing neurological function in the spinal cord, brain stem and cerebrum.  In the following paragraphs areas where evoked potentials have found or may soon find application in the evaluation of patients with neurological disorders are briefly reviewed.


### Visual Evoked Potential

The VEP's which have been described are all thought to arise in cerebral cortical elements.  Abnormalities in the VEP to diffuse light flash stimulation have been described in patients with visual loss due to optic nerve lesions (Richey et al 1971); Feisod et al 1973; Feinsod and Hoyt, 1975, Namerow and Enns 1972).  Abnormal responses have also been described in a large number of patients with multiple sclerosis when there is no clinical evidence of visual disturbance.  This suggests that this method is clinically useful. Nevertheless, it has not received widespread recognition in the clinic because these potentials vary considerably in waveform both within and across normal subjects which makes the definition of what is abnormal difficult.

The VEP to pattern reversal stimulation (alternating black

and white checkboard or gratings) is much more stable than the
flash evoked response.  Halliday et al (1972; 1973 a,b) employed
this method in patients with multiple sclerosis and found that the
prominent positive potential which peaks at about 100 msec is
delayed in most of these patients, including the majority of patients without clinically evident visual disturbances (Fig. 1).
These findings have been confirmed (Asselman et al 1975;  Celesia
and Daly 1977).  Other optic nerve lesions including tumors also
produce abnormalities of this potential.  Response latency is
primarily affected by demyelinating lesions whereas tumors chiefly
affect response amplitude and configuration (Halliday et al 1976).

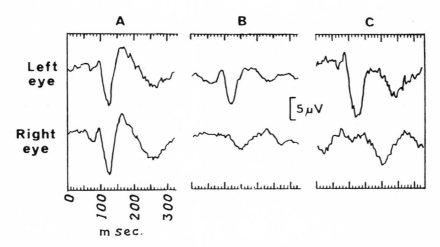

Figure 1.  Pattern-evoked responses to stimulation of the left eye
           and right eye recorded from a midline occipital electrode
           in a healthy subject (A) and 2 patients who were recover-
           ing from acute attacks of optic neuritis in the right eye
           with onset four weeks (B) and three weeks (C) previously.
           Relative positivity at the occipital electrode results
           in a downward deflection.  Note the delayed peak of the
           prominent positive potential from the affected eye and
           its smaller peak to peak amplitude (from Halliday et al
           (1972).

Pattern evoked VEP's are now being employed in many clinical laboratories in the evaluation of patients with optic nerve dysfunction. This method is also useful in measuring refractive errors. Insertion of the proper lens yields potentials of greater amplitude than those recorded when improper lenses are inserted (Harter and White 1968). This method is particularly useful in uncooperative patients such as young children. Similar methods have been employed in the evaluation of patients with color blindness and astigmatism (Regan and Spekreifse 1974; Regan 1976).

The VEP has not yet proven to be sensitive or reliable in the evaluation of patients with retrochiasmal involvement of the visual pathways. Differences in flash evoked potential amplitude between the two occipital poles have been observed in patients with homonymous defects (Vaughan et al 1963; Vaughan and Katzman 1964). However, there is normally considerable variability in the amplitude of these potentials on the two sides and symmetrical potentials have been observed in some patients with hemianopias (Asselman 1975). It is possible that the use of "steady state" potentials may prove to be of greater utility in the assessment of patients with retrochiasmal lesions. Using this method, stimuli are delivered at increasing rates and a series of oscillations are evoked which are related to the stimulus frequency. This technique has the disadvantage that special equipment and data processing is required but the advantage that recording time is very brief. Abnormal hemispheric distributions of steady state potentials have been observed in patients with retrochiasmal lesions which produce visual field defects (Regan and Heron 1969; Bodes-Wollner 1977).

## Auditory Evoked Potentials

Sohmer and Pratt (1976) recorded averaged evoked cochlear microphonics and eighth nerve action potentials from electrodes placed in the ear canal or over the mastoid region ipsilateral to the stimulated ear. These methods provide accurate information in the evaluation of cochlear function and peripheral hearing deficits.

The early scalp-recorded AEP's (latency less than 10 msec) to click stimulation consist of a series of 7 potentials or components (Jewett et al 1970)(Fig.2). These potentials are sometimes referred to as "far field potentials" because they are volume conducted events which are recorded at considerable distances from their generator sources. Studies in animals (Buchwald and Huang 1975) and man (Starr and Hamilton 1975; Stockard and Rossiter 1977) suggest that component 1 arises in the eighth nerve, component II from the region of the cochlear nucleus, component III from the area of the superior olive and trapezoid body and components IV and V from the midbrain. The sources of components VI and VII are unknown. Abnormalities of these potentials are judged primarily on the basis of prolonged latencies between component peaks and differences in the relative amplitudes of the different components. There is evidence which suggests that the site of a lesion in the cochlear nerve or brain stem can be localized in many patients using this method. Abnormalities in these potentials have been described in patients with acoustic neuromas, brainstem tumors, infarcts and demyelinating disease (Thornton and Hawkes, 1976; Sohmer et al 1974; Starr and Achor 1975; Robinson and Rudge 1975, Stockard and Rossiter 1977). These potentials have also been used to evaluate brainstem function in coma and brain death (Starr 1976; Greenberg et al 1977).

The middle and long latency AEP's (latency greater than 10 msec) do not yet have application in the neurology clinic. The reasons for this include their variability, their contamination by evoked myogenic potentials, the uncertainty regarding the neural substrate which underlies these potentials and the lack of specific criteria for what constitutes an abnormal response.

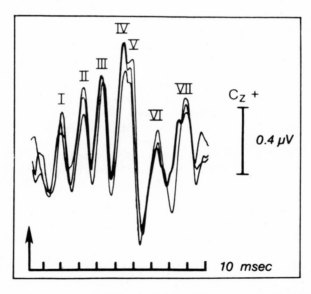

Figure 2. Vertex scalp-left mastoid reference recordings of auditory evoked brain stem potentials in a normal subject. Three individual recordings of 2,048 averaged responses to 60 d BSL left monaural clicks are superimposed. Relative positivity at grid 1 (scalp electrode) results in an upward deflection. Seven positive peaks can be discerned (From Stockard and Rossiter 1977).

## Somatosensory Evoked Potentials

In scalp-ear reference recordings, the SEP to median nerve stimulation consists of a series of potentials lasting several hundred msec (Fig.3). This response is thought to be mediated by dorsal column and lemniscal pathways (Halliday and Wakefield 1963). The first component is a positive potential which is widespread in its distribution over the scalp and peaks at about 15 msec. This potential may arise in the thalamus and thalamo cortical radiation(Cracco 1972; Allison et al 1974). Over the somesthetic scalp contralateral to the side of stimulation this potential is followed by a negative potential peaking at about 20 msec, an inconstant small positive inflection peaking at 25 msec and a positive potential peaking at 30 msec. These potentials are most prominent over somesthetic scalp regions and are thought to arise in specific somatosensory cortex (Allison et al 1974). The generator sources of the later potentials have not yet been defined.

All components of the SEP may be increased in peak latency and duration and decreased in amplitude in patients with peripheral neuropathy (Alajouanine et al 1958; Giblin 1964: Bergamini et al 1965). This can be explained by the decreased number of functioning sensory nerve fibers, the reduced conduction velocity of other affected fibers and the resultant increased temporal dispersion of impulses. Although these findings are of interest, this technique is of limited value in these patients since peripheral nerve function can usually be better evaluated by performing peripheral nerve conduction studies. Nevertheless, averaging techniques may find some application in evaluating patients with brachial plexus lesions or cauda equina syndromes where the precise site of involvement may be difficult to assess with conventional methods.

Scalp-recorded SEP's are decreased in amplitude over the affected hemisphere in patients with focal destructive cerebral lesions (Giblin 1964; Liberson 1966; Laget et al 1967; Williamson et al 1970; Kazaki et al 1971). In these patients the degree of SEP alteration generally correlated well with the severity of sensory impairment but exceptions have been noted. Abnormal but inconsistent alterations in SEP amplitude and waveform have also been observed in epileptic patients (Dawson 1947; Halliday, 1965; Halliday and Halliday 1970; Broughton 1969). For the most part, however, these findings in patients with cerebral dysfunction add little to the information that can be obtained from the clinical evaluation or the electroencephalogram and for this reason this method has not yet received much enthusiasm in the neurology clinic. It seems likely that the recording of these potentials will have clinical application after the neural generators of the many components are better understood and after criteria for what constitutes an abnormal response are clearly defined.

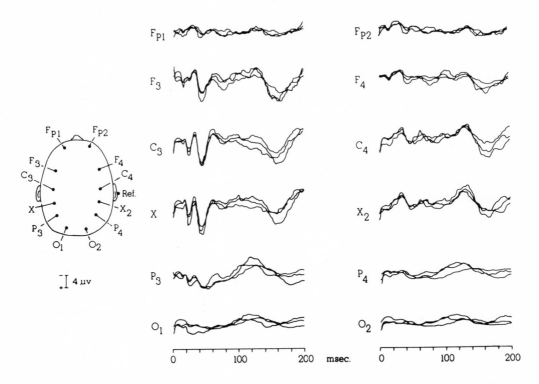

<u>Figure 3.</u> Distribution of the scalp recorded somatosensory evoked response to right median nerve stimulation in right ear reference recordings. The X scalp electrode lies over somatosensory cortex. Early components are most prominent overlying somesthetic scalp regions contralateral to the side of stimulation. Later components are more generalized (from Calmes and Cracco 1971).

The scalp recorded SEP to lower extremity peripheral nerve stimulation has been found useful in the evaluation of patients with spinal cord trauma (Perot 1973). The presence of a scalp-recorded response indicates that there is transmission of the ascending volley across the site of spinal cord injury. This provides another parameter in the estimation of the completeness of physiological transection of the spinal cord and is particularly useful in patients who are unconscious or uncooperative. Evoked

potentials to lower extremity peripheral nerve stimulation which
arise in spinal cord afferent pathways can also be recorded from
surface electrodes placed over the spine (Cracco 1973; Cracco et al
1975)(Fig.4). These potentials are not transmitted rostral to
clinically evident complete spinal cord lesions(Fig. 5). These
potentials are recorded with difficulty, particularly over rostral
cord segments because of their small signal size (less than 0.5 uV)
but this method has the advantage that it is possible to localize
the site of a lesion within the spinal cord. A good correlation
between abnormalities in the spinal evoked potentials and the
clinical status of infants and children with myelodysplasia has
been demonstrated (Cracco et al 1974).

Recently, using special recording methods, scalp recorded
median nerve evoked far field potentials have been described
(Cracco and Cracco 1976). This response consists of three short
latency positive potentials, the third of which is sometimes
bilobed (Fig. 6). These potentials may arise in (A) proximal
segments of stimulated median nerve fibers and spinal cord
(B) medial lemniscus, and (C) thalamus and thalamocortical radia-
tions, respectively. Similar potentials arising in these pathways
have been described in rats (Wiederholt and Iraqui Madoz, 1977).
Like the auditory evoked far field potentials, these potentials
may prove useful in the evaluation of patients with brain stem
and diencephalic dysfunction.

## Operating Room Applications

VEP's to flash stimuli have been used to monitor surgical
removal of orbital or chiasmatic lesions (Wright et al 1973;
Feinsod et al 1976; Allen and Starr 1977). Scalp recorded SEP's
have also been employed in monitoring surgery on the spinal cord
and AEP brainstem potentials in monitoring posterior fossa surgery.
An increase in evoked potential amplitude or the occurrence of
previously non existant evoked potentials have been described following removal of tumors. However the effects of anesthesia and
changes in blood pressure on these potentials must still be investigated and much more experience with this method will be required
before its value in monitoring neurosurgical procedures can be
assessed.

## Conclusion

At the present time pattern VEP's are useful in the evaluation
of patients with refractive errors, color blindness, astigmatism and
patients with optic nerve dysfunction, particularly those with multiple sclerosis. Cochlear microphonics and the recording of eighth
nerve action potentials provide a reliable method for evaluating

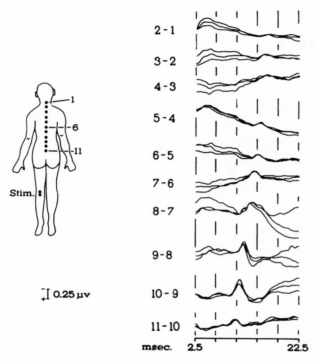

Figure 4.   Bipolar recordings of the spinal evoked response to left peroneal nerve stimulation. Interelectrode distance is 4.5 cm. Electrode 11 is placed over the second lumbar spine and electrode 1 over the third cervical spine. 8192 responses were summated in each recording. Three recordings are superimposed in each trace. There is a delay of 2.5 msec between the shock and the sweep onset. The analysis time is 20 msec. Relative negativity at grid 1 (caudal electrode) results in an upward deflection. The response progressively increases in latency rostrally (from Cracco 1973).

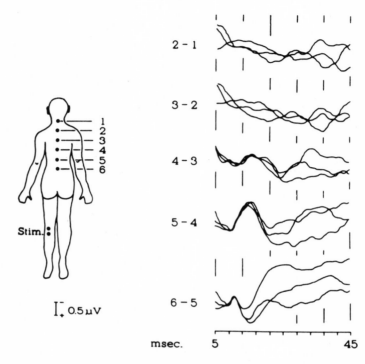

<u>Figure 5.</u>  Bipolar recordings of the spinal response to left
peroneal nerve stimulation in a patient with a clinically
evident complete spinal cord lesion at $T_8$.  There is a
delay of 5 msec between the shock and the sweep onset.
The analysis time is 40 msec.  Interelectrode distance
is 8 cm.  Responses caudal to the lesion (bottom 3
traces) are similar to those recorded in normal subjects.
No response is apparent in the lead in which the caudal
electrode is placed over the 6th thoracic spine
(2nd trace from top) in relation to the lesion or in
the more rostral lead (top trace).  (From Cracco 1973).

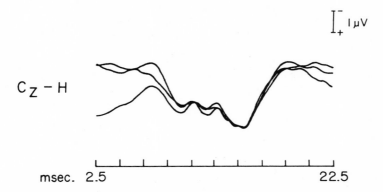

$C_Z - H$

msec. 2.5                          22.5

Figure 6. Far field somatosensory evoked potentials to right
median nerve stimulation recorded from the scalp vertex
in left hand reference recordings. 2048 responses were
summated. Three averaged responses are superimposed.
Relative positivity at scalp electrode results in
downward deflection. Three positive potentials are
apparent with peak latencies of about 9.0, 11.5 and
14.5 msec.

patients with peripheral hearing problems. The auditory brain
stem potentials are useful in patients with eighth nerve and brain
stem dysfunction and the somatosensory far field potentials may
provide another method for evaluating brain stem and diencephalic
dysfunction. The scalp-recorded SEP to lower extremity peripheral
nerve stimulation is useful in patients with spinal cord lesions
and the spinal evoked response should provide information concerning the level of the lesion in some of these patients.

It seems that later SEP's (latency $>$ 30 msec) and AEP's
(latency $>$ 10 msec) will provide clinically useful information
in patients with cerebral dysfunction after more is known about
the generator sources of the individual components and after
specific criteria for what constitutes an abnormal response are
defined. The late potentials which are related to attention and
central processing may prove to be of value in the evaluation of
patients with mental retardation and CNS degenerative disease and
the investigation of event related potentials which precede and
accompany motor behavior in patients with movement disorders may
provide greater insight into the nature of these disorders.

## REFERENCES

Alajouanine, T.; Scherrer, J.; Barbizet, J.; Calvet, J. and Verley,
R.: Potentiels evoques corticaux chez des subjets atteints de
troubles somesthetiques. Rev. Neurol., 98: 757-761, 1958.

Allen, A., and Starr, A. Sensory evoked potentials in the operating
room. Neurology, 27: 358, 1977.

Allison, T., Goff, W.R., Williamson, P.D. and Van Gilder, J.C. On
the neural origin of early components of the human somatosensory
evoked potential. Proc. Int. Symp. Cerebral Evoked Potentials in
Man, Belgium, 1974(In press).

Asselman, P., Chadwick, D.W. and Marsden, C.D. Visual evoked responses in the diagnoses and management of patients with multiple
sclerosis. Brain, 98: 261-282, 1975.

Bergamini, L.; Bergamasco, B. Fra, I.; Gandiglio, G.; Mombelli, A.M.
and Mutani, R.: Somatosensory evoked cortical potentials in subjects with peripheral nervous lesions. Electromyography, 5: 121-
130, 1965.

Bodis-Wollner, I. Recovery from cerebral blindness: evoked potential and psychophysical measurements. Electroenceph. clin. Neurophysiol., 42: 178-184, 1977.

Broughton, R.; Meier-Ewert, K. and Ebe, M.:  Evoked visual, somatosensory and retinal potentials in photosensitive epilepsy.  Electroenceph. clin. Neurophysiol., 27:  373-386, 1969.

Buchwald, J.S. and Huang, C.M.  Far Field acoustic responses:
origins in the cat.  Science, 189: 382-384, 1975.

Celesia, C.G. and Daly, R.F.  Visual electroencephalographic
computer analysis: a new electrophysiological test for the diagnosis
of optic nerve lesions.  Neurology, 1977 (in press).

Calmes, R.L. and Cracco, R.Q.  Comparison of somatosensory and
somatomotor evoked responses to median nerve and digital nerve
stimulation.  Electroenceph. clin. Neurophysiol.,31: 547-562, 1971.

Cracco, R.Q.  The initial positive potential of the scalp recorded
somatosensory evoked response.  Electroenceph. clin. Neurophysiol.,
32: 623-629, 1972.

Cracco, R.Q.  Spinal evoked response: peripheral nerve stimulation
in man.  Electroenceph. clin. Neurophysiol., 35: 379-386, 1973.

Cracco, J.B., Cracco, R.Q. and Graziani, L.J.  The spinal evoked
response in infants with myelodysplasia, Neurology, 4: 359-360,
1974.

Cracco,J.B., Cracco, R.Q., and Graziani, L.J.  The spinal evoked
response in infants and children.  Neurology, 25: 31-36. 1975.

Cracco, R.Q. and Cracco, J.B.  Somatosensory evoked potential in
man: far field potentials.  Electroenceph. clin. Neurophysiol,
41: 460-466, 1976.

Dawson, G.D.: Investigations on a patient subject to myoclonic
seizures after sensory stimulation.  J. Neurol. Neurosurg. Psychiat.
10: 141-162, 1947.

Feinsod, M. Abramsky, O. and Auerbach, E.  Electrophysiological
examination of the visual system in multiple sclerosis.  J. Neurol.
Sc., 20: 161-175, 1973.

Feinsod, M. and Hoyt, W. Subclinical optic neuropathy in multiple
sclerosis.  J. Neurol. Neurosurg. Psychiat. 38(2): 1109-1114, 1975.

Feinsod, M., Selhorst, J.B., Hoyt, W.F. and Wilson, C.B.  Monitoring optic nerve function during craniotomy.  J. Neurosurg., 44:29-
31, 1976.

Giblin, D.R.:  Somatosensory evoked potentials in healthy subjects
and in patients with lesions of the nervous system.  Ann. N.Y.
Acad. Sci. 93-142, 1964.

Greenberg, R.P., Becker, D.P., Miller, J.D. and Mayer, D.J.
Evaluation of brain function in severe head trauma with multimodal-
ity evoked potentials.  J. Neurosurg.,(in press) 1977.

Halliday, A.M.  The incidence of large cerebral evoked responses
in myoclonic epilepsy.  Electroenceph. clin. Neurophysiol.,
19: 102, 1965.

Halliday, A.M. and Halliday, E.: Cortical evoked potentials in
patients with benign essential myoclonus and progressive myoclonic
epilepsy.  Electroenceph. clin. Neurophysiol. 29: 106, 1970.

Halliday, A.M. and Wakefield, G.S.: Cerebral evoked potentials
in patients with dissociated sensory loss. J. Neurol. Neurosurg.,
Psychiat. 26: 211-219, 1963.

Halliday, A.M., Halliday, E., Kriss, A., McDonald, W.I. and Mushin,
J.  The pattern-evoked potential in compression of the anterior
visual pathways.  Brain, 99(2): 357-374, 1976.

Halliday, A.M. McDonald, W.I. and Mushin, J. Delayed visual evoked
response in optic neuritis.  Lancet, 1:982-985, 1972.

Halliday, A.M., McDonald, W.I. and Mushin, J.  Delayed pattern-
evoked responses in optic neuritis in relation to visual acuity.
Trans. Opthalmol.  Soc. VK., 93: 315-324, 1973a.

Halliday, A.M. McDonald, W.I. and Mushin, J. Visual evoked response
in diagnosis of multiple sclerosis.  Br. Med. J. 4:661-664, 1973b.

Harter, M.R. and White, C.T.  Effects of contour sharpness and check
size on visually evoked cortical potentials.  Vision Res. 8:701-711,
1968.

Jewett, D.L., Romano, M.N. and Williston, J.S.  Human auditory
evoked potentials: possible brain stem components detected on the
scalp.  Science, 167: 1517-1518, 1970.

Kazaki, A.; Shiota, K.; Terada,C.; Utsumi, S. and Hori, P.: Clinical
studies on the somatosensory evoked response in neurosurgical
patients.  Electroenceph. clin. Neurophysiol., 31: 184-191, 1971.

Laget, P.; Mamo, H. et Houdart, R.,4: De l'interet des potentials
evoques somesthesiques dans l'etude des lesions due lobe parietal
de l'homme. Etude preliminaire. Neuro-chirurgie. 13:841-853, 1967.

Liberson, W.T.:  Study of evoked potentials in aphasics.  Amer.J. Phys. Med. 45: 135-142, 1966.

Namerow, N. and Enns, N.  Visual evoked responses in patients with multiple sclerosis.  J. Neurol. Neurosurg. Psych. 35: 829-833, 1972.

Perot, P.L., Jr.  The clinical use of somatosensory evoked potentials in spinal cord injury.  Clin. Neurosurg. pp. 367-382, 1973.

Regan, D., Milner, B. and Heron, J.R.  Delayed visual perception and delayed visual evoked potentials in the spinal form of multiple sclerosis and in retrobulbar neuritis.  Brain, 99(1): 43-66. 1976.

Regan, D. and Spekreijse, H.  Evoked potential indications of color blindness.  Vision Res., 14: 89-95, 1974.

Richey, E.T., Kooi, K.A. and Tourtellotte, W.W.  Visually evoked responses in multiple sclerosis.  J. Neurol. Neurosurg. Psych. 34: 275-280, 1971

Robinson, K. and Rudge, P. Auditory evoked responses in multiple sclerosis.  Lancet, 1:1164-1166, 1975.

Sohmer, H., Feinmesser, M. and Szabo, G.  Sources of electrococh-leographic responses as studied in patients with brain damage. Electroenceph. clin. Neurophysiol., 37:663-669, 1974.

Sohmer, H. and Pratt, H.  Recording of cochlear microphonic potential with surface electrodes.  Electroenceph. clin. Neurophysiol., 40: 253-260, 1976.

Starr, A. Auditory brain stem responses in brain death.  Brain, 99: 543-554, 1976.

Starr, A. and Hamilton, A.E. Correlation between confirmed site of neurological lesions and abnormalities of far field auditory brain stem responses.  Electroenceph. clin. Neurophysiol., 4:595-608, 1976.

Starr, A. and Achor, L.J. Auditory brain stem responses in neurological disease.  Arch. Neurol., 32:761-768, 1975.

Stockard, J.J. and Rossiter, V.S.  Clinical and pathological correlates of brain stem auditory response abnormalities.  Neurology, 24:316-325, 1977.

Thornton, A.R.D. and Hawkes, C.H.  Neurological applications of surface recorded electrocochleography.  J. Neurol. Neurosurg. Psych. 39: 586-592, 1976.

Vaughan, H., Jr. and Katzman, R. Evoked responses in visual disorders.   Ann. New York Acad. Sci., 112:305-319, 1964.

Vaughan, H., Jr., Katzman, R. and Taylor, J.   Alterations of visual
evoked response in the presence of homonymous visual defects.
Electroenceph. clin. Neurophysiol., 15:737-746, 1963.

Wiederholt, W.G. and Iraqui-Madoz, V.J.   Far-field somatosensory
potentials in the rat.   Electroenceph. clin. Neurophysiol., 42:
456-465, 1977.

Williamson, P.D., Goff, W.R. and Allison, T.:   Somatosensory evoked
responses in patients with unilateral cerebral lesions.   Electroenceph. clin. Neurophysiol.   28: 566-576, 1970.

Wright, J.E., Arden, G. and Jones, B.R.   Continuous monitoring of
the visually evoked response during intra-orbital surgery.   Trans.
Opthalmolol.   Soc. VK, 93: 311-4. 1973.

Section III

# PSYCHOPATHOLOGY AND EVOKED POTENTIALS

# AUDITORY EVOKED POTENTIALS IN CHILDREN

# AT HIGH RISK FOR SCHIZOPHRENIA

David Friedman, Allan Frosch, and L. Erlenmeyer-Kimling

New York State Psychiatric Institute, Medical Genetics

722 West 168 Street, New York City, New York 10032

## INTRODUCTION

Many methods of attempting to determine the etiology of schizophrenia have been utilized, but, until recently, the antecedents of this disorder were sought in retrospective information from parents, school records, therapists' accounts, and other such information sources. The use of the longitudinal, prospective, high-risk method of research eliminates many of the biasing problems encountered in obtaining information using retrospective reports (Erlenmeyer-Kimling, 1968; Mednick and McNeill, 1968; Pearson and Kley, 1957). Two obvious advantages that high-risk studies have over other approaches are that: 1) they permit life history events and the impact of such events to be observed directly, and 2) they make it possible to distinguish psychobiological characteristics that are present before the onset of overt disturbances in functioning from those that appear later. Comprehensive reviews of high risk methodology and descriptions of ongoing studies exist, and we will not go into detail here (see Erlenmeyer-Kimling, 1975; Garmezy and Streitman, 1974).

Researchers have chosen the children of schizophrenic parents for study because they are considered to be at greater than usual statistical risk for developing the schizophrenic psychosis. Empirical risk estimates of becoming schizophrenic average about eleven percent for the children of one schizophrenic parent, and do not differ as a function of the sex of the parent (cf., Erlenmeyer-Kimling, 1977; Zerbin-Rüdin, 1967). This contrasts with a one percent risk estimate in the general population.

While it is possible that this eleven percent of the high risk group could raise or lower their group's mean value on some measures, causing group differences to be significant, it is relatively improbable that this would occur in most circumstances. For example, Hanson et al. (1976) were unable to find significant mean differences between high risk and matched normal control samples on a number of measures including pregnancy and delivery complications, physical growth variables, and psychological and neurological test items. However, they were able to identify a subgroup of five children, all of whom were at risk, who were deviant on three indicators, including poor motor skills, large intra-individual cognitive test scatter and observations of schizoid-like behaviors. The number of subjects "hitting" on all three indicators corresponded to seventeen percent of the high risk sample, a figure that agrees well with the empirical risk estimates.

This research strategy has been followed in our group (Erlenmeyer-Kimling, 1970; 1975) as demonstrated in a recent paper by Fein et al. (1974). Although significant group differences were not found, a high-risk subgroup was identified whose psychophysiologic profile was characterized by 1) high absolute threshold, 2) low uncomfortable threshold, 3) fast heart rate during uncomfortable stimuli, and 4) high amplitude skin conductance responses to uncomfortable stimuli. The auditory sensitivity pattern observed in this subgroup was similar to that reported by Levine and Whitney (1970) in research with adult schizophrenic subjects.

## Averaged Evoked Potentials in High-Risk Samples

Many investigators of the schizophrenias share the view that these disorders are a manifestation of brain dysfunction. Thus, the averaged evoked potential recorded from scalp, which has been shown to be an index of brain functioning in the normal subject, might be a useful tool in discriminating potential schizophrenics from both their normal control and their high-risk counterparts, who are not actually at genetic risk for schizophrenia. Few studies using this technique with high-risk samples have been reported, and it will, therefore, be an easy job to summarize the findings to date: In a small sample of subjects, Herman et al. (1977) tested six high-risk and six matched controls, between the ages of seven and ten, using a continuous performance test of visual attention. This task required a response to the letter X, the signal, and witholding of the response to non-signal letters. There were no group differences in percent correct or correct rejections. However, Herman et al. (1977) reported a marked between-groups difference, with much larger N100-P200 amplitudes and longer component latencies to both signal and non-signal stimuli in the high-risk group than in the normal control group. These authors concluded that their data suggested a maturational lag in visual stimulus processing in the high risk sample. However, the absence of a behavioral difference, coupled with small sample sizes, makes this interpretation premature.

In two papers, based on a preliminary and a later analysis with more subjects, Itil and his colleagues (1974) and Saletu et al. (1975) reported on auditory evoked potentials from high risk and normal control subjects. In the later of the two reports, 62 controls and 62 high risk children between the ages of ten and twelve were studied. No significant amplitude differences between the groups were found, but Saletu et al. (1975) did report finding significantly shorter latencies for the high risk children in peaks P200, P300 and N400. These latency differences were significant at modest levels (p < .05 for most; p < .01 for P300) and were small, varying from a mean difference of seven milliseconds to one of sixteen milliseconds. More than twenty-four separate tests of peak latency differences were performed, which could result in some small number of them turning out significant by chance. These factors detract from the forcefullness of the authors' conclusions regarding a hyper-arousal mechanism in the children at risk.

We have recorded averaged evoked potentials from a vertex electrode to repetitive tones presented to high risk (HR) and normal comparison (NC) children, who are part of a prospective, longitudinal study begun in 1971 (Erlenmeyer-Kimling, 1970). Our emphasis is on detecting significantly deviant subjects from both groups, although we do investigate between group differences as well.

METHODS

Subject Selection

The "at risk" children were obtained through their parents in a screening of consecutive admissions between June, 1971 and December, 1972 at six psychiatric hospitals in the greater New York Metropolitan Area. Criteria for this first step of inclusion were that the patients be: white, English-speaking, married at the time of admission, and still living with the spouse, and have two or more children between the ages of seven and twelve. The hospital records of patients meeting these criteria were evaluated for schizophrenia independently by two senior psychiatrists and a resident at New York State Psychiatric Institute without knowledge of the hospital diagnoses or the medications prescribed. No family was taken for study without a unanimous diagnosis of schizophrenia in the patient. Children of patients who have diagnoses other than schizophrenia are also studied as a comparison group, as are a group of children of two schizophrenic parents. Data on both of these groups are not available for the present report.

NC subjects were obtained through the cooperation of the Nassau and Rockland County school systems.

In these school districts, letters were sent to families with two or more children between the ages of seven and twelve. The names of both parents of a NC child were checked against the Department of Mental Hygiene files. Any child with a parent who had a history of psychiatric hospitalization was eliminated from the study. Parental criteria for inclusion were the same as those for the HR sample.

## Laboratory Procedures

The first time they were seen (in 1971-1972), the children were given a large battery of psychologic, psychophysiologic, psychiatric and neurologic tests. The auditory evoked response procedure, which is the subject of this report, was not given until the second round of testing, which occurred two years later. Some of the children tested during the first round were not available for the second round, resulting in some attenuation of sample size. In all aspects of the testing procedures, the experimenters had no knowledge as to whether a given child was HR or NC.

## Auditory Evoked Response Recording and Stimulating Procedures

EEG was recorded from vertex, midline occipital, and right eye supra-orbital locations, all referred to the left earlobe, amplified at a gain of 20,000 by Beckman pre- and power-amplifiers set to a frequency response of .03 to 30 hz. Data were recorded on FM analog tape with trigger pulses, and stored for off-line analysis. The data were digitized at two msec intervals for a 500 msec epoch following tone onset via a PDP-12 computer, averaged on an IBM 360 computer, and written out on a Hewlett-Packard X-Y plotter. Responses with movement artifacts and eye-movement contamination were eliminated by the averaging program, and from the remaining responses the first 200 "good" potentials were included for averaging. For each subject, then, 200 artifact-free epochs were averaged and standard deviations at each of the 250 time points were computed. Only the data from the vertex electrode will be reported.

The stimuli were 360, click-free, 1000 hz, 500 msec duration tones presented over a set of Sharpe headphones. The tones were generated by a Heathkit Sine-Square Audio Generator (Model IG-18) with an inter-stimulus-interval that varied randomly from 1 and 3/4 to 3 seconds. Subjects were instructed to try and ignore the tones. A fixation point was used to reduce eye movements.

## Age and Group Analyses

In each group, the subjects were divided into age bands, 8 - 10, 10 - 12, 12 - 14 years. HR children were age-matched with their NC

TABLE 1

Demographic Characteristics of the HR and NC Subjects

| | Mean Age | #Males | #Females | #SF | #SM |
|---|---|---|---|---|---|
| 8-10 | | | | | |
| HR | 9-4 | 6 | 1 | 2 | 5 |
| NC | 9-2 | 5 | 2 | | |
| 10-12 | | | | | |
| HR | 10-11 | 3 | 5 | 4 | 4 |
| NC | 10-11 | 3 | 5 | | |
| 12-14 | | | | | |
| HR | 13-6 | 2 | 4 | 3 | 3 |
| NC | 13-5 | 3 | 3 | | |
| Totals | | | | | |
| HR | 11-3 | 11 | 10 | 9 | 12 |
| NC | 11-2 | 11 | 10 | | |

counterparts, and, where possible, with a same-sexed comparison subject. This resulted in a total of 42 subjects, 21 in each group.
Table 1 presents some demographic characteristics of the 42 subjects.
As can be seen, age and sex are well-balanced between the groups.
The two far-right columns refer to the number of children of schizophrenic fathers (SF) and mothers (SM) in each age band for the HR
group.

## Data Analyses

The mean values and the standard deviations at each time point
were averaged by threes for each subject (250 time points divided
by 3) yielding 83 values at six msec per value, resulting in a total
epoch of 498 msec. This was done to allow us to use the BMD series
of computer programs (Dixon, 1975). In all of the BMD analyses, the
time points were entered as "variables" and the waveform for each

subject was considered a "case". Thus, the evoked potential data matrix consisted of 83 variables by 42 cases.

To determine if the two groups could be discriminated on the basis of their averaged responses or their background variability, stepwise linear discriminant function analyses (see Donchin, 1969; BMDP2M) were performed on the averaged values and the standard deviations at each time point. Principal Components factor analysis with varimax rotation (BMDP4M) was performed to determine the minimum number of waveshapes that could account for the variance in the evoked potential data matrix. Factor scores were then computed for each subject for each factor, and age by group analyses of variance were performed on the extracted factors.

## RESULTS AND DISCUSSION

The peak latency values reported here are mean values across groups obtained from the grand mean waveforms. The auditory evoked response elicited by the tones consisted of a series of negative and positive deflections beginning with an early negativity at 55 msec, followed by a positive wave at 95 msec, a negative wave at 125 msec, a positivity at 190 msec, a late negativity at 225 msec, and a late positive complex consisting of a peak at 285 msec and a later peak at 400 msec. A good deal of variability in both amplitude and latency of these later peaks was seen across subjects.

Figure 1 presents the grand mean responses averaged according to age and group, with grand means collapsed across age bands for each group appearing at the bottom of the figure, and grand means collapsed across groups for each age band appearing at the far right of the figure. Differences between the HR and NC groups are visible, but these are variable and not consistent in favoring one group over the other. That is, while the 8-10 year old HR subjects show larger N125-P190 amplitude than their NC counterparts, the 10-12 year old NC subjects show the same advantage over their HR counterparts, while in the 12-14 year olds differences are more difficult to discern. The grand means for the two groups seen at the bottom of the figure show very few areas of difference (with the exception of a somewhat larger N125-P190 component in the HR group, and very late positive activity in the HR group) while averaging according to age shows more prominent late positive activity for the youngest age band than for the two older age bands.

## Discriminant Analyses

Stepwise linear discriminant function analysis was performed on the mean values at each of the time points between the two groups using an F to enter value that would select a mean difference as

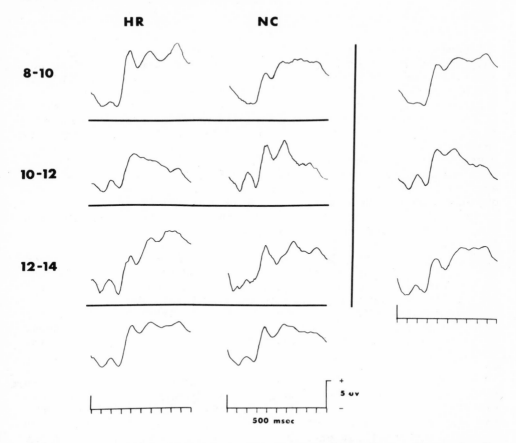

Figure 1. Grand mean auditory evoked potentials for each age band and group. Ns in each cell correspond to Table 1. Grand means at the bottom, below the heavy line are averaged across age bands for each group, while grand means to the right of the vertical line are averaged across groups for each age band.

significant at the .05 level. The discriminant function yielded no significant areas of difference, supporting our conclusion based upon visual inspection, that no differences existed between the grand means of the two groups. To determine if background variability could significantly discriminate the groups, the standard deviations across the epoch were subjected to discriminant analysis, and, again, no significant areas of difference between the groups were found.

## Principal Components Factor Analysis

Gross group differences of a consistent nature do not appear in this sample of subjects. However, as stated earlier, according to empirical morbidity risk estimates, one percent of the NC subjects and eleven percent of the HR subjects are expected to develop the schizophrenic psychosis. Thus, while group differences can yield important information, some method for identifying deviant subjects in the absence of group differences is needed. We were interested in developing a metric which would measure the degree to which a given subject's waveform differed from some "centroid" waveform. For this purpose, we used factor analysis (cf., Donchin, 1966) as an exploratory technique for analyzing the sources of variance in the evoked potential data matrix. Since we wanted to describe a subject's evoked response relative to some "normative" response, we were most interested in analyzing the between-subjects variance. Therefore, each subject's averaged values from a single vertex electrode were entered into the factor analysis and the correlations between the values at each time point were subjected to the Principal Components analysis. The first six factors accounted for ninety percent of the variance and, therefore, only these six factors were varimax rotated. Since we had used only one electrode and one averaged response per subject, the resultant factors can be considered to be the waveshapes that account for the variance in the data matrix.

Figure 2 presents the factor loadings of each of the six factors across the 83 time points. These loadings represent the degree of association of the factor and a given time point. These plots show the regions of time over which a given factor is active, and, in general, represent rather remarkably the components present in the grand mean waveforms. For example, factor 1 has high negative loadings peaking at 120 and 200 msec, and high positive loadings peaking at 360 msec, corresponding to negative components in the grand means at approximately 125 and 225 msec, and a positive component at approximately 350 msec.

For each of these factors, a factor score was derived for each subject. This score is a standard score with a mean of zero and a standard deviation of one, and indicates quantitatively the degree to which a subject's waveform is represented by a given factor. As an example, figure 3 presents the averaged waveform for a female NC subject whose age is 11 years, 5 months. This subject's highest score is on factor 6, a factor with negative loadings peaking at 120 and 210 msec, and positive loadings peaking at 162 and 288 msec. Inspection of her averaged evoked potential shows negative peaks at approximately 120 and 200 msec, and positive peaks at 170 and 275

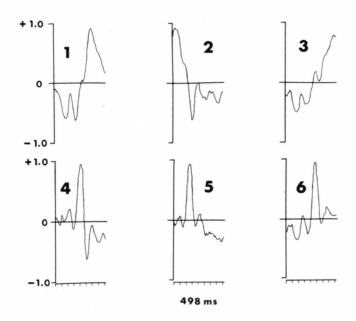

+1.0

0

−1.0

+1.0

0

−1.0

498 ms

Figure 2. Rotated factor loadings for the six factors obtained from Varimax rotation of the principal components. These loadings represent the correlations of each of the 83 time points ("variables") with the factors. Time scale is 498 msec (6 msec per point times 83 points)

msec. The correspondence between her evoked potential component latencies and the latencies to the peak loadings of factor 6 account for her high score on factor six.

Two by three ANOVAs with group and age band as the main variables were performed on each factor using the factor scores. Factor 3 was significantly affected by age ($F(2,36) = 3.82$, $p < .03$), with mean factor scores being highest for the youngest group of subjects.

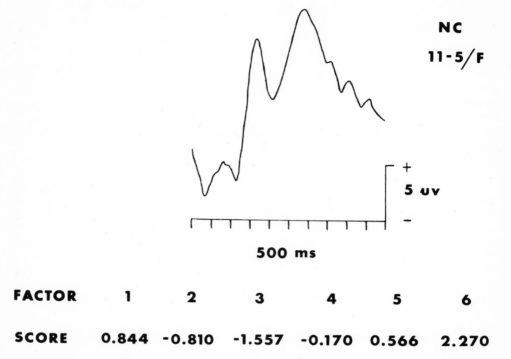

FACTOR        1        2        3        4        5        6

SCORE    0.844  -0.810  -1.557  -0.170  0.566   2.270

Figure 3. A typical averaged auditory evoked potential recorded from
a female (aged 11-5) normal comparison subject. Her scores on the six
factors are indicated. These scores quantify the degree to which her
evoked potential is represented by each of the six factors.

The youngest subjects' grand mean waveform was characterized by
prominent late positive activity, thus accounting for their higher
mean scores on factor 3, which had high positive loadings in the very
late portions of the response epoch. No group, age, or group by age
effects were significant for any of the other factors.

### Deviance Analyses

The results of the discriminant function analyses and the factor
score analyses agree well with previous reports (e.g., Hanson et al.,

1976; Fein et al., 1974) on measures other than the averaged evoked potential, in showing no gross differences between the HR and NC samples. To determine the number of significantly deviant subjects in both groups we used the mean factor scores of the NC sample on all factors as the centroid from which we computed Mahalanobis distances (a measure of multivariate distance) for each of the NC and HR children. These distances can be tested for significant departure from the centroid using the chi-square distribution and six degrees of freedom. Using this method, we identified five members of each group as significant outliers at the five percent level or better. The distribution of outliers across age bands was roughly equivalent for both groups.

This was an encouraging first step. We then wanted to determine if the averaged evoked potential measure of deviance was related to these childrens' scores on other measures used in this study. During the first round of testing, the full sample of subjects (of which the present subsample was a part) was given a battery of test procedures including a number of cognitive measures. These measures were subjected to multiple regression analysis controlling for age, sex and IQ. Five of these scores (further analyses are currently being performed using additional measures: Erlenmeyer-Kimling et al., in preparation) which showed significant group differences after application of such controls were retained and were entered into a discriminant function analysis between the HR and NC groups. In the resultant discriminant score distributions, a score which cut off five percent of the NC group was used as an index of deviance. Based on this cut-off score, 29 percent of the HR sample were identified as deviant. Using the measure of averaged evoked response deviance, we went back to the list of children who were seen as deviant on the discriminant score measure to determine if there was an association between the two deviance measures. Two of the HR and one of the NC children who were examined for averaged evoked response deviance were not included in the discriminant function analysis, thus reducing the number that could be compared on the two analyses to 19 HR and 20 NC subjects. Of the five HR children identified as evoked response outliers, three were also outliers on the discriminant score measure for the cognitive tests. A two by two contingency analysis resulted in a phi coefficient of .57 ($X^2(1) = 3.42$), which falls just short of the five percent level of significance. No such association was seen for the NC outliers, not one of which was seen as deviant on the discriminant score measure. The percentage of HR children "hitting" on both measures of deviance is 15.7, a figure in consonance with the empirical risk estimates for children of one schizophrenic parent.

Figure 4 presents the grand mean averages for the outliers of each group and the residual grand means after the outliers have been removed. It is clear that the outliers have been selected on the

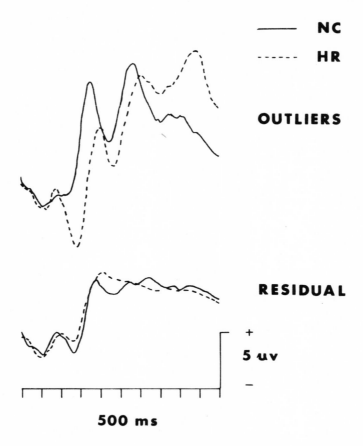

Figure 4. Grand mean evoked potentials averaged across outliers of both groups (N = 5 in each). The outliers were identified using the Mahalanobis $D^2$s. The residual waveforms were obtained by subtracting the outliers from the grand means of their respective groups.

basis of both amplitude and waveshape. The amplitudes of the major components of the outliers are roughly twice that of the component amplitudes of the residual waveforms, and, in addition, the outlier waveforms are composed of prominent positive activity in the later portions of the response. The residual waveforms of the two groups are remarkably similar, and are more similar with the outliers removed than with them in the average (see figure 1). With the outliers removed, very little late positive activity is seen in the residual waveforms.

The two groups of outliers had different mean factor score profiles. A consistent difference was seen for factor 5, on which all the HR outliers had negative factor scores and all the NC outliers had positive factor scores. This factor had high positive loadings peaking at 162 msec, and was identified with the P190 component. The major differences between the two groups of outliers are seen in the amplitude of N125, which is larger for the HR subjects, in the latencies of P190, N225 and P285, which are longer for the HR outlier group, and in very late positive activity which is more prominent and longer in latency in the HR outlier grand mean. Thus, the two outlier grand means begin to diverge at P190 (accounting for the consistent difference on factor 5), with all remaining peaks being longer in latency for the HR outliers.

Significance of differences between the outlier groups was assessed using the t-test, and alpha levels were corrected for the number of tests using the Bonferroni criterion (see Friedman et al., 1975 for a discussion of this test in an evoked potential setting). Thus, for six tests (factor scores) and significance at the .05 level, a p value of .008 is necessary; for five tests (peak latencies) a p value of .016 is necessary. Only the mean difference on factor 5 was significant using the conventional level of significance, and fell short of significance using a corrected level ($t(8) = 2.83$, p <.02). Mean peak latency differences were also tested: the mean difference for P190 with mean latency of 165 msec (SD = 9.35) for the NC outliers and 193 msec (SD = 17.88) for the HR outliers was significant ($t(8) = 3.10$, p <.005), as was the mean difference for P400, with a mean of 388 msec (SD = 12.60) for the NC outliers and 437 msec (SD = 14.40) for the HR outliers ($t(5) = 4.69$, p <.01; only four of the HR and three of the NC outliers produced this late positive component). None of the peak amplitude differences was significant, even at an uncorrected alpha level of .05. There were no significant differences (even at uncorrected alpha levels) between the two groups of subjects that comprised the residual grand means.

The differences between the outlier groups and the association between the averaged evoked potential and discriminant score measures of deviance in the HR outlier subgroup are encouraging. It is clear that both subgroups of outliers differed from their respective groups in both amplitude and waveshape, while the differences between the two outlier subgroups occurred mainly in peak latency, with the peaks in the HR subgroup occurring significantly later than in the NC subgroup. With no task imposed on the subject, and, therefore, with subject option uncontrolled (see Sutton, 1969), it is difficult to interpret these differences: are they due to a breakdown in sensory information processing or in the later, cognitive stages of information processing? It will be necessary to repeat the procedure for assessing deviance with measures derived from tasks that permit the investigator to specify which types of processing the subject is engaged in. We are currently performing such experiments, where the emphasis is on the cognitive aspects of information processing.

Our data point up the importance of the detection of outliers in high-risk research as an alternate methodology, in addition to searching for group differences. Unfortunately, the high-risk researcher does not know whether his detection measures will, after follow-up of those subjects at risk, prove to be predictive of schizophrenia. This, of course, remains to be seen.

## ACKNOWLEDGEMENTS

The authors would like to thank the following people for their aid in technical work related to this project: Dr. George Fein and Mr. Allan Barroni for data collection; Ms. Rebecca Jacobsen and Ms. Annette Zaffos for preparation of the data for analysis; Mr. Jim Hollenberg, Mr. John Nee, and Ms. Henrietta Wolland for computer programming; Ms. Barabara Cornblatt and Dr. Yvonne Stellingwerf for their valuable contributions; Drs. Rainer, Stone, and Cowan provided the diagnoses of the parents of our high-risk children, and Drs. Joseph Fleiss and Donald Ross provided statistical advice. We thank Dr. Herbert Vaughan, Jr. for his discussion and constructive criticism of this paper at the conference at which it was presented. Supported by Grant MH-19560 to the third author and by the Department of Mental Hygiene of New York State.

## REFERENCES

Dixon, W.J., (Ed): BMDP Biomedical Computer Programs., Berkeley: University of California Press, 1975.

Donchin, E. A multivariate approach to the analysis of average evoked potentials., IEEE Transactions Biomedical Engineering, 1966, BME-13, 131-139.

Donchin, E. Data analysis techniques in evoked potential research., in Donchin, E., and Lindsley, D.B. (Eds): Average Evoked Potentials: Methods, Results, and Evaluations., Washington, D.C., NASA SP-191, 1969, 199-236.

Erlenmeyer-Kimling, L. Studies on the offspring of two schizophrenic parents, in Rosenthal, D., and Kety, S.S. (Eds): The Transmission of Schizophrenia., New York: Pergamon Press, 1968.

Erlenmeyer-Kimling, L. A prospective study of children of schizophrenic parents., USPHS Grant MH-19560, 1970.

Erlenmeyer-Kimling, L. A prospective study of children at risk for schizophrenia: methodological considerations and some preliminary findings., in Wirt, R.D., Winokur, G., and Roff, M. (Eds): Life History Research in Psychopathology, Vol. 4, 1975, Minneapolis: University of Minnesota Press, 23-46.

Erlenmeyer-Kimling, L. Issues pertaining to prevention and intervention in genetic disorders affecting human behavior., in Albee, G.W., and Joffe, J.M. (Eds): Primary Prevention in Psychopathology., Hanover: Univ. Press of New England, 1977, in press.

Erlenmeyer-Kimling, L., Cornblatt, B., and Fleiss, J.L. Cognitive test data on children of schizophrenic parents., in preparation.

Fein, G., Tursky, B., and Erlenmeyer-Kimling, L. Stimulus sensitivity and reactivity in children at high risk for schizophrenia. Psychophysiol., 1975, 12, 226.

Friedman, D., Simson, R., Ritter, W., and Rapin, I. Cortical evoked potentials elicited by real speech words and human sounds., Electroenceph. clin. Neurophysiol., 1975, 38, 13-19.

Garmezy, N., and Streitman, S. Children at risk: the search for the antecedents of schizophrenia. Part 1 Conceptual models and research methods., Schiz. Bull., 1974, 8, 14-90.

Hanson, D.R., Gottesman, I.I., and Heston, L.L. Some possible childhood indicators of adult schizophrenia inferred from children of schizophrenics., Brit. J. Psychiat., 1976, 129, 142-154.

Herman, J., Mirsky, A.F., Ricks, N.L., and Gallant, D. Behavioral and electrographic measures of attention in children at risk for schizophrenia., J. Abn. Psychol., 1977, 86, 27-33.

Itil, T.M., Hsu, W., Saletu, B., and Mednick, S. Auditory evoked potential investigations in children at high risk for schizophrenia., Amer. J. Psychiat., 1974, 131, 892-900.

Levine, F.M., and Whitney, N. Absolute auditory threshold and threshold of unpleasantness of chronic schizophrenic patients and normal controls., J. Abn. Psychol., 1970, 75, 74-76.

Mednick, S.A., and McNeill, T.F. Current methodology in research on the etiology of schizophrenia: serious difficulties which suggest the use of the high-risk group method., Psychol. Bull., 1968, 70, 681-693.

Pearson, J.S., and Kley, I.B. On the application of genetic expectancies as age-specific base rates in the study of human behavior disorders., Psychol. Bull., 1957, 54, 406-420.

Rutchmann, J., Cornblatt, B., and Erlenmeyer-Kimling, L. Report on a continuous performance test of sustained attention in children at risk for schizophrenia., Arch. Gen. Psychiat., 1977, 34, 571-575.

Saletu, B., Saletu, M., Marasa, J., Mednick, S., and Schulsinger, F. Acoustic evoked potentials in offsprings of schizophrenic mothers ("High Risk" children for schizophrenia)., Clin. Electroenceph., 1975, 6, 92-102.

Sutton, S. The specification of psychological variables in an average evoked potential experiment., in Donchin, E., and Lindsley, D.B. (Eds): Average Evoked Potentials: Methods, Results, and Evaluations., Washington, D.C.: NASA SP-191, 1969, 237-297.

Zerbin-Rüdin, E. Endogene psychosen., in Becker, P.E. (Ed): Humangenetik, (Handbuch, Vol. 2), Stuttgart, Thieme, 1967.

# AN EVOKED POTENTIAL STUDY OF ENDOGENOUS AFFECTIVE DISORDERS IN ALCOHOLICS[1]

Donald C. Martin

Departments of Biostatistics and Psychiatry

Joseph Becker, Veronica Buffington

Department of Psychiatry and Behavioral Sciences

SC-32, University of Washington, Seattle WA 98195

## ABSTRACT

This study investigated the hypothesis that some alcohol abusers have variations in neurophysiological response patterns akin to those found in endogenous affective disorders. VERs were obtained from three groups of alcohol abusers using procedures developed by Buchsbaum and Silverman (1968). The groups consisted of alcohol abusers with 1) a family history of bipolar affective disorder 2) a negative family history of affective disorders and 3) a family history of unipolar depression. Changes in VER with variation in stimulus intensity analogous to those reported for bipolar (augmenters) and unipolar (reducers) depressives were expected and obtained for Groups 1 and 3 respectively.

This interim report is based upon a sample of 43 (7,22 and 14 respectively). Two global VER amplitude measurements taken over 500 milliseconds, the mean absolute deviation and the mean squared deviation, showed significant differences (p=.02 and .01 respectively) in the predicted direction. Although none of the

[1] This study was supported by Grants 63-0625 from the Alcoholism and Drug Abuse Institute at the University of Washington , AA01881 from the National Institute on Alcohol Abuse and Alcoholism,and Public Health Service Grant 5 R01 MB 00184-03.

groups were VER reducers, Group 1 showed the largest VER augmentation and Group 3 the least. Two specific VER amplitude measurements, (P90-N140) and (P200-N140), failed to show significant differences although the latter measurement showed some trend in the hypothesized direction.


## INTRODUCTION

Clinical observers have often noted a high concordance between alcoholism and affective disorders within individuals and within families (Fox, 1967; Freed, 1970). While some writers speculate that a predisposition to depression may underly alcoholism (Mendels, 1970; Ostow, 1970), others argue that depression in alcoholics is due largely to an overlap in physical symptoms, and to the psycho-social repercussions of their drinking (Button, 1956; Hewett, 1943; Milam, 1976).

Since there are no well validated genetic markers of a predisposition to alcoholism or to depression, investigators have relied on family concordance studies to support their contention of a linkage between the two. Winokur and his associates (1970, 1971) and Woodruff, et al. (1973) report a very high rate of unipolar depression among the first-degree female relatives of male alcoholic subjects. No other psychiatric disorder occurs beyond population expectancies within these families except for alcoholism and sociopathy in other male kin.

Psychopharmacological studies also suggest a possible linkage between alcoholism and predisposition to depression. For example, although detoxified alcoholics resemble anxious reactive depressives clinically, they respond better to medications that are most effective with more endogenous like affective disorders (Butterworth, 1971; Butterworth & Watts, 1971; Overall, et al., 1973; Wren, 1974). Endogenous affective disorders are thought to have a heavier genetic loading than reactive depression though the issue is controversial (Eysenck, 1971; Gershon, et al., 1971).

In sum, it could be hypothesized that alcoholism sometimes partly masks an underlying predisposition to depression. The difference in the sex-specific frequency of expression of depression (females overt - males masked) could be due, of course, to sex linked genetic factors or to cultural expectancies. The overt expression of the hopelessness and helplessness characteristic of depression is regarded as unmanly in most cultures (Zetzel, 1965). Hence, males with a depressive diathesis which is relieved by alcohol might be especially susceptible to alcoholism.

A leading problem in much clinical research is the reduction of heterogeneity within diagnostic categories; unaccounted for variance can be considerably reduced if meaningful, homogeneous, subgroups can be identified (Garmezy & Rodnick, 1959). The evidence reviewed suggested that it might be possible to discriminate alcoholics with a predisposition to depression from those not so predisposed. This discrimination could have implications for etiology, treatment, and prevention.

Further validation of a construct like alcoholics predisposed to affective disorders requires a supportive "nomothetic net" of relations (Cronbach & Meehl, 1958). We turned to visual evoked potentials because distinctive averaged visual evoked response patterns for unipolar and bipolar affective disorders have been reported (Buchsbaum, 1976). Clinically, depressed unipolars (those with depressive episodes only) have been identified as "reducers", whereas bipolars (those with manic and depressive episodes) have been identified as "augmenters." Normal controls display intermediate or mild augmenter tendencies. With clinical remission, the evoked potentials of patients with affective disorders reputedly normalize (Buchsbaum, et al., 1971).

However, our pilot work suggested that if male alcoholics were divided into three groups: 1) those with a positive family history of bipolar affective disorder, 2) those with a negative family history of affective disorder, and 3) those with a positive family history of unipolar depression, the order effects of response magnitude (bipolars, normals, unipolars) obtained in the Buchsbaum, et al. (1971) findings with affectively disordered patients could be replicated. This study was designed to investigate the presence and stability of such anomalies irrespective of the alcoholic's present clinical status vis a vis depression and/or alcohol abuse (though data are being obtained on these variables). We were interested in attempting to identify a relatively stable neurophysiological marker that might further validate the existence of affectively predisposed subgroups of alcoholics. The findings presented here provide an interim report on this work.

Flash intensity measures of averaged evoked potentials were used in line with Soskis and Shagass' (1974) conclusions that such measures have yielded promising psychiatric, though variable personality correlates (Coursey et al., 1975; Rust, 1975; Zuckeman, 1974). Such data yield relatively good reliabilities, can be computer analyzed, and seem to be relatively uninfluenced by ocular factors.

Previous work on the visual cortical evoked potentials of alcoholics (ably summarized in Soskis and Shagass, 1974) suggest that alcohol evokes an inhibitory-like response in the CNS designed to prevent overstimulation (Buchsbaum, 1975). Alcohol reputedly suppresses the amplitude of the evoked response (Gross, et al., 1966), reduces the amplitude-intensity slope (Spilker & Calloway, 1969) and averaged evoked response (AER) asymmetries (Rhodes et al., 1975), as well as hemispheric amplitude differences (Lewis et al., 1970). Support for the hypothesis of an inhibitory-like CNS response to alcohol is provided by the findings of Coger, et al. (1976) on the REM rebound-like effects of withdrawal on AERs. Both alcoholics who had been withdrawn from alcohol for 3 weeks and those who were in the process of withdrawal consistently had greater AER intensity-amplitudes than non-alcoholic controls.

To summarize: since both AERs (Buchsbaum, 1974) and depressive disorders appear to be strongly influenced by genetic factors (Gershon, et al., 1971; Winokur, 1975) and unipolar and bipolar affective disorders are associated with distinctive AER patterns, our hypothesis was that the AERs of alcoholics with a positive family history of unipolar disorder would have reducer tendencies; alcoholics with a negative family history of affective disorder would be intermediate augmenters; and alcoholics with a positive family history of bipolar affective disorder would be relatively strong augmenters.


                                    SUBJECTS


Forty-three male subjects, recruited largely from the Alcoholism Treatment Unit at the Seattle Veterans Administration Hospital, participated in the study. The subjects consisted of male alcohol abusers who met the Guze Drinking Inventory (1965) criteria for being designated as alcoholic. These subjects had first-degree relatives living within the Seattle area who were also interviewed.

All subjects participated in two sessions. At the interview session, subjects and family members received a standard psychiatric interview ,the research diagnostic criteria (personal and family histoy versions) (Endicott & Spitzer, 1973),and the Beck Depression Inventory (1967). If any indication of a personal or family affective disorder was elicited, a determination was made of whether it was primary or secondary (Robins, et al., 1972), unipolar or bipolar (Winokur, et al., 1971a) and more endogenous or reactive (Carney & Sheffield, 1972). The interviewer classified the subjects into three groups: 1) subjects with a family history of bipolar affective disorder;, 2) subjects with a negative family history of affective disorder, 3) subjects with a family history of unipolar depression. Age, socio-economic status (Hollingshead, 1957),and competence data (Phillips & Zigler, 1961) were obtained on all subjects interviewed. Table 1 summarizes the age characteristics of the sample.

TABLE 1

MEAN AGE

| GROUP | N | AGE | | |
| | | MEAN | (SD) | RANGE |
| UNIPOLAR | 14 | 43.8 | (10.0) | 27-59 |
| NEGATIVE | 22 | 43.8 | (11.5) | 22-62 |
| BIPOLAR | 7 | 48.7 | (12.2) | 30-65 |

Three estimates of past and current patterns of reported alcohol consumption were derived from a quantity-frequency-variability interview of the subjects drinking history and practices.Cahalan al.'s (1969) Quantity- Frequency-Variability (QFV) categories for current consumption are presented in Table 2. The QFV classified all subjects as "heavy drinkers" based on their past consumption.

The second estimate , Cahalan et al.'s (1969) Volume Variability (VV) score divides subjects according to eleven non-ordered categories that reflect individual differences in the massing and spacing of drinking. It is a particularly useful system for separating out binge drinkers from drinkers who consume alcohol on a more regular basis. As is shown in Table 2, subjects current drinking behavior was clustered in categories representing abstainer, binge, and heavy drinking patterns. All subjects were classified as heavy drinkers (Hi Volume, Hi Maximum) for their past drinking behavior.

The third estimate, derived from Jessor et al. (1968), is a continuous variable that represents average ounces of absolute alcohol consumed per day. It is a composite score of all types of alcohol consumed and is calculated according to the amount of absolute alcohol in each drink. Mean, standard deviation, and range of Jessor scores for past and current alcohol use are presented in Table 3.

TABLE 2

CAHALAN'S CURRENT ALCOHOL USE CATEGORY BY GROUP

|               | GROUP    |          |         |
|---------------|----------|----------|---------|
| ALCOHOL USE   | UNIPOLAR | NEGATIVE | BIPOLAR |
| QFV           |          |          |         |
| ABSTAINER     | 8        | 15       | 6       |
| INFREQUENT    | 1        | 1        |         |
| LIGHT         |          |          |         |
| MODERATE      | 1        | 1        | 1       |
| HEAVY         | 4        | 5        |         |
| VV            |          |          |         |
| ABSTAINER     | 8        | 15       | 6       |
| INFREQUENT    | 1        | 1        |         |
| LOW VOL,HI MAX |         | 1        |         |
| MED VOL,HI MAX |         |          | 1       |
| HI  VOL,MED MAX |        | 1        |         |
| HI  VOL,HI MAX | 5       | 4        |         |

TABLE 3

JESSOR'S ALCOHOL USE BY GROUP
( AVERAGE OUNCES OF ABSOLUTE ALCOHOL PER DAY)

|          |    | PAST AA SCORE |       |          | CURRENT AA SCORE |       |         |
|----------|----|------|-------|----------|------|-------|---------|
| GROUP    | N  | MEAN | (SD)  | RANGE    | MEAN | (SD)  | RANGE   |
| UNIPOLAR | 14 | 4.1  | (1.9) | 0.4-7.4  | .9   | (1.5) | 0.0-4.6 |
| NEGATIVE | 22 | 4.8  | (2.3) | 1.0-8.7  | .6   | (1.1) | 0.0-3.4 |
| BIPOLAR  | 7  | 5.7  | (3.5) | 1.4-12.4 | .1   | (0.2) | 0.0-0.4 |

VER PROCEDURE

At the beginning of the laboratory session, subjects were questioned about their current use of medication, caffeine, nicotine, handedness, and recency of last drink. Current affective state was assessed by the Beck Depression Inventory and the Today form of the Multiple Affect Adjective Check List.

Visual evoked responses were obtained using procedures detailed by Buchsbaum and Silverman (1968). Subjects were seated in a reclining chair in a semi-darkened quiet room. Visual stimuli were generated by a Grass PS 22 photostimulator located 50 cm in front of the subject's eyes. The subject was instructed to keep his eyes closed during stimulus presentation. Blocks of stimulus flashes consisted of a randomized sequence of 10 or 11 flashes at one of four flash intensities. A one second interval separated each flash within the block and a three second interval separated the blocks. Three groups of 16 blocks were presented with a three minute rest period between each group. A total of 504 flashes, 126 for each of the 4 intensities, was presented. The EEG was recorded from Cz, Pz, and Oz referenced to the right ear with the left wrist used as ground. Only the EEG data from Cz is discussed in this paper. Eye movement was recorded between the outer corner and just above center of the right eye. Both EEG and eye movement were amplified (bandwidth .3 and 100 Hz) by a Grass polygraph and recorded along with a flash marker channel on a Vetter Model A tape recorder.

## ANALYSIS OF EEG DATA

The recorded data were digitized on a PDP 11/20 minicomputer with 128 samples per 500 millisecond sweep. Each of the 504 sweeps was saved for an editing program. This program computed the power in the eye channel and a measure of the high frequency noise in the EEG channel. The latter statistic is based upon the sum of squares of the first differences and was proposed by Morse and Grubbs (1947). A listing of stimulus times and simple bar graphs of the statistics was printed for each sweep. When either of these statistics exceeded a threshold value a small plot was made of that sweep. Sweeps that were seriously contaminated by eye movement, noise spikes, false markers due to switching the tape recorder off or on, etc. were deleted.

The averaging program computed the mean and standard deviation for each time point across sweeps. Each sweep was adjusted to have a zero mean across all 128 samples in the sweep. Variability thus would be reduced between sweeps if a large time constant had been used and the signal had contained very low frequency components. This adjustment would not change the shape of the AER. An on-line CRT displayed amplitudes and latencies of selected peaks of the AER. The selected peak values and the AER for each of the four flash intensities were then plotted with a two standard deviation confidence interval and the standard deviation.

The means and standard deviations for all intensities and leads were also saved in a summary computer file. A pooled mean evoked response was then computed across the four flash intensities and plotted on a single page with the four average evoked responses for each intensity. An example of this plot is shown in Figure 1.

Two additional graphical data presentations were computed. The first is the standardized deviation from the pooled mean for each flash intensity. This plot was a useful display of the differences between intensities but not as useful as an indicator of systematic change as a function of intensity. The second plot was developed to display systematic change with emphasis on the linear trend. The procedure is to fit each time point across the four intensities by orthogonal polynomials and then plot the standardized coefficients.

The polynomials are in terms of the logarithms of the four flash intensities (1, 2, 4, and 16). Because these points are unequally spaced on a log scale, it was necessary to compute the values of the orthogonal polynomials. These are:

| constant | linear | quadratic | cubic |
|----------|-----------|-----------|-----------|
| 0.5 | -0.591608 | 0.564076 | -0.286039 |
| 0.5 | -0.253546 | -0.322329 | 0.762770 |
| 0.5 | 0.084515 | -0.644658 | -0.572078 |
| 0.5 | 0.760639 | 0.402911 | 0.095346 |

where each column is a polynomial. Let $a_i(t)$ and $s_i(t)$ denote the AER and standard deviation. For the i-th flash intensity at the t-th time point where the average is based upon $n(i)$ sweeps, the polynomial decomposition is computed by

$$c_j(t) = \sum_{i=1}^{4} p_{ij} a_i(t)$$

where the p's are from the above table. The variance of these terms is estimated by

$$v_j(t) = \sum_{i=1}^{4} p_{ij}^2 s_i^2(t)/n_i$$

The z scores are computed for the 128 time points and i=1...4 flash intensities by

$$z_j(t) = c_j(t)/\sqrt{v_j(t)}$$

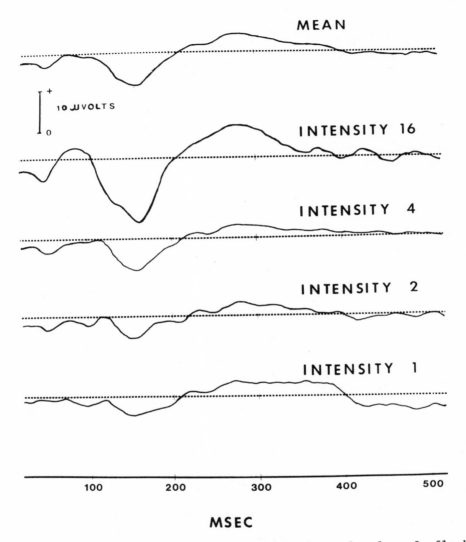

Figure 1.  Average Evoked Responses for four levels of flash
intensity and the pooled mean.

The z scores are then plotted for each   degree.   An   example   of
this   plot   is   shown   in   Figure   2.     The  linear term is of the
greatest interest.  This example shows   about   a   three   standard
deviation  positive  trend  near   90   milliseconds,   a very large
negative trend from about 140 to 175 milliseconds and a   positive
trend   again from 225 to 325 milliseconds as well as a suggestion
of   a   pair   of   late   positive   trends   between   400   and   500
milliseconds.     The   quadratic   and   cubic   plots   indicate small
departures from linearity except for a slight departure after 400
milliseconds on the quadratic plot.

      Two   global   measures   of   evoked   response   amplitude   were
computed.   The first was the standard deviation of the amplitudes
of the AER for each   intensity.     This   is   proportional   to   the
square   root   of   the   power.     The   second   measure was the mean
absolute deviation:

$$d_i = \sum_{t=1}^{128} |a_i(t) - m_i| /128$$

where

$$m_i = \sum_{t=1}^{128} a_i(t)/128.$$

These two measures of global amplitude are very similar  but  the
mean   absolute   deviation   is less sensitive to short high voltage
peaks.   The orthogonal polynomial decomposition   was   applied   to
both   of   these   global   measures and the linear trend terms have
been used in the analysis.

      Three VER components, P90, N140, and  P200    were identified
by   two   individuals  .    Differences  in peak identification were
resolved   and   a   reliability   score   was   assigned  based    upon
disagreements.     This   procedure   was   not   very satisfactory.  A
significant number of   subjects   had   waveforms   that   made   peak
identification   doubtful   at best.   The P90 peak was particularly
troublesome.   For some subjects, the number of peaks changed as a
function of intensity.  Nonetheless, trend measures were computed
for the P90–N140 as well as the P200– N140 measurements.

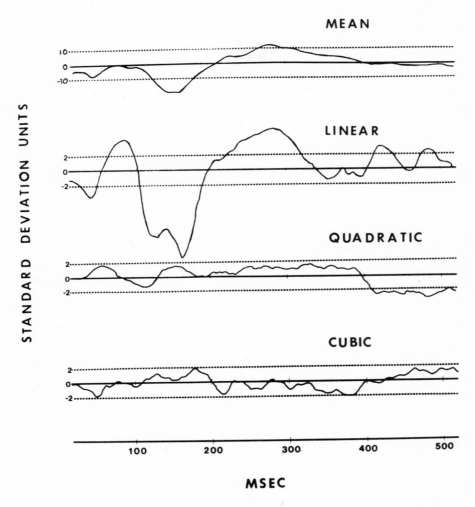

Figure 2.   Polynomial decomposition of VERs from Figure 1.

RESULTS AND DISCUSSION

This study investigated the hypothesis that some alcoholism masks an endogenous affective disorder. The disorder may initially be alleviated by drinking and impulsive behavior. It was assumed that the hypothesis would more likely be valid in families with a high incidence of affective disorder. If the hypothesis was valid, a sizable proportion of male alcoholics from such families should have the distinctive anomalous VER's characteristic of unipolar depressives and bipolar affectives respectively.

The four VER slope measures for the alcoholics with bipolar family histories were expected to be larger than slopes for alcoholics with a negative family history which, in turn, should have tended to have been larger than the slopes for alcoholics with unipolar family histories.

The Jonkheere-Terpstra test (Hollander and Wolf, 1973) is a nonparametric analog of a one way analysis of variance for ordered alternatives. The means, standard deviations and tail probabilities for Jonkheere's test of the four VER slope measures are given in Table 4.

TABLE 4

JONKHEERE-TERPSTRA TEST FOR GROUP DIFFERENCES IN SLOPE MEASURES

| | GROUP | | | |
| --- | --- | --- | --- | --- |
| | UNIPOLAR | NEGATIVE | BIPOLAR | |
| SLOPE MEASURES | MEAN (SD) | MEAN (SD) | MEAN (SD) | P |
| P90 TO N140 | 10.8(12.7) | 4.5(15.1) | 6.5(18.5) | 0.921 |
| N140 TO P200 | 9.0(10.1) | 13.7(16.1) | 16.7(12.0) | 0.093 |
| MEAN ABSOLUTE DEVIATION | 1.6( 1.8) | 2.2( 1.9) | 5.2( 3.0) | 0.021 |
| MEAN SQUARED DEVIATION | 2.2( 2.4) | 3.2( 2.3) | 5.2( 3.0) | 0.009 |

The mean slopes for VER slope measures based upon the P90 - N140 measurements were not in the order specified by the alternative hypothesis and the null was not rejected. The problem of consistent P90 identification may account for this result. Although the mean slope for the three groups based upon the measure are in the right order, the P200-N140 variability was great enough to prevent rejection.

The two global VER amplitude measurements, the mean absolute deviation and the mean squared deviation, showed significant differences (p = .02 and .01 respectively) in the predicted direction. Although none of the groups were VER reducers in these measures, Group 1 showed the largest VER augmentation and Group 3 the least.

Figure 3 shows the medians, quartiles and extremes of the slope of the mean squared deviation measure for the three groups. The observations become progressively more skewed as well as increasing both the means and medians. While family history of affective disorder may be assumed to identify subjects at risk for unipolar or bipolar depression, it is quite possible that any individual subject might not reflect the corresponding depressive disorder. These "false positives" would tend to fall at the low end of the distribution of bipolars and the high end of the unipolar group. This is consistent with the increasing skewness and larger dispersions of the unipolar and bipolar groups.

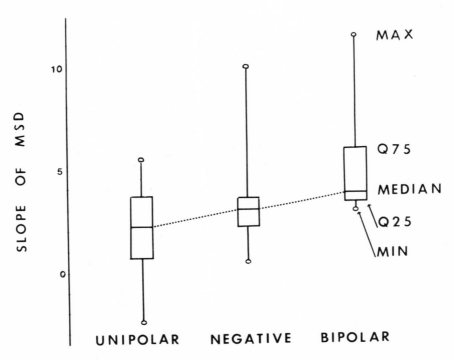

Figure 3.  Medians, Quartiles and extremes of the mean squared deviation slope measure for alcoholics with a family history of unipolar depression, bipolar affective disorder, or a negative affective history.

These findings support the hypothesis that some alcohol abusers have variations in neurophysiological response patterns akin to those found in endogenous affective disorders.

BIBLIOGRAPHY

Beck, A.T. Depression: Clinical, experimental, and theoretical aspects. New York: Harper & Row, 1967.

Buchsbaum, M. Self-regulation of stimulus intensity: Augmenting/reducing and the average evoked response. In G.E. Schwartz and D. Shapiro (Eds.), Consciousness and self-regulation. Advances in research. New York: Plenum Press, 1976.

Buchsbaum, M. Average evoked response augmenting/reducing in schizophrenia and affective disorders. D.X. Freedman (Ed.), The biology of the major psychoses: A comparative analysis. New York; Raven Press, 1975.

Buchsbaum, M. Average evoked response and stimulus intensity in identical and fraternal twins. Physiological Psychology, 1974, 2, 365-370.

Buchsbaum, M., Goodwin, F., Murphy, D. & Borge, G. AER in affective disorders. American Journal of Psychiatry, 1971, 128, 19-25.

Buchsbaum, M., & Silverman, J. Stimulus intensity control and the cortical evoked response. Psychosomatic Medicine, 1968, 30, 12-23.

Butterworth, A.T. Depression associated with alcohol withdrawal: Imipramine compared with placebo. Quarterly Journal of Studies in Alcohol. 1971, 32, 343-348.

Butterworth, A.T. & Watts, R.D. Treatment of hospitalized alcoholics with doxepin and diazepam. Quarterly Journal Studies on Alcohol,, 1971, 32, 72-81.

Button, A.D. A study of alcoholics with the MMPI. Quarterly Journal of Studies on Alcohol, 1956, 17, 263-281.

Cahalan, D., Cisin, I.H. & Crossley, H.M. American drinking practices. New Brunswick, N.J.: Rutgers Center of Alcohol Studies, Monograph No. 6, 1969.

Carney, M.W.P., & Sheffield, B.F. Depression and the Newcastle Scales: Their relationship to Hamilton's Scale. British Journal of Pyschiatry, 1972, 121, 35-40.

Coger, R.W., Dymond, A.M., Serafetinides, E.A., Lowenstam, I. Alcoholism: Averaged visual evoked response amplitude-intensity slope and symmetry in withdrawal. Biological Psychiatry, Vol. 11, No. 4, 1976.

Coursey, R.D., Buchsbaum, M. and Frankel, B.L. Personality measures and evoked responses in chronic insomniacs, Journal of Abnormal Psychology, 1975, 84 (3), 239-249.

Cronbach, L. & Meehl, P.E. Construct validity in psychological tests, Psychological Bulletin, 1955, 52, 281-302.

Endicott, J., & Spitzer, R.I. What! Another rating scale? The psychiatric evaluation form. Journal of Nervous and Mental Disease, 1972, 154, 88-104.

Eysenck, H.J. The classification of depressive illness. British Journal of Psychiatry, 1970, 117, 241-271.

Fox, R. Alcoholism and reliance upon drugs as depressive equivalents. American Journal of Psychotherapy, 1967, 21, 585-596.

Freed, E.X. Alcoholism and manic-depressive disorders: Some perspectives. Quarterly Journal of Studies on Alcohol. 1970, 31, 62-89.

Garmezy, N. & Rodnick, E.H. Premorbid adjustment and performance in schizophrenia: Implications for interpreting heterogeneity in schizophrenia. Journal of Nervous and Mental Disease, 1959, 129, 450-466.

Gershon, E., Dunner, D., Goodwin, F. Toward a biology of affective disorders. Archives of General Psychiatry, 25, 1971, 1-15.

Gross, M.M., Begleiter, H., Tobin, M., & Kissin, B. Changes in auditory evoked response produced by alcohol. Journal of Nervous and Mental Disease. 1966, 142, 493-499.

Guze, S.B., Goodwin, D.W., & Crane, J.B. Criminality and psychiatric disorders. Archives of General Psychiatry, 1965, 20, 583-591.

Hewitt, C.C. A personality study of alcohol addiction. Quarterly Journal of studies on Alcohol. 1943, 44, 368-386.

Hollingshead, A.B. Two factor index of social position. New Haven: Yale Universiity, 1957.

Hollander,Myles and Wolfe,Douglas A. Nonparametric Statistics. New York: Wiley, 1973.

Jessor, R., Graves, T.D., Hanson, R.C., & Jessor, S.L. Society, personality and deviant behavior: A study of a tri-ethnic commmunity. Holt, Rinehart and Winston, Inc., New York, NY, 1968.

Morse, A.P. Grubbs F.E. . The estimation of dispersion by differences. Annals of Mathematical Statistics 1947, 18, 194-213.

Mendels, J. Concepts of Depression. New York: Wiley, 1970.

Milam, J.R. The emergent comprehensive concept of alcoholism. Kirkland, Wash: ACA Press, 1976.

Ostow, M. The psychology of melancholy. New York: Wiley, 1970.

Overall, J.E., Brown, D., Williams, J.D., & Neill, L.T. Drug treatment of anxiety and depression in detoxified alcoholic patients. Archives of General Psychiatry, 1973, 29, 218-221.

Perris, Carlo EEG techniques in the measurement of the severity of depressive syndromes. Neuropsychobiology, 1975, 1, 16-25.

Phillips, L., & Zigler, E. Social competence: The action-thought parameter and vicariousness in normal and pathological behaviors. Journal of Abnormal Psychology. 1961, 63, 137-146.

Rhodes, L.E., Obitz, F.W. and Creel, D. Effect of alcohol and task on hemispheric asymmetry of visually evoked potentials in man. Electroencephalography and Clinical Neurophysiology. 1975, 38 (6), 561-568.

Robins, E., Munoz, R.A., Martin, S., & Gentry, K.A. Primary and secondary disorders. In J. Zubin, & F.A. Freghan (Eds.), Disorders of mood. Baltimore: John Hopkins Press, 1972, 33-56.

Rust, J. Cortical evoked potential, personality, and intelligence. Journal Comprehensive Physiological Psychology, 89 (10), 1220-1226, 1975.

Rust, J. Genetic effects in the cortical auditory evoked potenntial: A twin study. Electroencephalography and Clinical Neurophysiology. 1975, 39, 321-327.

Salamy, A. The effects of alcohol on the variability of the human evoked potential. Neuropharmacology, 1973, 12,1103-1107.

Soskis, D.A. Shagass, C. Evoked potential tests of augmenting-reducing. Psychophysiology, 1974, 11, 1975-190.

Spilker, B., & Callaway, E. "Augmenting" and "reducing" in averaged visual evoked responses to sine wave length. Psychophysiology, 1969, 6, 49-57.

Winokur, G. Heredity in the affective disorders. In E.J. Anthony & T. Benedek (Eds.) Depression and human existence. Boston: Little, Brown 1975, 7-21.

Winokur, G., Reich, T., Rimmer, J., and Pitts, F.N. Alcoholism III. Diagnosis and familial psychiatric illness in 259 alcoholic probands. Archives General Psychiatry. 23, 1970, 104-111.

Winokur, G., Rimmer, J., and Reich, T. Alcoholism IV. Is there more than one type of alcoholism? British Journal Pscychiatry. 1971, 118, 525-531.

Winokur, G., Cadoret, R.J., Dorzab, J., & Baker, M.    Depressive
    disease:    A genetic study.    Archives of General Psychiatry,
    1971, 24, 135-144.    (a)
Woodruff, R.A., Guze, S.B., Clayton, P.J., & Carr, D.    Alcoholism
    and depression.    Archives of General Psychiatry, 1973, 28,
    97-100.
Wren, J.C., Kline, N.S., Cooper, T.B., Varga, E., & Canal, O.
    Evaluation    of    lithium therapy    in    chronic    alcoholism.
    Clinical Medicine.    1974, 81, 33-36.
Zetzel, E.R.    Depression and the capaciity to bear it.    In M.
    Schur    (Ed.)  Drives, affects, behavior.    Vol.    2.   New York:
    International University Press, 1965.
Zuckerman, M.    The Sensation Seeking Motive.    In Maher, B.A.
    (Ed.), Progress in Experimental Personality Research, 1974.

# AUDITORY EVOKED POTENTIALS AND PSYCHOPATHOLOGY*

Kenneth Lifshitz,  Samuel Susswein and Kai Lee

Rockland Research Institute

Orangeburg, New York  10962

## INTRODUCTION

Based on accumulated scientific knowledge it appears reasonable to assume a functional relationship between the scalp recorded electroencephalogram (EEG) and brain processes.  One can further reasonably expect that EEG would, in some way, reflect the altered mental state associated with serious psychopathology. As evidenced by this conference and the large number of articles published on this topic, event-related potentials are viewed as a potentially fertile area for the study of EEG-psychopathology relationships. Background issues concerning event related potentials have been well covered in books by Shagass (1), Regan (2) and Calloway (3), as well as in various review papers.

This report deals primarily with issues relating to the diagnosis of "schizophrenia".  As commonly used, "schizophrenia" is a somewhat nebulous diagnostic label which, despite its nonspecificity, is associated with one of the major causes of human suffering. Generally, medical science has been better able to deal with illnesses in which agreed upon instrumental measurements are significantly involved in the definition of the illness.  In the hope of finding such measurements we are studying EEG derived parameters for useful relationships to the diagnosis of schizophrenia.

In studying event related potentials from severely ill psychiatric patients auditory stimuli (events) have a unique advantage.  Subject cooperation required for controlling pupil size

*This study supported in part by N.I.M.H. Grant MH 24908.

and eye position is absent and there is no need to attach electrical or other transducers to the subject, thereby simplifying both psychological and legal factors. Reports on auditory averaged evoked potentials (AAEPs) in schizophrenic subjects note a tendency towards a decrement in the amplitude of the auditory AEP, e.g. Saletu et al. (4) and Levitt et al. (5). Jones et al. (6) noted this decrease in amplitude and a subsequent increase in amplitude for those patients who improved clinically. Levitt comments on a less marked decrease in auditory AEP amplitude in severely depressed subjects than in schizophrenics. A number of papers report an increase in the variability is not due to an increase in the variability of the ongoing ability of the auditory evoked potential in schizophrenics (7,8,9 and 10). This increase in variability is possible related to the diminished amplitude of the auditory AEP. Calloway et al. (7) present evidence that the increased AEP variability is not due to an increase in the variablity of the ongoing EEG. However, this conclusion is based upon analysis of the prestimulus EEG leaving open the possibility of post-stimulus artifact. An increase in the variability of the visual AEP reported by Lifshitz (11) on further analysis appears to have been related to difficulty in maintaining visual fixation with schizophrenic patients.

Considerable interest in the "late" components of the AEP has been generated due to their sensitivity to psychological state. Particular attention has been paid to the vertex positive components of the auditory AEP occurring at about 300 msec. This component increases in amplitude with the significance and uncertainty of the stimulus (12). The $N_1$ peak (about 100 msec) is increased in size with heightened attention; worth noting is that long interstimulus intervals abolish this effect (13). Auditory AEP components are also markedly affected by stages of sleep. Except for REM sleep there is a general tendency towards increase in amplitude and an increase in the latency of $N_2$ and later peaks with increasing depth of sleep (14). These reports indicate that, in general, levels of arousal affect the AEP.

A number of theories have postulated altered states of arousal in schizophrenic subjects. Broen (15) in his review of schizophrenia notes, in summary, "the evidence we have discussed indicates that, in situations that are relatively low-stress situations for normals, schizophrenics tend to be abnormally aroused on a number of physiologic measures..." Drug models of schizophrenia which depend upon the effect of amphetamines have also lead to speculation about pathological states of arousal. Because the issue of arousal or level of consciousness is pertinent to our studies a measure of this characteristic is desirable. In clinical electroencephalography an increase of low frequency EEG activity is commonly recognized as being associated with pathological states

of decreased awareness or consciousness.  In the nonpathological
alterations of arousal and consciousness that occur with sleep, the
studies of Lubin et al. (16) and Johnson et al. (17) have indicated
that for normal male subjects the single most consistent discrimina-
tor of stages ranging from wakefulness to deep sleep is the increase
of power in the 0.2 to 3.8 Hz (delta) EEG band.  Increased reaction
times are also associated with increased delta band power in normal
and schizophrenic subjects (18).  We have therefore used the amount
of delta band power as an indicator of arousal in our studies.

In this paper we report on selected auditory AEP findings
derived from a study in which a larger number of instrumentally
measured variables are evaluated for their relationship to psychopathology.

## METHOD

Results are reported based on data from 47 male, chronic
schizophrenic inpatients with a mean age of 41 $\pm$ 9 years, with
at least one year (mean 17 years) of hospitalization.  At
least three psychiatrists, including the senior author, agreed
upon the diagnosis of schizophrenia and our analysis of clinical
records substantiated this diagnosis in the usual clinical sense.
Subcategorization of diagnoses is unrealistic except, perhaps, for
the 13 patients diagnosed as paranoid.  Portions of our data
analysis use a random subset of 30 of these patients.  A group of
22 non-schizophrenic hospitalized patients were used as controls.
They had a mean age of 42 $\pm$ 9 years and a mean hospitalization
time of 8 years.  Ten of these subjects were diagnosed as chronic
alcoholics, 6 as mental retardates, 4 as having an organic brain
syndrome and 2 as severe neurotics.  Nineteen were receiving
medication equivalent to an average 600 mg of thorazine per day.
Thirty normal individuals with a mean age of 39 $\pm$ 9 years were
used as healthy controls.  These were principally Institute
employees, the majority personally known for several years with
no history of psychiatric hospitalization, neurologic illness or
the use, within one month, of medication considered psychotropic.

The EEG was recorded using drilled silver-silver chloride
electrodes from 4 scalp and 1 paraorbital derivation, as indicated
in Figure 1.  Symmetrical locations over the dominant hemisphere,
as determined by handedness, were used.  $C_z$ is two centimeters
lateral to the usual 10-20 designation, $0_1$ ($0_2$) is located at the
usual 10-20 site; both of these leads were referenced to balanced
ears.  Channels A and B were determined by our interest in electric
field configurations and the fact that the auditory evoked
potential tends to be maximum in the region of the vertex;

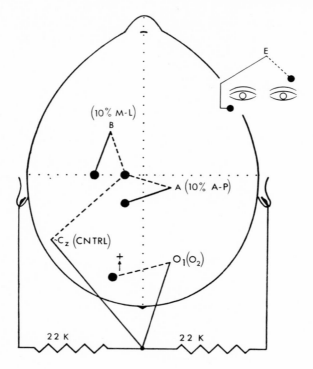

Figure 1

    Placement of electrodes for EEG recording.  Electrodes
for A are 2 cm from the midline.  For left handed individuals
the mirror image application is used.  The resistors are used
to minimize and unbalanced contribution from "active" ears
with unequal electrode impedances.


contamination from cranial muscles also tends to be minimal in this
area.  Channel A was taken as 10% of the inion to nasion distance
and parallel to the anterior-posterior plane; Channel B was taken
as the same distance and lying in the medial-lateral plane.  The
paraorbital channel was recorded from electrodes above the left
and below the right lateral canthus of the eyes.

    Measurements were made with the subject supine in an electri-
cally shielded room.  A ventilating fan provided a constant low
level background noise.  Tone stimuli, one second in length, of
700 Hz fundamentally frequency and moderate intensity (70db) were
randomly presented with a separation of at least 8 seconds.  The
EEG in each channel was digitized at 180 samples per second. For
each channel 512 data points (2.8 seconds) were collected before
and after the onset of stimulus.  Data was stored on IBM compatable

magnetic tape.  Before further processing each 1024 point block of
data had the best fit, least squares, regression line subtracted.
The subjects were told before and during the initial presentation
of the tone stimuli, that throughout the measurements the tone
stimuli would continue to occur, that they did not mean anything,
and required no response.  A light weight was placed over the
subjects eyes, in order to minimize blink artifacts.  At least
the first 12 data blocks were not utilized in analysis as they
were considered to be atypical due to habituation effects.  Artifact signals were initiated either by the technician (observing
both the paper record and the subject over closed circuit TV) or
instrumentally by a signal greater then 15 microvolts and over
100 Hz (muscle artifact) or by signal amplitudes above 100 to 167
microvolts.  Such an artifact signal discarded the data block and
started a new one.  EEG amplification was 3 db down at 0.16 Hz
and 50 Hz, rolloff at 50 Hz was 12 db per octave.

Valid responses to 150 stimuli were collected.  Delta band
power for the 2.8 seconds preceding each stimulus was calculated
for the Cz derivation (19), offline by using a Fast Fourier
Transform (20).  Averaged evoked potentials for each subject were
calculated by selecting the 50 responses preceded by EEG of the
lowest delta power, 50 intermediate delta power responses and the
50 high delta power responses.  Additionally, all 150 responses
were used for computing an AEP without delta power sorting.


## RESULTS AND DISCUSSION

The delta band power sorting results in low, medium and high
values for the different subject groups.  Pairwise comparisons by
Mann-Whitney U-Test shows no significant difference in these
values.  However, the schizophrenic subjects show a narrower range
of values than do the two control groups.  Thus the mean of the
power in the 0.35 to 3.8 Hz band is 18 microvolts sq. for the
low 1/3 of the normal control epochs and 100 microvolts sq. for
the high 1/3 of the delta epochs; the equivalent values for the
chronic schizophrenic subjects are 21 $\mu v$ sq. and 85 $\mu v$ sq.  This
sorting procedure makes a difference in the associated auditory
AEP, which may be noted by comparing Figures 2 and 3.  In these
figures the data for the $C_z$ and A EEG derivations are shown.
Curves are shown for 30 normal controls and 30 matched chronic
schizophrenic patients.  For the grand mean auditory AEP shown
in Figure 2, for channel $C_z$, the $N_1$-$P_2$ amplitude is larger in the
controls.  The equivalent curves in Figure 3 (not equated for
delta power) show a similar difference.  In Figure 3 the higher
2/3 of the delta power epochs are added and we note that the
control subjects show a negative deflection peaking at about 0.7
seconds.  Also from the curve immediately below the top one we may

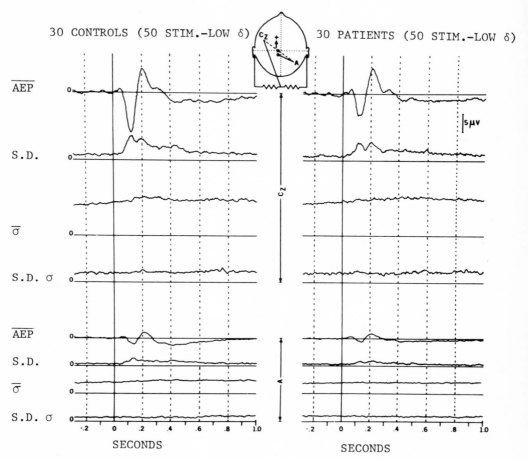

## Figure 2

AEP is the grand mean auditory AEP, calculated in each
subject from the 50 (of 150) EEG epochs with the lowest delta
band power. S.D. is the standard deviation of the 30 individual AEPs. σ̄ is the grand mean of the standard deviations of
the 50 EEG epochs used in each subject to compute their AEP.
S.D.σ̄ is the standard deviation of the 30 subjects' σ.

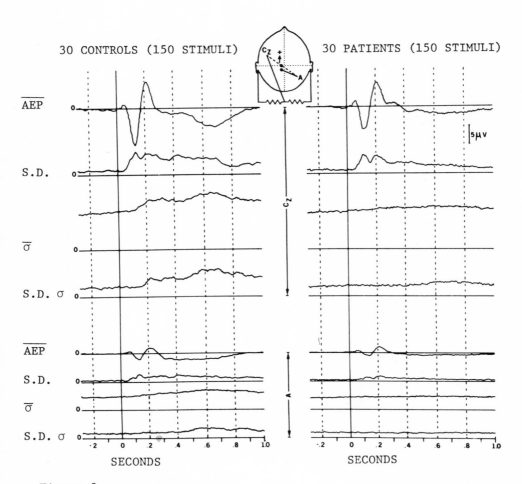

30 CONTROLS (150 STIMULI)    30 PATIENTS (150 STIMULI)

$\overline{AEP}$

S.D.

$\overline{\sigma}$

S.D. $\sigma$

$\overline{AEP}$

S.D.

$\overline{\sigma}$

S.D. $\sigma$

SECONDS    SECONDS

Figure 3

Vertical axis labels as in Figure 2. The underlying data differs from Figure 2 in that 150 unsorted EEG epochs are used to calculate the subjects' AEP and σ. Scale indicated by 5μv calibration at upper right of figure.

see in <u>Figure 3</u> a greater amount of variation between subjects
indicated in the standard deviation (S.D.). Similarly the third
curve down (σ), the mean of all the individual subjects standard
deviation curves for their AEP, is larger especially for the
control subjects. The fourth curve down (S.D.σ) shows the
standard deviation of subjects from the curve above. The lower
four curves present similar data for channel A. Channel $C_Z$ and A
are presented at the same scale.

   <u>Table 1</u> presents univariate and multivariate analyses of
variance, separately considered for the AEP derived from channel
A, $C_Z$ and E. Data selected from each subject on the basis of
50 low delta power epochs per AEP, presented in the rows indicated
by δ1, and for 150 unselected epochs per AEP in the row δ4. Taken
as the AEP variables are the average amplitude by tenths of a
second, after stimulus onset, for the first half second and by
quarters of a second for the last half second. Each row considers
the probability of the null hypothesis of equality for 30 chronic
schizophrenic patients, 22 chronic control patients and 29 normal
control subjects. The last column indicates the multivariate,
simultaneous, probability of equality across all time blocks. If
we look at the column for the time block 0.1 to 0.2 seconds we see
that for the vertex channel ($C_Z$), low delta power AEP s (δ1) that

<u>Table I</u>. Univariate (variables are average amplitude of AEP time
blocks) and multivariate probabilities of the null hypothesis of
equality between 30 chronic schizophrenic patients, 22 chronic
control patients and 29 normal controls. Separately considered
for localized vertex (A), vertex to ears ($C_Z$) and eye channels.
For 50 selected low delta power responses (δ1) or 150 responses
(δ4) per subject.

AEP TIME BLOCKS - ANOVA - P of $H_0$

| Channel | 0-.1S | .1-.2 | .2-.3 | .3-.4 | .4-.5 | .5-.75 | .75-1. | MANOVA |
|---------|-------|-------|-------|-------|-------|--------|--------|--------|
| A (δ1)  | .158  | .017  | .486  | <u>.001</u> | .003 | .026 | .192 | <u>.001</u> |
| A (δ4)  | .064  | .021  | .454  | <u>.001</u> | .015 | <u>.006</u> | .461 | <u>.001</u> |
| $C_Z$(δ1) | .210 | <u>.005</u> | .205 | .831 | .585 | .312 | .660 | .267 |
| $C_Z$(δ4) | .613 | .051 | .398 | .256 | .516 | .042 | .846 | .066 |
| E (δ1)  | .158  | .508  | .352  | <u>.009</u> | <u>.001</u> | .023 | .229 | .208 |
| E (δ4)  | .118  | .602  | .165  | <u>.010</u> | <u>.005</u> | .018 | .500 | .142 |

the probability of an equality between the three groups is 0.005.
This time block captures the swing between $N_1$ and $P_2$, the most
commonly measured peak amplitude of the vertex AAEP.  The difference
is due primarily to the smaller amplitude of the schizophrenic
population.  If we look across the rows we see the greatest probability of difference between the groups is for the .3 to .4 sec time
block in channel A.  For $\delta 1$ and $\delta 4$ $p \leq$ .001.  The average amplitudes
of the auditory AEP's from this channel and time block are -0.33 μv
for the schizophrenics, -1.18 μv for the other chronic patients and
-1.43 μv for the normal controls.  The multivariate analysis of
variance shows channel A to be the only one  differentiating  between
groups at $p \leq$ .001.  The data for the eye channel (E) is included
principally to indicate that the results do not arise from occular
artifacts.  It should be noted that in addition to occular artifacts
the eye channel records frontal EEG.

Figure 4 displays the results of analysis in a format which
permits more detailed evaluation by the reader.  The data consists
of a display of time point by time point probabilities (Mann-
Whitney U-Test) of the equivalence of the auditory AEP's for 30
chronic schizophrenic subjects and 30 normal control subjects, for
both low delta power selected epochs and unselected epochs.  The
responses from the 5 derivations indicated in Figure 1 are presented.
A more detailed explanation of the technique can be found in a paper
by Kohn and Lifshitz (21).  We may note that for low delta epochs
the region of maximal difference in channel $C_z$ is from 0.1 to 0.2
seconds.  When all evoked potential epochs are examined (in the
right column) the differentiating region shifts to 0.6 to 0.8 seconds.  Channel A may be noted to be the best differentiator
between the groups, showing both a broad time region of significant
difference, starting after 0.3 seconds, and very small probability
values.  Figure 4 indicates that the next best channel differentiating the two samples is the paraorbital one.  The temporal and
amplitude character of the data indicates that it is not the cause of
the results seen for channel A, though there may be a common
underlying phenomena.

The amplitude of the channel A auditory AEP between 0.3 and
0.4 seconds shows a correlation with age on the order of 0.5
(Pearson product moment), such that older people are more likely
to show the same findings as schizophrenics.  However, this is not
the source of the difference between our group.  A possible
important source of the noted AAEP difference is exposure of the
schizophrenic subject to antipsychotic medication.  To evaluate
this we separately examined three subgroups of schizophrenic
patients.  One consisting of 12 patients who had not received any
medication for more than 27 days (probably free of most proximal
effects), a group of 15 subjects who had not received medication

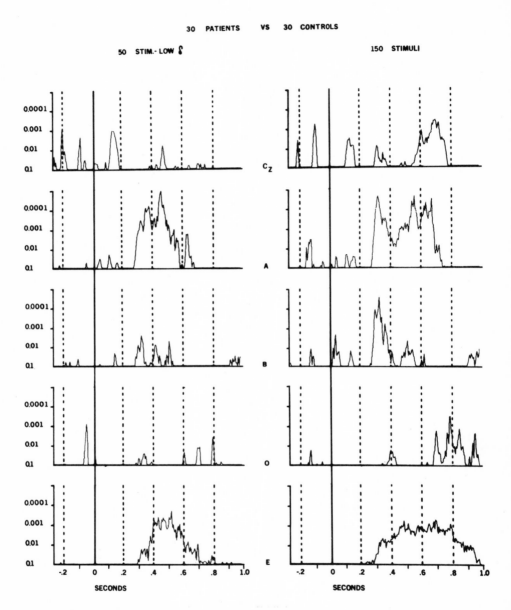

Figure 4. Point by point Mann-Whitney U-Test comparisons of the auditory AEP of 30 chronic schizophrenic patients versus 30 normal control subjects. EEG leads as indicated in Figure 1; for low delta power EEG epochs and unsorted EEG. Probability of ordinal equivalence of the two groups is scaled on the vertical axis.

for 6 to 27 days (probably continuing to show some antipsychotic
action and a group of 20 subjects on antipsychotic medication.
Of necessity the subjects who could be taken off medication for
the longest periods of time were, to some extent, self selected.
Table II presents a univariate and multivariate analysis of variance of these three groups presented in a manner analagous to
Table I. The table shows both univariate and multivariate
"significant" differences. Again, channel A and the 0.3 to 0.4
second segment of the AEP is the most "significantly" different.

Figure 5 shows the group grand mean auditory AEPs for the
data in the second row of Table II. All of these group AAEPs have
somewhat different characteristics. Group III, those patients on
medication, has the grand mean AAEP with the largest late negativity, which indicates that the effect of medication may be to
diminish the differences we have observed. The group longest
off medication shows the least amount of negative excursion after
the first quarter of a second. Interestingly, the group off
medication only a short time has an overall appearance most like
the normal control population.

As might be expected stepwise discriminant function analysis
presented with the variables we have been discussing selects
as the best differentiator the 0.3 to 0.4 second Channel A time
block. With this variable, unsorted by delta power, a discriminant
function program can distinguish between the chronic schizophrenic
patient and our other two groups combined, as indicated in
Table III, in better than 70% of the cases.

Table II. Univariate and multivariate (variables are average
amplitudes of AEP time blocks) probabilities of the null hypothesis
between chronic schizophrenic subjects off medication $\geq$ 28 days (N=12)
off medication 6 to 27 days (N=15) or on antipsychotic medication
(N=20). Separately considered for localized vertex (A) and vertex
to ears ($C_z$) channels. For 50 selected low delta responses ($\delta 1$) or
150 responses ($\delta 4$) per subject.

AEP TIME BLOCKS - ANOVA - P of $H_o$

| Channel | 0-.1S | .1-.2 | .2-.3 | .3-.4 | .4-.5 | .5-.75 | .75-1. | MANOVA |
|---------|-------|-------|-------|-------|-------|--------|--------|--------|
| A ($\delta 1$) | .179 | .665 | .363 | .003 | .032 | .229 | .075 | .007 |
| A ($\delta 4$) | .769 | .754 | .426 | .008 | .013 | .117 | .070 | .021 |
| $C_z(\delta 1)$ | .116 | .981 | .402 | .048 | .060 | .373 | .927 | .008 |
| $C_z(\delta 4)$ | .219 | .706 | .483 | .197 | .038 | .431 | .558 | .255 |

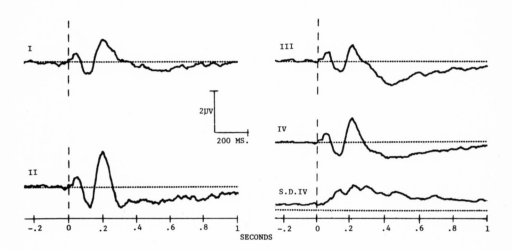

Figure 5

Group grand mean AEPs, channel A, 150 responses per subject. I= 12 chronic schizophrenics off medication $\geq$ 28 days; II= 15 chronic schizophrenics off medication 6 to 27 days; III= 20 chronic schizophrenics on medication; IV= I+II+III and associated standard deviation.

Table III. Discriminant Function Analysis

DISCRIMINANT CLASSIFICATION - channel A, 0.3 to 0.4 sec.

| Amplitude | % Correct | Schizophrenic Patients | Combined Controls |
|-----------|-----------|------------------------|-------------------|
| Patients  | 80.0      | 24                     | 6                 |
| Controls  | 64.7      | 18                     | 33                |
| Total     | 70.4      | 42                     | 39                |

Our data for lead $C_z$ is compatible to that in other reports on the auditory AEP recorded between the vertex and a distant electrode. The more interesting results, derived from channel A, cannot be directly compared to other studies because of unique electrode positioning. However, the field potentials which it measures is probably analogous to those alterations seen by $C_z$. In this context we may note that various studies have shown the absolute amplitude of the sound evoked, vertex negative wave occurring between 200-300 msec to be proportional to the reaction time at a significant level (22-25). In a study of autistic children during sleep (26) it was noted that during stage 2 sleep, the amplitude of the negative wave peaking about 275 msec was significantly smaller in autistic children, and that paradoxical sleep leads to a larger supression of this wave in controls than in autistic children. Negativity in this region of the auditory AEP has also been found to decrease amplitude with the unphysiological drowsiness produced by nitrous oxide (23). Under normal conditions the magnitude of this late negativity is contributed to by the presence of a continuous auditory stimulus, such as we use in our experimental paradigm. Jarvelehto and Fruhstoffer (27) feel, on the basis of its cranial distribution, that the continuous sound evoked DC potential recorded at the vertex is in fact a contingent negative variation. This response has been reported as abnormal in schizophrenic subjects, having a decreased amplitude and a prolonged reset time (28,29). Similar subjects have been noted as having a higher level of fixed anterior negativity by Cowen (30). These reports suggest that there may be a deficit in the mechanism generating low frequency, vertex region negative activity in chronic schizophrenic subjects, which may be related to an increased negative level of electrical bias over the frontal cortex.

Figures 2 and 3 permit a visual evaluation of the reports of increased variability in the auditory AEP of schizophrenics, upon which we have previously commented. The third tracing from the top, labelled $\sigma$ in each of the illustrations, shows the grand mean standard deviation associated with the auditory AEP in each subject. The individual subject's standard deviation contributing to this grand mean $(\overline{\sigma})$ is derived from the EEG time blocks contributing to his auditory AEP. The amount of variability which can be expected in repeated measures of the AEP for an individual is inversely proportional to the standard deviation of the associated EEG data blocks. Thus, the grand mean standard deviation $(\overline{\sigma})$ is approximately proportional to the amount of variability, at each AEP time point, that may be expected for the group. For selected low delta power data the standard deviation $(\sigma)$ of the patients AAEP is nonsignificantly larger than the normal controls for the first two tenth of second and nonsignificantly smaller for the last 8/10 of a second. In the data from all 150 EEG blocks for each subject

there is a significant difference in $\sigma$.  Table IV contains data
pertaining to this difference.  The columns indicate the time
blocks constituting the data variables; there is an additional
time block from 1/2 second before stimulus onset to stimulus
onset.  The values given in the rows for the patients and the
controls are the mean amplitudes of $\sigma$, in microvolts, over
time blocks indicated.  Univariate comparisons of these variables
indicate a "significantly" ($p \leq .05$) higher value for the normal
control subjects for 3 of the comparisons.  When the 8 variables
are considered simultaneously, in a multivariate analysis of
variance, the standard deviations of the AEP's from the control
subjects are significantly larger than the chronic schizophrenic
patient's at $p < 0.001$. The apparent difference of our results
from those of Calloway et al. (7), whose recording technique is
similar to ours, may be related to several differences.  Their
subjects were seated with eyes open and presented with stimuli
randomly separated by 1.75 to 3 seconds.  Our subjects were
lying, with eyes closed and presented with stimuli randomly
separated by more than 8 seconds.  The reference for their vertex
electrode is slightly different and, perhaps most consequentially,
they were dealing with acute rather than chronic schizophrenic
subjects.  However, it is also possible that their experimental
conditions were more conducive to the inclusion of stimulus locked
artifacts.

Table IV.  Ensemble mean of standard deviation for individual AEP
time blocks as indicated, for 30 chronic schizophrenic patients
and 29 normal control subjects, 150 stimuli per subject.

TIME BLOCKS OF AEP S.D. FOR CHANNEL $C_Z$

|       | -.5-0s | 0-.1  | .1-.2 | .2-.3 | .3-.4 | .4-.5 | .5-.75 | .75-1 |
|-------|--------|-------|-------|-------|-------|-------|--------|-------|
| Pts.  | 9.83   | 10.31 | 10.49 | 10.89 | 10.99 | 10.97 | 11.22  | 10.86 |
| Cont. | 9.68   | 10.25 | 11.41 | 13.13 | 13.16 | 12.91 | 14.19  | 12.89 |
| p <   | .84    | .93   | .27   | .04   | .05   | .09   | .04    | .10   |

FOR ALL DATA BLOCKS MUTLIVARIATE $p < .001$

SUMMARY

   Auditory averaged evoked potentials (AAEPs) were studied in
a group of chronic schizophrenic males (N=47), psychiatrically
hospitalized non-schizophrenic males (N=22) and normal male
subjects (N=30). Data for analysis was derived from 5 EEG leads.
Auditory stimuli, one second in duration, with interstimulus
intervals of over 8 seconds were used. Data was collected and
digitized under computer control. The AAEPs were calculated for
150 stimulus presentations. The 2.8 seconds of EEG prior to stimulus onset from lead $C_z$ was evaluated for delta band power in order
to equate the AAEPs for arousal level. The 50 EEG epochs with the
lowest delta power were used to calculate AAEPs which were also
analyzed. The AAEPs from lead Cz referenced to balanced ears
showed the previously reported $N_1$-$P_2$ amplitude decrement in
schizophrenic subjects as compared to normals, ascribable mainly
to N1 ($p \leq .01$); this was not a significant differentiator from
other patients. The reported increase in variability of the AAEP
was not substantiated in our sample of chronic schizophrenics. The
best differentiation between groups was obtained from the EEG
recorded from a closely spaced (about 3.2 cm) pair of electrodes
located parallel, and 2 cm lateral, to the mid-sagittal plane in
the region of the vertex. The late negativity (anterior electrode
active) measured between 0.3-0.4 second from this derivation
is decreased in our chronic schizophrenic subjects, $p \leq 0.001$
and can be used to differentiate them from the other two groups
(a posteriori) in 70% of the subjects. This late negativity was
evaluated in the schizophrenic subjects who were on antipsychotic
medication, off medication for 6 to 27 days and off medication for
more than 27 days. Antipsychotic medication appeared to act in a
manner so as to increase in magnitude the diminished late negativity.
Our findings may be related to others in which late, slow negative
event related potentials have been found to differ when brain
function was altered.

REFERENCES

1. Shagass, C. Evoked Brain Potentials in Psychiatry. New
      York: Plenum Press, 1972.
2. Regan, D. Evoked Potentials in Psychology, Sensory Physio-
      logy and Clinical Medicine. New York, Wiley-Interscience,
      1972.
3. Callaway, E. Brain Electrical Potentials and Individual
      Psychological Differences. New York, Grune & Stratton, 1975.

4. Saletu, B., Itil, T.M., & Saletu, M. Auditory Evoked Response, EEG and Thought Process in Schizophrenics. Amer. J. Psychiat. 1971, 128, 336-344.

5. Levit, R., Sutton, S. & Zubin, J. Evoked Potential Correlates of Information Processing in Psychiatric Patients. Psychol. Med., 1973, 3, 487-494.

6. Jones, R.T. & Callaway, E. Auditory Evoked Responses in Schizophrenia - A Reassessment. Biol. Psychiat., 1970, 2, 291-298.

7. Callaway, E., Jones, R.T. & Donchin, E. Auditory Evoked Potential Variability in Schizophrenia. Electroenceph. Clin. Neurophysiol. 1970, 29, 421-428.

8. Callaway, E. & Halliday, R.A. Evoked Potential Variability: Effect of Age, Amplitude and Methods of Measurement. Electroenceph. Clin. Neurophysiol., 1973, 34, 125-133.

9. Donchin, E., Callaway, E., & Jones, R.T. Auditory Evoked Potential Variability in Schizophrenia. II. The Application of Discriminant Analysis. Electroenceph. Clin. Neurophysiol. 1970, 29, 429-440.

10. Inderbitzen, L.B., Buchsbaum, M. & Silverman, J. EEG-Averaged Evoked Response and Perceptual Variability in Schizophrenics. Arch. Gen. Psychiat. 1970, 23, 438-444.

11. Lifshitz, K. An Examination of Evoked Potentials as Indicators of Information Processing in Normal and Schizophrenic Subjects. In: Average Evoked Potentials. (eds.) Donchin, E. and Lindsley, Washington, D.C.: NASA, 1966.

12. Sutton, S. The Specification of Psychological Variables in an Averaged Evoked Potential Experiment. In Average Evoked Potentials. (ed.) Donchin, E. and Lindsley, D.B., Washington, D.C.: NASA, 1969, pp. 237-262.

13. Schwent, V.L., Hillyard, S.A. & Gallambos, R. Selective Attention and the Auditory Vertex Potential. I. Effects of Stimulus Delivery Rates. Electroenceph. Clin. Neurophysiol. 1976, 40, 604-614.

14. Weitzman, E.D. & Kremen, H. Auditory Evoked Responses During Different Stages of Sleep in Man. Electroenceph. Clin. Neurophysiol., 1965, 18, 65-70.

15. Broen, W.E., Jr. Schizophrenia, Research and Therapy. New York: Academic Press, 1968.

16. Lubin, A., Johnson, L.C., & Austin, M.T. Discrimination Amongst States of Consciousness Using EEG Spectra. Psychophysiol., 1969, 6, 122-132.

17. Johnson, L., Lubin, A., Naitoh, P., Nute, C., & Austin, M. Spectral Analysis of the EEG of Dominant and Non-Dominant Alpha Subjects During Waking and Sleeping. Electroenceph. Clin. Neurophysiol., 1969, 26, 361-370.

18. Stevens, J.R., Lonsburg, B., & Goel, S. Electroencephalographic Spectra and Reaction Time in Disorders of Higher Nervous Function. Science, 1972, 176, 1346-1349.

19. Lifshitz, K. & Gradijan, J., Spectral Evaluation of the Electroencephalogram: Power and Variability in Chronic Schizophrenics and Control Subjects. Psychophysiol., 1974, 11, 479-490.

20. Bendat, J. & Piersol, A., Random Data: Analysis and Measurement Procedures. New York, Wiley-Interscience, 1971, 322-330.

21. Lifshitz, K. & Kohn, M. A Nonparametric Statistical Evaluation of Changes in Evoked Potentials to Different Stimuli. Psychophysiol. 1976, 13, 392-398.

22. Wilkinson, R.P. & Morlock, H.C. Auditory Evoked Response and Reaction Time. Electroenceph. Clin. Neurophysiol., 1967, 23, 50-56.

23. Jarvis, M.J. & Lader, M.H. The Effects of Nitrous Oxide on the Auditory Evoked Response in a Reaction Time Task. Psychopharmacologia (Berl.), 1971, 20, 201-212.

24. Bostock, H. & Jarvis, M.J. Changes in the Form of the Cerebral Evoked Response Related to the Speed of Simple Reaction Time. Electroencephal. Clin. Neurophysiol. 1970, 29, 137-145.

25. Lader, M. & Norris, J. The Effects of Nitrous Oxide on the Human Auditory Evoked Response. Psychopharmacologia (Berl.), 1969, 16, 115-127.

26. Ornitz, et al. The Auditory Evoked Response in Normal and Autistic Children During Sleep. Electroenceph. Clin. Neurophysiol. 1968, 25, 221-230.

27. Jarvelehto, T. & Fruhstoffer, H. Is the Sound Evoked DC Potential a Contingent Negative Variation? Electroenceph. Clin. Neurophysiol. Supplement 33, 105-108, 1973.

28. Timsit, M., Koninckx, N., Dargent, J., Fontaine, O. and Dongier, M. Variations Contingentes Negatives En Psychiatrie. Electroenceph. Clin. Neurophysiol. 1970, 28, 41-47.

29. Dongier, M., Timsit-Berthier, M., Koninckx, N. and Delaunoy, J. Compared Clinical Significance of CNV and Other Slow Potential Changes in Psychiatry. Electroenceph. Clin. Neurophysiol. 1973, Supplement 33, 321-326.

30. Cowen, M.A. and Cassel, W. Some Aspects of the Baseline Transcephalic D.C. Potential in Psychiatric Patients. J. Psychiat. Res. 1968, 6, 13-20.

# A NEUROPHYSIOLOGY OF MIND?

Herbert G. Vaughan, Jr.

Albert Einstein College of Medicine

1300 Morris Park Avenue, Bronx, New York   10461

The search for electrophysiologic correlates of mental illness must proceed in parallel with the investigation of the neurophysiologic basis of normal mental processes.  The difficulty and
complexity of the latter enterprise is apparent, yet most of our
efforts to examine relations between brain potentials and psychopathology have comprised rather simple approaches which seek
pathognomonic alterations in the electroencephalogram or in
event-related brain potentials.  This strategy rests upon two
principal assumptions.  First, that relatively homogeneous diagnostic groupings can be clinically defined which share some
common pathobiologic mechanism;  and second, that the underlying
neurobiological abnormality be reflected in some observable
aspect of scalp recorded potentials.  As I have pointed out
elsewhere (Vaughan, 1975, and in press), neither of these pre-
sumptions has a high probability of being correct.  Clearly,
the nosology of mental illness cannot pretend to the definition
of neurobiologically homogeneous entities.  Phenomenologically,
individual instances of deviant psychological function are not
only diverse in their behavioral manifestations but vary strik-
ingly over time, except perhaps in certain chronically institutionalized patients.  The notion of a pathognomic neurophysiologic index implies a stable manifestation of neural function
which must remain invariant in the face of major clinical variations both within and among individuals.  The evidence to date,
when repeated observations are made on the same patient, does
not support such stability.  Indeed, the main conclusion which
may be drawn from current experience with electrophysiologic
indices of psychopathology is that they tend to reflect the
severity of behavioral disturbance, rather than a specific

nosologic category.  Further advances in defining relationships
between electrophysiologic measures and specific aspects of
psychopathology will surely require far more detailed behavioral
and electrophysiological characterization of individual patients
studied over the dynamic evolution of their illnesses.  Only
then will the significance of electrophysiologic changes begin
to be apparent.  For this reason, the approach employed by
Friedman and colleagues (this volume) is promising.  Unlike most
electrophysiologic studies of psychopathology, high risk research
involves uncertainty as to which subjects will actually become
sick.  It is necessary, therefore, to examine the behavioral and
electrophysiologic characteristics of individuals within the
high-risk group in hope of differentiating those individuals who
will succumb from those who will remain healthy.  Efforts to
determine the behavioral and electrophysiologic features of
outliers may prove a fruitful innovation in research tactics.
There are difficulties here, however.  We do not know that any
premorbid electrophysiologic indices exist.  Indeed, the paucity
of electrophysiologic deviations in grossly psychotic patients
dictates considerable caution in the belief that these can be
readily observed, even if some basic neurobiologic abnormality
were present in the premorbid state.  The basic question facing
the search for neurophysiologic indices of psychopathology is -
what are we to look for?  What abnormal mechanisms exist which
are reflected in scalp recorded brain potentials?

    This question leads to the main thesis of this discussion,
namely, that the pathophysiology of mental illness must derive
from a sound neurophysiology of normal mental processes.  That
is not to say that we must understand the neurophysiologic basis
of mind before attempting to examine the pathoneurophysiologic
basis of mental illness.  Indeed, the deviant processes observed
in mental illness, like those associated with gross forms of
cerebral damage, may provide us with important leads to the
investigation of normal brain mechanisms.  The principal point
I wish to make is that research on psychopathology divorced
from the investigation of normal brain mechanisms is severely
handicapped in the search for neurobiologically significant
indicators of deviant mental function.

    We must now examine critically the possibilities for
effective analysis of neural processes which underlie human
experience and behavior.  Two decades of intensive study of event-
related human brain potentials have identified neuroelectric
phenomena associated with a variety of sensory, cognitive and
motor processes.  Yet, many difficulties have been encountered
in establishing quantitative relationships between psychological
variables on the one hand and ERP waveform measures.  In part,
these difficulties are an intrinsic part of early exploratory

investigations in a previously untapped area of knowledge. There
are few precedents from other disciplines to guide these investigations of human brain potentials. Indeed, some of the concepts
and approaches derived from neurophysiology, electroencephalography and various branches of psychology have been somewhat
counterproductive. The investigation of the neurophysiologic
correlates of human psychological processes is actually a new
scientific discipline which links psychology and neurobiology.
Since there are enormous voids in knowledge between these disciplines, a good deal of work is required to figure out how best
to effectively bridge these gaps. Since this new discipline
is neither solely psychological nor biological in its essence,
it must identify those concepts and methods which are relevant
and to exclude those which are extraneous to the main goal of
understanding the neurophysiologic basis of mental processes. It
is necessary to develop new operational procedures which are most
suitable for relating psychological and neurophysiological phenomena.

In evaluating the appropriate methods for relating biological
and psychological variables, it is important to identify dimensions
of covariation, wherein direct correlations of the two phenomena
can be sought. Clearly, the fundamental common dimension is
that of time: the concomitant variation of psychological and
neurophysiological processes. The basic problem is to develop
techniques for defining the temporal course of psychological
processes and for identifying their neurophysiological substrates.

If we consider first the psychological variables, it is
apparent that a simple behaviorist approach is not sufficient,
since all behaviors are consequent to the physiologic processes
that generate them. The only psychological phenomena that are
concurrent with brain events are experiential. Ritter (this
volume) develops the case that conscious processes have causal
significance for cognitive psychology. Although I concur with
his view, it is not necessary to agree with this position to
accept the fact that experience is the only psychological phenomenon which is concurrent with neurophysiologic ones.

But much of the brain's work undoubtedly never reaches consciousness. It is necessary, therefore, to distinguish between
the neurophysiologic correlates of experience and those physiologic events which represent unconscious processes. At the
extremes, this distinction is rather trivial. No one seriously
supposes that processes in retina which are necessary for visual
experience, themselves constitute a part of the neural substrate
of visual experience. More central processes cannot be so easily
differentiated. Only by establishing the temporal course of a
specific type of experience does it seem possible to circumscribe

its neurophysiologic substrate.

The fundamental ideas underlying modern information processing approaches to cognitive function were advanced by F.C. Donders
over a century ago.  His reaction time methods are paradigmatic
for a neurophysiology of mental functions.  An important elabora-
tion of Donder's processing stage concept of perceptual and cona-
tive processes is due principally to Sternberg, who introduced
the technique of varying the amount of processing within each
stage, an approach with great potential value for identifying
the electrophysiologic correlates of a specific psychological
process.

Currently, information processing approaches are well developed in cognitive psychology and are being applied to studies
of human ERP with increasing frequency.  However, reaction time
methods alone do not adequately define the temporal course of
the experiential aspects of sensory and cognitive processes.
Indeed, it may not always be the case that the experience elicited
by a stimulus precedes the behavioral response to it.  The use
of synchronization methods (e.g., Efron, 1970;  Haber and Standing,
1970) and masking techniques can approach perceptual timing more
directly.

Few electrophysiologic studies have utilized these methods,
so our present information on which ERP components might be concurrent with specific aspects of perceptual processing is scanty.
Until such identification has been accomplished, however, efforts
to relate evoked potentials to sensory experience will remain
less than satisfactory.  To date, there is no established quantitative relationship between perceptual magnitude and the size
of any evoked potential component.  This state of affairs permits
only the most tentative of speculations on the perceptual significance of variations in EP amplitude.  In the domain of psychopathology, much has been made of the possible significance of
variations in the stimulus intensity - EP amplitude function
with respect to "augmenting" and "reducing" of perceived stimulus
intensity.  At this point, there are no data to confirm this
postulated relation between EP amplitude and perceived magnitude
of the stimulus.  Clearly, major efforts must be devoted to establishing quantitative covariation of perceptual and cognitive
variables with ERP measures in order to determine the validity
of these relationships.

These studies will generally utilize measures of ERP amplitude as the principal index of the underlying physiologic processes.  At this point we must critically examine the notion that
ERP measures are meaningful reflections of underlying neural
mechanisms.  There are serious impediments to the acceptance of

this presumption.  Potentials recorded from the cortical surface
depict but a fraction of the complex field potentials recordable
within a given area.  These field potentials bear complex and
often indeterminate relationships to neural firing patterns.
The latter in turn vary widely from cell to cell within a given
cortical region.  Frequently dissociation of local field potentials and firing patterns of individual cells can be demonstrated.
Added to these unpromising circumstances, the potentials recorded
at the surface of the scalp are substantially influenced by the
nature of the source geometry and volume conduction characteristics of the intervening tissues, producing a degraded and
biased representation of intracranial potential fields.  All
of these facts could seriously compromise the assumption that
scalp recorded ERP provide valid indices of intracranial neural
processes.  How are these problems to be dealt with?  Indeed,
the first question is can they be dealt with?

     Two main positions have been taken to bolster confidence
in the validity of scalp potential recordings as indices of the
neural mechanisms underlying psychological processes.  Both of
these are, in my view, rather unsatisfactory.  The first position, which I have taken myself on occasion, is to insist that
the proof of the pudding is in the eating.  If reliable correlations between psychological and ERP measures are demonstrated,
then neurophysiology must come up with an explanation of these
observations.  This would be a reasonable position, if indeed
such correlations had been found.  The fact is that very few
quantitative relationships between ERP and psychological variables have been established.  In the area of sensory psychophysics,
where such relationships should be most readily demonstrated, if
present, there is an extensive list of failures to establish
a quantitative covariation between evoked potential amplitude
and perceived stimulus magnitude.  There are some exceptions,
however, and many of the failures reflect procedural short-
comings.  Nevertheless, it is hard to argue on the record that
EP - psychological correlations have been widely established.
The experience of Hillyard, Picton and their associates in
demonstrating an effect of selective attention on the amplitude
of the N100 auditory EP component illustrates the difficulties
in defining experimental conditions required to demonstrate reliable covariation between ERP and psychological variables.
My assessment of these problems is that we do not yet understand
what to measure in our physiological data, and that more knowledge of the relationships between the ERP and underlying neural
activity is required.

     The second position originally proposed by Wolfgang Köhler
asserts that field potentials (i.e., intracortical currents) in
and of themselves represent essential features of the neural

mechanisms underlying psychological processes.  This thesis
possesses some attractiveness, especially as regards the physiologic substrate of conscious experience.  Unfortunately, in the
absence of supporting psychophysiological correlations, this
notion degenerates into Eddingtonian mysticism, incapable of
empirical validation.

From a strictly pragmatic viewpoint, the recording of gross
field potentials provide data of greater utility for advancing
psychophysiologic correlations than the alternative technique
of unit recording, which is, of course, generally applicable
only in experimental animals.  First, field potentials directly
reflect postsynaptic activity.  By contrast, extracellular
action potential recording can be viewed as the neurophysiological
analog of motor behavior.  It can only reflect the all or nothing
output of the complex analog computations carried out within each
neuron.

It seems that only evidence of the sort obtainable at great
labor in behaving experimental animals will permit us to determine relationships between gross field potentials, neural firing
patterns and psychological processes.  Until recently there have
been few data on correlations between field potential and unit
activity in behaving animals.  With Joseph Arezzo and our students,
we have begun a systematic examination of intracortical field
potentials and patterns of neural firing in alert monkeys
implanted with multiple movable intracranial electrodes.  We
have examined patterns of activity throughout the brain in response to non-signal, visual, auditory and somatosensory stimuli.
Both the gross EP and patterns of multiple unit activity (MUA)
have been extensively mapped.  Two findings of relevance to
the present discussion have ensued.  Stimuli which require no
specific cognitive processing or behavioral response elicit
cortical responses limited to the modality specific regions of
parietal, temporal and occipital cortex and to limited posterior
frontal regions.  These animal studies support the conclusion
based upon human scalp EP topography (Vaughan, 1969;  Simson
et al., 1976; 1977), that the principal sources of human sensory
EP are within the primary and secondary cortical areas.  Since
these non-signal stimuli are perceived, it seems likely that
these cortical regions must in part subserve the elementary processes of sensory experience.  Other cortical regions, including
frontal and posterior association cortex are not implicated.  The
second finding of the animal studies is that gross field potentials show substantially more activity in the long latency range
which we presume to underlie the sensory experience than does
the action potentials.  This observation suggests that few
effects on intracortical neural output are occurring when information processing is not required.  On the other hand, large late

fluctuations in postsynaptic activity are present.  The time
course of the later field potentials (which are analogous to
the N100-P200 sequence in man) suggests that they could represent a neural substrate of sensory experience.  There are few
data in man which would validate the belief that these late potentials mediate sensory experience.  Of note, however, is the
estimate by Efron, derived from behavioral data, that the minimum
duration of visual and auditory percepts generated by brief stimuli are in the order of 200 msec.  Vaughan and Silverstein (1968)
also found that changes in visual EP related to  change in subjective brightness induced by metacontrast was limited to the
evoked activity between 150 and 300 msec after the target stimulus.  Simson et al. (1977) found a distinct negative potential
with similar timing and topography to the P200 VEP component
in the EP to target stimuli in a discrimination task.  Taken
together, these observations encourage the belief that field
potentials may, when studied more extensively, be found to correlate both in timing and possibly in magnitude, with sensory experience.

There are, as yet, no correlative field and unit activity
studies in animals trained to perform sensorimotor tasks.  It is
noteworthy that there are striking increases in firing of units
within the monkey's parietal association cortex when performing
goal directed motor tasks, as contrasted to their silence when
non-significant stimuli were presented (Mountcastle et al., 1975).
Nevertheless, long latency gross potentials are readily recorded
from the same cortical area in response to non-signal stimuli
(Arezzo and Vaughan, 1975).  Again, it appears that cellular
output, manifested by increase in firing, may occur only when the
cortical region under consideration is required to process data
beyond its obligatory response to input.  The gross field potentials give evidence, however, that the cortical region does respond over a prolonged period - a response which may have experiential but not behavioral consequences.  Further support for
the association of field potentials and firing patterns with
output requirements, is our finding (Arezzo et al., 1977) that
there is a close correspondence between the gross potentials and
multiple unit firing patterns in motor cortex of monkeys trained
to perform self-paced hand movements.  Under these conditions,
cortical output is necessary to drive the spinal motoneuron pool,
and a good correspondence is seen between the field potentials
which reflect postsynaptic activity and the firing pattern reflecting neuronal output.

We can hypothesize from the foregoing that the extent to
which neural firing patterns and gross field potentials show
some correspondence is determined by the requirements for output
from a particular cortical region.  As a corollary of this

hypothesis we would expect field potentials to be recorded from regions comprising the last step in a particular information processing sequence. Unit activity from that region would principally reflect afferent activation of that region whereas the post-synaptic activity is reflected in the more prolonged gross potentials. Thus, the field potentials provide a source of information on cortical processing not obtainable from unitary recordings alone. If it should turn out that good correlations between firing patterns and field potentials obtain when output from a region is required, then recordings of field potentials would be a valid index of neuronal firing under these specific conditions; conversely, dissociation of firing patterns and post-synaptic activity would be found when output is not required.

Having put forward this tentative formulation of the conditions under which a correspondence between overall firing patterns within a cortical region and gross potentials might occur, we must examine the extent to which local field potentials are accurately reflected at the scalp through volume conduction of extracellular current flows within the brain and its coverings. The elementary features of volume conduction were treated qualitatively by Lorente de No who introduced the concept of open and closed field generators. Only cellular configurations that possess axial asymmetry and radial symmetry can generate far fields recordable at the scalp. Such structures include cerebral and cerebellar cortex, hippocampus and large fiber bundles. The fields they set up are dipolar with their axis of maximum potential in the direction of the axial asymmetry. Generator characteristics are determined both by gross geometry and by the current flows set up by the individual elements within a source (viz., Vaughan, 1974; Goff, Allison and Vaughan, 1977). It is possible, given the gross geometry and current emission characteristics of intracranial sources, together with tissue conductance and the dimensions of the conductive media, to calculate surface field potential distributions. Even approximate calculations have proven useful for interpreting the topography of scalp-recorded ERP. They have shown us that potentials generated by circumscribed cortical sources have rather wide scalp distributions, but with smaller amplitudes than those produced by more extensive sources. For cortical generators of equal source current density the larger the source the greater the amplitude of the scalp recorded potentials. Thus, there is an intrinsic ambiguity in the interpretation of scalp potential amplitude variations - they may reflect either changes in amount of extent of neural activity, an ambiguity which can be resolved only by detailed mapping of the surface potential distribution.

It is evident therefore that quantitative analyses of the ERP must evaluate not only the magnitude and timing of their

components, but also their spatial distribution.  The interpretation of scalp recorded ERP topography in relation to intracranial
processes is often difficult, however, due to (1) the spatiotem-
poral overlap of components generated by different intracranial
sources;  (2) the non-unique inferences on gross source location
and configuration that can be drawn from surface potential
distributions;  and (3) the complex summation of extracellular
currents due to diverse neuronal activity within an active region.
These problems can only be overcome by extensive correlative investigations carried on in parallel in man and experimental
primates.  In the meantime, investigations of the ERP correlates
of normal and deviant psychological processes in human subjects
must recognize the limitations on the inferences on underlying
neural processes that can be drawn from these data.  We have not
yet achieved a neurophysiology of the mind -- but its prospects
as an emergent discipline appear bright.

## REFERENCES

Arezzo, J. and Vaughan, H.G., Jr.  Cortical potentials associated
with voluntary movements in the monkey.  Brain Research, 1975, 88,
99-104.

Arezzo, J., Vaughan, H.G., Jr. and Koss, B.  Relationship of neuronal activity to gross movement-related potentials in monkey
pre and postcentral cortex.  Brain Research, 1977, 132, 362-369.

Efron, R.  The minimum duration of a perception.  Neuropsychologia,
1970, 8, 57-63.

Goff, W.R., Allison, T. and Vaughan, H.G., Jr.  The functional
neuroanatomy of event related potentials.  In, E. Callaway (Ed.),
Proceedings of the Conference on Event Related Brain Potentials
in Man.  New York:  Academic Press, in press.

Haber, R.N. and Standing, L.G.  Direct estimates of the apparent
duration of a flash.  Canadian Journal of Psychology, 1970, 24,
216-229.

Mountcastle, V.B., Lynch, J.C., Georgopoulos, A., Sakata, H. and
Acuna, C.  Posterior parietal association cortex of the monkey:
command functions for operations within extrapersonal space.
Journal of Neurophysiology, 1975, 38, 871-908.

Simson, R., Vaughan, H.G., Jr. and Ritter, W.  The scalp topography of potentials associated with missing visual or auditory
stimuli.  Electroenceph. clin. Neurophysiol., 1976, 40, 33-42.

Simson, R., Vaughan, H.G., Jr. and Ritter, W.  The scalp topography of potentials in auditory and visual discrimination tasks. Electroenceph. clin. Neurophysiol., 1977, 42, 528-535.

Vaughan, H.G., Jr.  The relationship of brain activity to scalp recordings of event-related potentials.  In, E. Donchin and D.B. Lindsley (Eds.), Averaged Evoked Potentials:  Methods, Results, Evaluations.  Washington, D.C., National Aeronautics and Space Administration (NASA #SP-191), 1969.  Pp. 45-94.

Vaughan, H.G., Jr.  The analysis of scalp-recorded brain potentials.  In, R.F. Thompson and M.M. Patterson (Ed.), Bioelectric Recording Techniques, Part B:  Electroencephalography and Human Brain Potentials.  New York, Academic Press, 1974.  Pp. 157-207.

Vaughan, H.G., Jr.  Physiological approaches to psychopathology. In, M.L. Kietzman, S. Sutton and J. Zubin (Eds.), Experimental Approaches to Psychopathology.  New York, Academic Press, 1975. Pp. 351-363.

Vaughan, H.G., Jr.  Toward a neurophysiology of schizophrenia. In, L.C. Wynne (Ed.), Nature of Schizophrenia.  New York:  John Wiley & Sons, Inc., in press.

Vaughan, H.G., Jr. and Silverstein, L.  Metacontrast and evoked potentials:  A reappraisal.  Science, 1968, 160, 207-208.

# SIGNAL-TO-NOISE RATIO AND RESPONSE VARIABILITY IN AFFECTIVE DISORDERS AND SCHIZOPHRENIA

Monte S. Buchsbaum, Richard Coppola

Biological Psychiatry Branch

Nat. Inst. of Mental Health, Bethesda, Md.

## INTRODUCTION

Schizophrenic patients tend to have smaller and apparently more variable evoked potentials (EPs) than normal controls. The amplitude abnormality is consistent with a number of psychological theories of schizophrenia (e.g. Freud, Pavlov, Venables, Broen and Storms, Silverman) characterized by Epstein and Coleman (1970) as assuming that the "basic deficit in schizophrenia consists of a low threshold for disorganization under increasing stimulus input." While it is difficult to compare specific components in recordings made from different laboratories, there is general agreement that the P100-N140-P200 complex is smaller in schizophrenics, regardless of sensory modality (see review by Buchsbaum, 1977). As predicted by the various theories, reduction in amplitude is particularly marked for high levels of stimulation such as rapid rates of stimulus presentation, high intensity (Landau, 1975; Rappaport, 1975), novel (Roth and Cannon, 1972) or paired stimuli (Shagass, 1976).

Disorganized processing of sensory input might also be apparent as EPs varying more from trial to trial. Schizophrenics' responses to perceptual tasks do seem to vary more from trial to trial than those of normals. Inability to maintain a stable response set, postulated by Shakow (1963) to be a major

psychological deficit in schizophrenics, might also be
associated with variation in perceptual processing.
Indeed, studies have linked individual differences in
EP variability to perceptual response variability
(Callaway, 1975; Inderbitzen, Buchsbaum and Silverman,
1970), and a number of studies have reported greater
EP variability in schizophrenics (Borge, 1973; Cohen,
1973; Jones et al., 1965; Jones and Callaway, 1970;
Lifshitz, 1969; Rappaport et al., 1975; Saletu, Itil
and Saletu, 1971; and Saletu, Saletu, and Itil, 1973).
However, the average EP technique, while adequate for
examining the mean response to a sensory signal, is
quite ambiguous as to whether low amplitude of
individual EPs or high variability are responsible for
the low average EP amplitude observed in
schizophrenics (Figure 1).

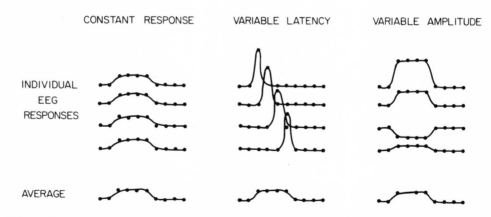

Fig. 1.   Low Amplitude and High Variability in the
          Average EP
Single Eps that have both constant latency and low
amplitude may produce a low amplitude average EP.
However, high amplitude variable EPs may produce
similar averages.

Trial to trial variation in the EP is difficult
to measure since each trial is embedded in background
EEG activity often with amplitude four or more times
greater than the EP. Averaging reduces the size of
this background relative to the EP but obscures trial
to trial variation. Thus, while examination of
multiple average EPs recorded on the same session
reveals more variation in EP size and shape in
schizophrenics than in normals (Saletu, Itil, and
Saletu, 1971) this might reflect changes in the ratio
of EEG background to EP amplitude (see Figure 2).
More variable appearing EPs in schizophrenics might
arise if their small EPs were embedded in normal
amplitude EEG. Since there is some agreement that
overall EEG amplitude is not reduced in schizophrenics
(Itil, Saletu and Davis, 1972; Shagass, 1976) whereas
EP amplitude is, this might well be the explanation of

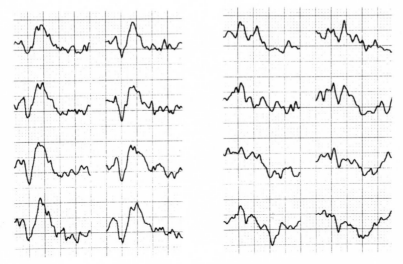

Fig. 2. Auditory Average EP Variation
Auditory EPs recorded from vertex; 500 msec, positive
up. A total of 512 tone bursts at 1 sec intervals
were presented to subjects and responses averaged at
random into sets of n=64. Right - Subject shows
constant waveform. P100-N120-P200 complex clearly
seen. Left - Schizophrenic patient shows variable
average.

the apparently high variability reported.  It
therefore seemed appropriate to quantify the
relationship between EP signal size and EEG
background, and study this relationship in patients
with schizophrenia and affective illness.  In this
preliminary report, we present a comparison of a
variety of techniques for assessing EP amplitude,
background EEG amplitude, signal-to-noise ratio and
its variation.

## Signal-to-Noise Ratio Techniques
## for Average EPs

The overall size of any signal can be
conveniently measured by computing its variance over n
discrete time points.  Thus, an average EP and an EEG
sample recorded in the computer can be compared in
size by computing the ratio of their two variances.
This ratio of the variance of a signal to the variance
in background noise may be termed the signal-to-noise
ratio or SNR.  Conventionally in the measurement of
electrical signals the variance is termed "power" and
is widely used.

The variance of the background EEG during the EP
may be estimated by first removing the EP signal from
each trial.  This is conveniently done by alternately
adding and subtracting successive EP trials (the
plus-minus average or $\pm$AEP).  The variance calculated
across on the resulting sum (Schimmel, 1967) is then a
power measure of background EEG.  To compute the
signal-to-noise ratio, the variance of the average EP
is divided by the quantity 1/M times the variance of the
plus-minus sum.  (If the sum EP is used, its variance
must be divided by $M^2$).  If widely aberrant or
artifactual single trials might greatly influence the
average EP, it is possible that computation of the
median EP instead of the average would reduce their
impact and give both a higher and more reliable
signal-to-noise EP estimate.

## Signal-to-Noise Ratio Techniques
## for Single EP Trials

Since the EP amplitude cannot be estimated from a
single stimulus presentation, the plus-minus average
technique cannot yield a trial by trial estimate of
signal-to-noise ratio.  Two new techniques, based on

comparing pairs of EP trials, were developed by
Bershad and Rockmore (1974) and their application to
EP data is presented elsewhere (Coppola, Tabor, and
Buchsbaum, submitted for publication).  In this
report, we have used an empirical technique, based on
simulation studies of synthetic EPs at known
signal-to-noise ratios.  First, a synthetic data base
was created.  Synthetic EEG was generated from
Gaussian random noise low pass filtered to give a
frequency spectrum closely resembling EEG.  A
synthetic EP waveform, consisting of a signal whose
frequency increased from 1.5 to 5 Hz over 0.5 sec, was
used.  Using the synthetic EEG and EP, single "EP
trials" consisting of the EP and synthetic EEG were
formed.  Each single trial consisted of 50 data
points, representing 400 msec after stimulus onset.
Since the variance of the EP and the variance of the
EEG generator were known, single trials of any
signal-to-noise ratio could be produced by multiplying
the synthetic EEG by an appropriate factor.  Fifty
sets of 32 trials per set were generated for each of
12 SNRs ranging from 0.08 to 4.13.  Thus we had the
equivalent of 50 synthetic subjects with 32 raw EEG
trials at each of 12 SNRs.

For each set of 32 trials we calculated:
1) the average EP
2) the z-transforms of the product moment
   coefficients between the average EP
   and each of the 32 trials
3) the mean and variance of these z-transforms

The means and variances were averaged over the 50
sets, giving an estimate at each of the 12 SNRs.
Least squares curve fits were then performed to
establish the relationship between the given SNR and
the averaged z-transform measure (ZA) and its
variance.  The relationship between ZA and the SNR
allows us to estimate the SNR on new actual data.  The
expected variance of ZA may also be compared to the
observed variance to estimate trial to trial variation
in SNR.  Specific equations are given in the Appendix.


METHODS


Subjects


Psychiatric inpatients from the NIH Clinical
Center were studied, off all psychoactive medications

and usually after two weeks of admission.  The
patients were 14 schizophrenic patients (7 men and 7
women) and 32 (11 men and 21 women) bipolar affective
disorder patients.  Of the 14 patients admitted with a
diagnosis of schizophrenia, 12 met Research Diagnostic
Criteria (RDC) (Spitzer, Endicott, and Robins, 1975).
A group of normal volunteers (26 men and 45 women)
were recruited to age and sex match the psychiatric
patient population.  Twenty-nine of these normal
volunteers were tested twice on two occasions 2 or
more weeks apart to assess reliability of the
procedure.  Most patients were also tested twice and
the mean of the two values obtained used in various
group comparisons.

## Evoked Response Recordings

     Vertex to right ear recordings were made using an
EEG amplifier with a low frequency 3 dB point at 0.5
Hz followed by an active low pass filter flat to 40 Hz
and down 42 dB at 60 Hz.  Stimuli were either a 0.5
sec light flash at 80 foot lamberts (experiment LV) or
a 0.5 sec tone burst at 500 Hz (experiment TV).  They
were presented at a rate of one per 2 seconds.
Responses to the first 10 stimuli were ignored, then
32 single trial responses were collected.  Each trial
was checked for saturation on the A/D converter and
stimuli were presented until 32 good trials were
achieved.  Amplication was set so that eye or movement
artifacts generally caused system saturation and
relatively uniform trial editing was thus achieved.
EEG was sampled every 8 msec for 32 msec before the
stimulus and 484 msec after the stimulus.  Stimulus
presentation and EEG sampling were controlled by a
PDP-11 computer (Coppola, 1977).

     Subjects were instructed to relax, sit still and
observe the stimuli.  The order of presentation of LV
and TV was randomized.

## DATA ANALYSIS

### ZA SNR Technique

     EP trials were analyzed in the same manner as the
synthetic data.  The first 50 time points after the'

stimulus for each of the 32 good trials were used. For the ZA method, the mean EP was formed and this wave form correlated with each of the 32 single trials, as detailed in the Appendix. The resulting 32 product moment correlation coefficients were z-transformed to normalize the distribution and then the mean and variance of the distribution were calculated. The mean z-transformed correlation was then entered into the empirical equation (7) derived from the simulation to yield the estimated SNR and empirical equation (8) to yield the expected variance. The ratio of observed to expected variance could then be calculated (Table I).

## Plus-Minus SNR Technique

Using the same 400 msec data base and mean EPs, the ±SNR was calculated by alternate adding and

## Table I
### Mean SNR and SNR Variability in Patient and Control Groups

|  | Light Stimuli | | | Tone Stimuli | | |
|  | Schiz. | Norm. | BP | Schiz. | Norm. | BP |
|---|---|---|---|---|---|---|
| ZA SNR | .22** | .43 | .33 | .15 | .16 | .17 |
| Obs/Exp Variance | 2.14 | 1.87 | 1.90 | 2.13* | 1.31 | 1.65* |
| + SNR AEP | .20* | .36 | .25 | .08* | .14 | .11 |
| + SNR MEP | .22* | .37 | .27 | .09* | .15 | .11 |

Signal to noise (SNR) ratio and ratio of observed to expected variance of SNR in normal, schizophrenic (Schiz.) and bipolar affective disorder patients (BP).

* $p < 0.05$, different from normal controls.
+ $p < 0.05$, different from schizophrenics.
** $p < 0.001$, different from normal controls.

subtracting of the 32 raw EP trials. This yielded a ±
average for each set. A median EP was formed by
finding the median value for each time coordinate.
The variance across the 50 time points for the average
EP (AEP) plus minus EP (±EP) and median EP (MEP) was
then calculated to yield a measure of signal power
(variance of AEP or MEP) and noise power (variance of
±EP). The SNR ratios for the AEP and MEP could then
be calculated. All SNR ratios were then expressed as
$\log_e$ for statistical comparisons to normalize the
distributions and the mean values retransformed back
for tabular presentation.


## Peak Measurement Technique

EP peaks were identified visually on a digital
CRT and amplitudes measured from a 32 msec
pre-stimulus average. N140 was identified as the most
negative point 100-150 msec post stimulus. P200 was
the first following major positive peak; P100 was the
preceding positive peak. If two adjacent positive
peaks were available, the largest was identified as
P100 or P200. Peaks were measured without reference
to any previous run on the same subject. An effort
was made to identify peaks close to 100, 120 and 200
msec if possible.

EP amplitude was also assessed using an area
measure (Buchsbaum, 1974). We calculated the mean
absolute deviation from zero baseline over three time
bands corresponding to mean peak latencies; P100
(76-112 msec), N140 (116-152 msec) and P200 (168-248
msec). The baseline was established by removing the
mean of the entire 512 msec recording epoch (including
32 msec prestimulus baseline). This baseline was used
because we have found higher test-retest reliabilities
over time using this baseline rather than a
prestimulus baseline (Buchsbaum, 1976). It might be
argued that the mean value over the entire EP epoch
might rise and fall due to the occurrence of late
(i.e. P300) events, thus distorting measurements of
earlier amplitudes. However, with minimal task
demands P300 may not appear or, if it does, P300
duration is minimal and the EP is usually at or below
baseline by 400-450. Further, since late positive
components are quite variable, it seems unlikely that
they could increase test-retest reliability.

# RESULTS

## Range of Signal-to-Noise Ratios

Normal individuals showed SNRs ranging from below 0.13 up to 2.5 for visual EPs and for auditory EPs up to 0.6. The distribution showed many low values and a few high ones, so all statistics were done on $\log_e$ transformations of the SNR. Low SNR individuals had visual EPs which were neither uniformly small nor indistinct, as can be seen in Figure 3.

## Signal to Noise Ratio (SNR) Reliability

Both EPs and background EEG amplitude range widely from individual to individual. In our data, EP amplitude appears to be a more stable individual characteristic than EEG amplitude however, with the ratio of the two (the SNR) having the highest reliability (Table II). For nearly every measure, visual EPs appear more reliable than auditory EPs, perhaps because of their larger size. The ZA SNR measure is more reliable than the +SNR technique (p <0.10, Fisher Test) perhaps because it is based on 32 estimates rather than a single determination using the average. The + average, a measure of background EEG amplitude has quite low reliability indicating that EEG amplitude during EP trials is not a reliable trait variable under the resting, non-task conditions used here. Single aberrant trials, perhaps containing artifacts, seem not to be contributing to the ZA SNR or its variance since when the +SNR or variance measures are based on the median EP no significant change in reliability is seen. Indeed, although the median EP technique was expected to reject outliers and thus improve the EP estimate, the reliabilities of both area integral and hand measured peaks were also generally slightly lower for median EP than the average EP. Further, as can be seen in Table III, median EPs had essentially the same SNR as average EPs.

## Amplitude Measurement Reliability

It is noteworthy that the area integration technique, first adopted by Shagass (1972), yielded

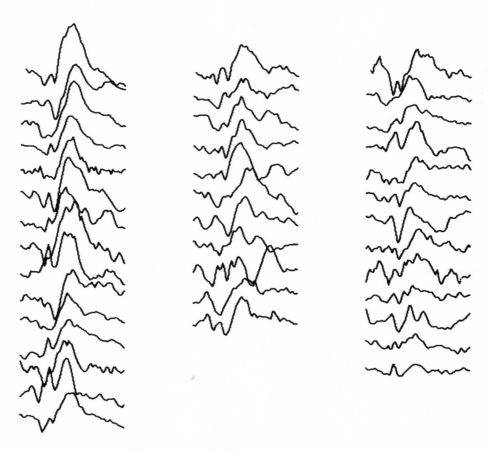

Fig. 3.   EP Waveform and SNR
Visual EP waveforms (400 msec epoch, positive up)   for
39  randomly  selected normal adults shown in order
of  computed  signal-to-noise  ratio  (ZA  technique).
Left column EPs show SNR from 2.5 at   top   to   0.5   at
bottom;  center  column  from  0.5  at  top to 0.25 at
bottom; right column from 0.25 at top to 0.13 or lower
at bottom.   Note that while high SNR individuals   tend
to  have  large  amplitude,  amplitude  varies widely.
Typical triphasic EP waveforms with the P100-N120-P200
complex are clearly seen even in individuals with  low
SNRs  (e.g.  individual  third from bottom, right-hand
column).

Table II
Test-Retest Reliability of Signal-to-
Noise Ratio (SNR) and
Amplitude Measures in 29 Normal Controls

| | Light Stimuli | Tone Stimuli |
|---|---|---|
| **EP SNR** | | |
| ZA SNR | .823 | .573 |
| Observed ZA variance/ Expected ZA variance | .711 | .418 |
| + SNR AEP | .597 | .260 |
| $\mp$ SNR MEP | .636 | .344 |
| **EP Variance** | | |
| Variance AEP | .736 | .420 |
| Variance MEP | .703 | .349 |
| Variance $\pm$AEP | .344 | .134 |
| **EP Amplitude** | | |
| Area 76-112 (P100) | .809 | .722 |
| Under 116-152 (N120) | .768 | .257 |
| Curve 168-244 (P200) | .650 | .427 |
| Baseline P100 | .679 | .125 |
| to N120 | .456 | .558 |
| Peak P200 | .568 | .170 |

Product moment correlation coefficients calculated between values obtained on two separate
recording sessions two or more weeks apart.

(p <0.05, 1 tailed for r >0.30)


higher reliabilities for peaks P100, N140 and P200
than visual identification techniques. We have
achieved higher visual identification test-retest
values when the judge is able to see both pairs of EPs
together, or when many examples of a person's EPs are
available: nevertheless the low reliability achieved
here illustrates the problems that may result with
visual peak identification even if fairly stringent

rules are used.  Reliabilities for visual peak
identification in the auditory EP were low especially
for P100 which may vary widely in latency and appear
as several wavelets from 50 to 100 msec stimulus.
Area measurement is thus particularly useful for this
component.  As can be seen by the relatively high
reliability (Table II) and patient group differences
(Table III) the 76-112 msec band appears empirically
useful.

## Amplitude Measurement and SNR

Given a SNR of 0.4 for individual visual EPs in
normal subjects, averaging 32 trials yields an average
EP with a SNR of 32 x 0.4 or 12.8.  It should be noted
that the SNR is a power measure, based on the
variance.  Amplitude measures are proportional to the
square root of power (the standard deviation) and the
ratio of EP amplitude to background EEG mean amplitude
would be $\sqrt{32}$ x $\sqrt{0.4}$ or 3.58.  This SNR is observed
when examining the amplitude measures.  For example
we obtained a mean amplitude in 72 subjects for peak
N120 of 5.3 microvolts using the area under the curve
technique (Table III).  We also applied the same area
technique to the plus-minus average EP, obtaining 1.48
microvolts; 5.3/1.48=3.58.

However, for auditory stimuli, the SNR of 0.16
for single trials yields an average EP for 32 trials
with a SNR of 5.12; the ratio of amplitude to
background EEG would be $\sqrt{32}$ x $\sqrt{.16}$ or only 2.26.  This
may be too low to allow reliabile peak identification
and may explain low reliability in identifying
component landmarks in the auditory EP (Table II).

When EP components are identified by visual
inspection, local maxima or minima are selected as
peaks.  This tends to increase EP amplitude slightly
since unidirectional random variation is taken
advantage of.  Thus, in individuals with low SNRs,
baseline to peak or peak-to-trough amplitudes will be
systematically overestimated.  The low amplitude EPs
reported in schizophrenics below and elsewhere cannot
therefore result from poor SNRs.

Table III

Evoked Response Amplitude in Patient

and Normal Control Groups

| | | Light Stimuli | | | Tone Stimuli | | |
|---|---|---|---|---|---|---|---|
| | | Schiz. | Norm. | Bipolar | Schiz. | Norm. | Bipolar |
| Area | 76-112 P100 | 3.4** | 4.9 | 4.5* | 2.9* | 4.1 | 5.2*,+ |
| Under | 116-152 N120 | 4.5 | 5.3 | 5.0 | 2.8 | 3.5 | 4.2*,+ |
| Curve | 168-244 P200 | 6.9 | 8.6 | 8.3 | 4.3 | 4.3 | 3.5* |
| Baseline | P100 | 2.2 | 1.6 | 1.2 | 2.4 | 1.7 | 2.1 |
| to | N120 | -4.0 | -5.4 | -5.8 | -4.4* | -6.5 | -7.3+ |
| Peak | P200 | 12.0* | 15.2 | 13.4 | 6.6 | 6.6 | 4.7* |
| Variance | AEP | 29.3 | 40.8 | 39.9 | 14.9 | 14.9 | 16.8 |
| " | MEP | 31.7 | 44.0 | 42.0 | 16.1 | 16.4 | 18.0 |
| " | +AEP | 141.9 | 114.8 | 177.3 | 197.0 | 131.9 | 170.0 |

All values given in microvolts. Area measure is mean deviation over fixed time periods. Baseline to peak is level of visually identified peak above (positive values) or below (negative values) prestimulus baseline. Variance calculated across the 50 coordinates in the average (AEP), median (EP) or plus-minus (+AEP, estimate of background EEG) curves.

* p <0.05, different from normal controls.
+ p <0.05, different from schizophrenics.
** p <0.01, different from normal controls.

## Signal-to-Noise Ratio in Patient and
## Control Groups

For both visual and auditory stimuli, schizophrenics had lower SNRs. The ZA SNR measure on visual EPs differentiated the groups the most clearly (t of 4.24), showing an almost 2-fold difference in mean SNR. Using the median SNR of the 72 normals and 14 schizophrenics (0.350) as a dividing criterion would identify 13 of 14 schizophrenics but produce 34 false positive normals ($\chi 2$, $p < 0.05$). The $+$SNR measure also differentiated the schizophrenic and $\overline{n}$ormal controls, although at slightly lower significance levels. Bipolar affective disorder patients, although having slightly lower SNR levels than normal controls showed no significant differences. SNR variability was also increased in the schizophrenic group, although this effect was only significant for tone stimuli. In all groups and for both modalities, the expected variance was significantly lower than the observed variance ($p < 0.01$). Bipolar patients were also more variable in SNR from trial to trial than normal but significantly less variable than the schizophrenic group.

## EP Amplitude

Consistent with earlier reports (see Buchsbaum, 1977) schizophrenics tended to have smaller EPs (Table III). Overall measures of EP size (e.g. variance of average EP or median EP) did not significantly differentiate either schizophrenics or bipolars from normal. Individual components, especially P100, did however. The area measure showed P100 significantly diminished both for visual and auditory stimuli in schizophrenics and significantly elevated in bipolars for auditory stimuli.

## DISCUSSION

Individual differences in SNR appear to be a stable individual trait and mean levels of SNR differ between a small population of off medication schizophrenic patients and normal controls. These differences arise more from differences in size of the EP than size of background EEG. In our data not only do measures of background EEG ($+$AEP) have low test-retest reliability, but background EEG amplitude

is only marginally (-0.15) correlated with SNR.
Zerlin and Davis (1967) also noted that EEG background
was insufficient "to account for more than a small
part of the wide fluctuations in amplitude" in a
subject with an unusually high SNR.  However, the fact
that background EEG is somewhat larger than normal in
schizophrenics and that their EPs are somewhat smaller
enlarges normal/schizophrenics' differences.

The ZA SNR measure had two advantages over the $\pm$
average SNR.  First, it had higher test-retest
reliability for both visual and auditory stimuli.
Second, it yielded a variance measure, not obtainable
with the +SNR.  The variance measure also differed
significantly in both bipolar and schizophrenic
patients.  The ZA SNR was superior to merely measuring
overall EP size (e.g. the variance of the average EP);
no variance measure showed either patient group to be
significantly different from normal controls.

Do the individual differences in SNRs observed
merely represent the proportion of poor quality
artifact-filled EEG in each subject's data?  The
programming steps to eliminate bad trials on line
should have minimized this problem.  The fact that
SNRs were no higher for the median EP than average EP
also tends to indicate that artifacts are not a
primary contributor.  Artifact-filled EEG should also
extend across both visual and auditory stimulus
recording.  Yet, the visual and auditory ZA SNRs
correlate only 0.152 in 72 normal subjects -- whereas
the background EEG (as measured by the variance of the
+ average) correlates 0.42 (p<0.05) across modalities.
Thus it appears that electrophysiological SNR more
than EMG, eye blink or other noise artifacts is being
reported.  The finding of increased variation of
schizophrenics' SNRs from trial to trial is of special
interest since apparent variability of schizophrenics'
EPs has been widely reported.  In fact, every group
showed significantly more variability in SNR than
expected on the basis of our simulation.  This
increased variability could come from greater
minute-to-minute changes in average EEG amplitude than
normal.  However, schizophrenics have been reported to
show diminished variation in EEG activity across 20
second epochs in comparison with normals (Goldstein,
1963).  This result was supported by results of Itil,
Saletu and Davis (1972), although sex differences were
reported by Shagass (1976).  Thus with SNR levels, EP
variation itself may well be implicated in this
result.

Acknowledgments:

The authors wish to thank Cathy King and Gail
Schechter for technical assistance, Arlene Ammerman
for secretarial help, Frederick Goodwin, Dennis Murphy,
Robert Post and Daniel van Kammen for support of this
project with patients on their research wards.

References

1.   Bershad, N.J. and Rockmore, A.J., On estimating signal to
     noise ratio using the sample correlation coefficient.   IEEE
     Trans. on Information Theory  20:   112-113, 1974
2.   Borge, G.F., Perceptual modulation and variability in psychia-
     tric patients.  Arch. Gen. Psychiatry 29:   760-763, 1973
3.   Buchsbaum, M.S., Average evoked response and stimulus inten-
     sity in identical and fraternal twins.  Physiological Psy-
     chology 2:   365-370, 1974
4.   Buchsbaum, M.S., Self-regulation of stimulus intensity:
     augmenting/reducing and the average evoked response,   in:
     Consciousness and Self Regulation. (Eds) Schwartz, G.E. and
     Shapiro, D.  Plenum Press, New York, 1976, pp. 101-135
5.   Buchsbaum, M.S., The middle evoked response components and
     schizophrenia.  Schizophrenia Bull. 3:   93-104, 1977
6.   Callaway, E., Brain Electrical Potentials and Individual
     Psychological Differences.  Grune & Stratton, New York, San
     Francisco, London, 1975
7.   Cohen, R., The influence of task-relevant stimulus variations
     on the reliability of auditory evoked responses in schizo-
     phrenia, in:  Average Evoked Responses and Their Conditioning
     in Normal Subjects and Psychiatric Patients.  (Eds.) A.
     Fessard and G. Lelord, Inserm, Paris, 1973, pp. 373-388.
8.   Coppola, R., A table driven system for stimulus-response
     experiments.  Proc. of the Digital Equipment Users Soc.,
     1977.
9.   Epstein, S. and Coleman, M., Drive theories of schizophrenia.
     Psychosom. Med. 32:   113-140, 1970.
10.  Goldstein, L., Murphree, H.B., Sugerman, A.A., Pfeiffer, C.C.
     and Jenney, E.H., Quantitative electroencephalographic
     analysis of naturally occurring (schizophrenic) and drug-
     induced psychotic states in human males.  Clin. Pharmacol.
     Ther. 4: 10-21, 1963.
11.  Inderbitzen, L.B., Buchsbaum, M.S. and Silverman, J., EEG-
     averaged evoked response and perceptual variability in
     schizophrenics.  Arch. Gen. Psychiatry 23:   438-444, 1970
12.  Itil, T.M., Saletu, B. and Davis, S., EEG findings in chronic
     schizophrenics based on digital computer period analysis and
     analog power spectra.  Biol. Psychiatry 5:   1-13, 1972

13.  Jones, R.T., Blacker, K.H., Callaway, E. and Layne R.S., The
     auditory evoked response as a diagnostic and prognostic
     measure in schizophrenia. Am. J. Psychiatry 122:  33-41,
     1965
14.  Jones, R.T. and Callaway, E., Auditory evoked responses in
     schizophrenia--a reassessment. Biol. Psychiatry 2:  291-298,
     1970
15.  Landau, S.G., Buchsbaum, M.S., Carpenter, W., Strauss, J. and
     Sacks, M., Schizophrenia and stimulus intensity control.
     Arch. Gen. Psychiatry 32:  1239-1245, 1975
16.  Lifshitz, K., Intra and inter individual variability and the
     averaged evoked potential in normal and chronic schizophrenic
     subjects. Electroenceph. Clin. Neurophysiol. 27:  686-689,
     1969.
17.  Otnes, R.K. and Enochson, L.  Distal Time Series Analysis.
     John Wiley, New York, 1972
18.  Rappaport, M., Hopkins, H.K., Hall, K., Belleza, T. and Hall,
     R.A., Schizophrenia and evoked potentials:  maximum ampli-
     tude, frequency of peaks, variability and phenothiazine
     effects. Psychophysiology 12:  196-207, 1975
19.  Roth, W.T. and Cannon, E.H., Some features of the auditory
     evoked response in schizophrenics. Arch. Gen. Psychiatry 27:
     466-471, 1972
20.  Saletu, B., Itil, T.M. and Saletu, M., Auditory evoked res-
     ponse, EEG, and thought process in schizophrenics. Am. J.
     Psychiatry 128:  336-344, 1971
21.  Saletu, B., Saletu, M. and Itil, T.M., The relationships be-
     tween psychopathology and evoked responses before, during,
     and after psychotropic drug treatment. Biol. Psychiatry 6:
     46-74, 1973
22.  Schimmel, H., The (+) reference:  accuracy of estimated mean
     components in average response studies. Science 157:  9294,
     1967
23.  Shagass, C., Evoked Brain Potentials in Psychiatry. Plenum
     Press, New York, 1972
24.  Shagass, C., An electrophysiological view of schizophrenia.
     Biol. Psychiatry 11:  3-30, 1976
25.  Shakow, D., Psychological deficit in schizophrenia. Behav.
     Sci. 8:  275-305, 1963.
26.  Spitzer, R.L., Endicott, J.E. and Robins, E., Research
     Diagnostic Criteria (RDC) for Selected Group of Functional
     Disorders. New York, Biometrics Research, New York State
     Psychiatric Inst., 1975.
27.  Zerlin, S. and Davis, H., The variability of single evoked
     vertex potentials in man. Electroencephalogr. Clin. Neuro-
     physiol. 23:  467-474, 1967

## Appendix


### Simulation of the EP Trials

The Gaussian noise simulation of EEG was generated by averaging 12 uniformly distributed (0 to 1.0) random numbers, subtracting the mean value, and multiplying by a desired factor. The resulting noise values were digitally low pass filtered to give a frequency spectrum more closely resembling EEG. The individual successive Gaussian noise points $(x_i')$ were transformed into new $(x_i)$ simulated EEG points by the equation (Otnes and Enochson, 1972).

$$x_i = Gx_{i-1} + x_i'(1-G) \tag{1}$$

where

$$G = \exp(-\Delta t/RC) = \exp(-0.008/0.04) \tag{2}$$

$\Delta t$ being our sampling interval, .008 sec and RC being the time constant
The synthetic EP, $S(t)$, was generated by

$$s(0.4-t) = 60\exp(-3.5t)\sin(2\pi(1.5+8.2t)t) \tag{3}$$

to generate a swept frequency at 50 values of t 0, 0.008, 0.016.... 0.400 sec

The sum of $s(t)$ and $x(i)$ produced a single EP trial, simulating activity from 0 to 400 msec.

Next, the average evoked potential is calculated

$$AEP(i) = \frac{1}{M} \sum_{k=1}^{M} EP_{ki} \quad ; \quad i=1...n \tag{4}$$

where M equals the total number of trials (32 in our case) and
where n equals the number of time samples (50 in our case)
and k equals trial number

Next, product moment correlation coefficients are calculated between each of the 32 individual EP trials and the AEP. Each r is thus based on the 50 pairs of

AEP(i) and x(i) values: the z transform of each of the 32 correlations is then obtained:

$$Z_k = \tfrac{1}{2}\log_e \left((1+r_k)/1-r_k)\right) \; ; \; k=1\ldots M \qquad (5)$$

The average correlation is then

$$ZA = \frac{1}{M} \sum_{k=1}^{M} Z_k \qquad (6)$$

Least squares curve fits were performed to establish a relationship between SNR and the averaged z-transform measure (ZA) and between the variance of $Z_k$ (calculated over the 32 trial values) and the SNR (MLAB program, Knott and Reece, 1972).

Empirical SNR equations

The SNR is related to ZA by

$$Log_e SNR = 2.66-1.56\exp(-1.16ZA+1.56) \qquad (7)$$

The expected value (EV) of the variance of ZA

$$EVZA = -0.04ZA+0.098 \qquad (8)$$

Given new sets of EP data and the average EP, ZA can be calculated from the set of correlation coefficients (Eq. 5 and 6) and then values of ZA entered into equation 7 to yield the signal-to-noise ratio and into equation 8 to yield the expected variance. It should be noted that equations 7 and 8 can yield negative values for both SNR and EVZA if ZA is sufficiently negative. In the current study, we used a cutoff of 0.13 for SNR, entering this value for subjects with lower computed values. EVZA would not fall below 0 under usual circumstances.

# SENSORY EVOKED POTENTIALS IN PSYCHOSIS

Charles Shagass, M.D.

Temple University Health Sciences Center
Eastern Pennsylvania Psychiatric Institute
Philadelphia, Pennsylvania

Three decades have elapsed since Dawson (1947) demonstrated that the averaging method can be used to extract sensory evoked potentials (EPs) from the electroencephalographic (EEG) rhythms in which they are embedded. During the first half of this thirty year period, the development of apparatus for accomplishing averaging was the prime concern of the few investigators in the field. Following introduction of commercially produced equipment in the early 1960s, the volume of EP studies quickly expanded. Although EP recording was applied to clinical psychiatric research relatively early (Shagass and Schwartz, 1961), the number of psychiatric studies has grown quite slowly. The lack of faster progress can probably be attributed mainly to methodological difficulties inherent in studying psychiatric problems. At present, however, the slowly accumulated body of data bearing on EP correlates of mental illness may have reached the stage of beginning to justify optimism that it will be possible to realize one of the ultimate goals of such research, namely, to establish useful, objective neurophysiological indicators of psychopathology. The purpose of this paper is to review the principal findings obtained in EP investigations of the major psychoses.

A second major goal of EP research in psychiatry is to furnish clues as to deviant brain mechanisms in mental illness. In this connection, it should be noted that the EP approach offers one of the few feasible avenues for bridging the gap between clinical psychiatric phenomena and those detailed neuronal events, such as unit discharges and neurotransmitter levels, that can be studied directly only in the brain tissue of experimental animals. Three facts give rise to the bridging role of the EP approach: (1)

There are no convincing animal models of major mental illnesses; they must be studied in man. (2) EP recording is a noninvasive procedure. (3) The same kinds of EP phenomena can be recorded in both humans and animals. Consequently, EP correlates of psychiatric disorders can provide the basis for neurophysiological animal models of such illnesses, and the underlying mechanisms can be explored in experimental animals.

## METHODOLOGY

Application of EP methods to psychiatric investigations requires control of a number of factors, such as age, sex, level of alertness, and extracerebral contaminants (Shagass, 1972). Drug status requires special attention, as psychoactive drugs can alter EPs, and may continue to do so for some time after medication is stopped (Saletu et al, 1973); consequently, to evaluate research findings, the current and past drug history of subjects must be considered. The issue of interactions between age, sex, and diagnosis needs particular consideration in psychiatric investigations, because EP differences related to age and sex have been found in patient groups, although absent in normal controls (Shagass et al, 1974a). The spectre of unreliability in diagnostic criteria also haunts all psychiatric research, although different observers seem to agree well with respect to gross categories, particularly of the major psychoses (Spitzer et al, 1974).

In designating evoked potential (EP) peaks, the polarity-latency notation will be used here wherever possible, e.g., P100 would indicate a scalp-positive peak usually occurring 100 msec post-stimulus.

Clinical psychiatric groups have been compared with respect to several kinds of EP measurements. The amplitudes and times of occurrence (latency) of EP peaks provide quantitative descriptors of EP characteristics. Although hand measurements are still commonly used, they are often replaced or supplemented by automatic computer techniques, which are more satisfactory for amplitude measurements than for detecting peak latencies. Variations of amplitude or latency with stimulus strength provide intensity-response functions; when such curves are made linear, the slope of the regression line can be used to characterize the individual. As the slope tends to be correlated with mean level, it may be desirable to adjust the slope for mean level by covariance. Variability of EP wave shape over time has received considerable study; a commonly used means of quantifying temporal variability has been by computing product-moment correlation coefficients between corresponding data points in EPs taken at different times. Recovery functions have also been compared in clinical groups. Recovery procedures involve the use of one or more stimuli (conditioning) to modify responsiveness, followed by a constant (test) stimulus; by varying interstimulus interval (ISI), the time course of recovery of responsiveness can be determined. We have also employed a modified recovery procedure in which only one ISI was used, but conditioning stimulus intensity was varied (Shagass, 1972).

## EP FINDINGS IN SCHIZOPHRENIA

### Somatosensory Evoked Potentials (SEP)

Amplitudes of early SEP components (before 100 msec post-stimulus) were found to be greater than normal in schizophrenics over a range of stimulus intensities; however, the finding was not specific to schizophrenia (Shagass and Schwartz, 1963a). More recently, similarly elevated amplitudes over several stimulus intensities were observed only in chronic schizophrenics; in acute and latent subtypes, the results were like those of normals (Shagass et al, 1974a). Ikuta (1974) has also reported increased early amplitude in schizophrenics. Compared to chronic patients, acute schizophrenics tend to have lower intensity-amplitude slopes, and thus to be "reducers" if one applies the concept underlying Buchsbaum and Silverman's (1968) test of Petrie's (1967) augmenting-reducing dimension (Shagass et al, 1974a). When SEP measurements were related to Brief Psychiatric Rating Scale symptom ratings within a heterogeneous schizophrenic population, early amplitudes were greater in the more floridly psychotic patients with low depression ratings than in those who were more depressed and less psychotic (Shagass et al, 1974b).

In our recent studies, we randomly intermingle left and right median nerve stimuli with auditory click and visual checkerboard pattern flashes. In an initial analysis of the results in schizophrenia, we found that, compared to 16 matched healthy controls, SEP peaks after 100 msec, i.e., N130, P180, and P280, were attenuated in 32 schizophrenics (Shagass et al, 1977a). The group mean SEPs in Fig. 1 illustrate this finding for left median nerve stimuli. The right hand portion of Fig. 1 shows the results of t-test comparisons between individual data point means; the display is arranged so that the curve rises above base line only when the .05 significance level was achieved. Similar results were obtained with right median nerve stimuli. In apparent contradiction of previous results, Fig. 1 does not reveal important early SEP amplitude differences and even suggests that P30 was of lower amplitude in the schizophrenics. However, it should be noted that, since 22 of 32 patients were males, and since female schizophrenics tend to have higher than normal amplitudes, whereas the reverse trend is

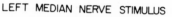

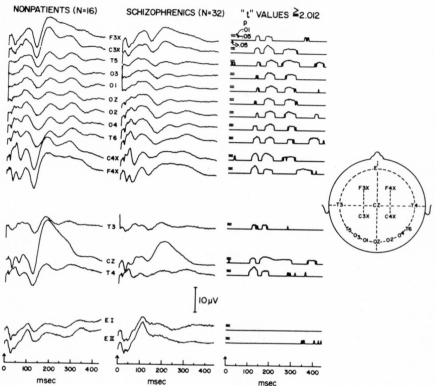

Fig. 1 - Group mean somatosensory evoked potentials (left median nerve stimuli) for 16 non-patients and 32 schizophrenics matched for age and sex. C and F leads are displaced 2 cm behind conventional 10-20 system locations and are, therefore, designated C3X, F3C, etc. Linked ear reference. Positivity at scalp gives upward deflection. Column of "t" values at right arranged so that the deflection from base line occurs only when .05 level of significance reached. Two lead montages were used, with EOG lead in each; EI and EII are spearate recordings from the EOG lead.

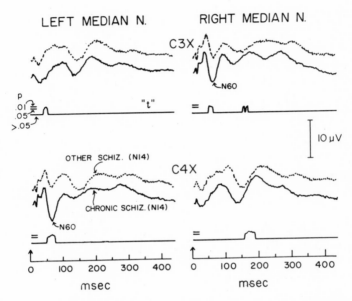

Fig. 2 - Comparison of mean SEPs for the C3X and C4X leads with right and left median nerve stimulation in 14 chronic (paranoid, undifferentiated, simple) schizophrenics and 14 schizophrenics of other types (acute, catatonic, schizo-affective) matched for age and sex. Corresponding "t"-tests below as in Fig. 1. Note that N60 is clearly negative in the chronic patients and not in the others.

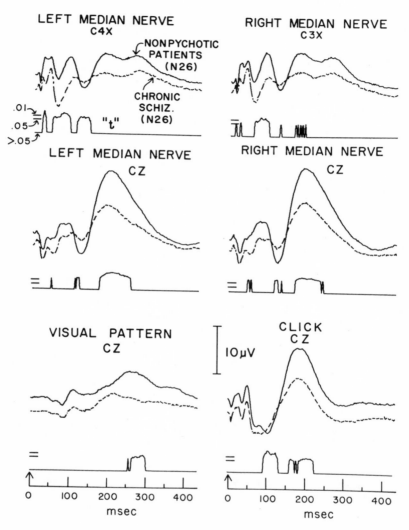

Fig. 3 - Comparison of mean evoked potentials of 26 chronic schizophrenics and 26 age and sex matched nonpsychotic patients (14 personality disorders, 12 neurotics) in selected leads for 4 stimulus modalities. Note pronounced N60 in C4X and C3X leads and generally reduced later activity of schizophrenics.

found in males, the SEP results are not necessarily discordant with previous findings (Shagass et al, 1972).

The schizophrenic patients were then subdivided into two age and sex matched groups, each containing 14 patients of the following subtypes: A - chronic undifferentiated, chronic paranoid, simple; B - catatonic, schizoaffective, acute. The main SEP difference found between these two groups was that peak N60 was more negative at the C4X or C3X leads in group A (chronic, Fig. 2). The patients in subtypes suggesting a persistent, chronic disorder showed negativity at 60 msec in the SEP from the lead over the post-central gyrus, whereas those with more acute or episodic disorders did not. More recently, comparison of SEPs in a larger sample of 26 chronic schizophrenics with those of 26 age and sex matched nonpsychotic patients (psychoneuroses and personality disorders) has again revealed greater posterior N60 peaks in the schizophrenics, as shown in Fig. 3 (Shagass et al, 1977b). Since N60 is normally negative in SEPs from a lead anterior to the central sulcus (F4X in Fig. 1), the increased posterior negativity in chronic schizophrenics suggests that this normal component is unusually distributed in these patients. This could result from deviant anatomy, but more probably reflects impairment of some mechanism that normally restricts the spread of activity.

## Auditory Evoked Potentials (AEP)

Several investigators have found that AEP amplitude is reduced from normal in schizophrenic patients (Jones and Callaway, 1970; Saletu et al, 1971; Cohen, 1973). The published observations concern mainly the amplitude of the N100-P200 peaks. Our recent data have confirmed these results (Shagass et al, 1977a). AEP latencies P60, N100, and P180 have been reported as faster than normal in schizophrenics (Saletu et al, 1971); however, so far, we have not been able to confirm this observation.

## Visual Evoked Potentials (VEP)

Studies of VEP amplitude in schizophrenia have produced variable results. However, the recent study by Schooler et al (1976) suggests that, within a schizophrenic population, VEP amplitudes (P100-N140) tend to be greater in the more chronic patients. In an early study of VEP to flash, we found that P45 latency tended to be faster in schizophrenics than in other subjects; also, there was less after-rhythm in schizophrenics than in any other group except chronic brain syndromes (Shagass and Schwartz, 1965). Rappaport et al (1975) found that schizophrenics had lower amplitudes and more VEP peaks up to 400 msec than normal subjects.

Landau et al (1975) reported that the VEP intensity-amplitude function in "reactive" schizophrenics tended to be of reducing type, i.e., to show less amplitude increase, or even amplitude reduction, with increasing stimulus intensity; the comparison groups were matched normals and bipolar depressives. Reducing was greatest in patients with good prognosis.

## Wave Shape Variability

Correlation coefficients, computed over the corresponding data points of the entire wave form (500 msec) of VEPs and AEPs taken at different times, have regularly indicated that variability is greater than normal in schizophrenics (Callaway et al, 1965; Lifshitz, 1969; Cohen, 1973; Rappaport et al, 1975). However, for SEP at least, the results pertain only to events after 100 msec. We found that variability of SEP wave-shape before 100 msec was less in chronic schizophrenics than in acute or latent patients or normals; variability was also lower in patients who were less depressed and more floridly psychotic (Shagass et al, 1974a, 1974b). In contrast, the sicker schizophrenic patients tended to have greater SEP variability after 100 msec.

Spatial variability can also be assessed with the correlation method; the correlation is run between EPs from two different leads, rather than between EPs from the same lead taken at different times. Rodin et al (1968) found that VEP spatial wave shape variability was greater than normal in schizophrenics.

## Recovery Functions

Utilizing paired, equal intensity, electrical stimuli to ulnar or median nerves in early studies, we found that SEP amplitude recovery was reduced from normal in schizophrenics (Shagass and Schwartz, 1963b). The reduction occurred mainly in the first recovery phase, which normally shows return to pre-conditioning stimulus responsiveness at some ISI before 20 msec. Although only the N20-P30 peaks were measured in the first studies, subsequent work indicated that other peaks up to 100 msec also showed generally reduced recovery in schizophrenic patients (Shagass, 1968). The same results as in schizophrenia were also obtained in several other disorders. In contrast to reduced SEP amplitude recovery, SEP latency recovery was found to be accelerated in schizophrenics, and this has recently been confirmed (Shagass et al, 1974a).

Reduced recovery in schizophrenics, as compared to normals, has also been found with auditory stimuli (Cohen, 1973). Several workers have found that VEP amplitude is attenuated in schizophrenic

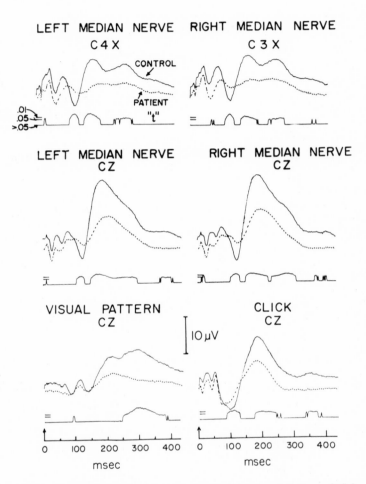

Fig. 4 - Comparison of mean evoked potentials of 16 non-patients and 32 schizophrenic patients in selected leads for 4 stimulus modalities. Note marked attenuation of activity from 250 to 400 msec with visual stimuli.

patients (Speck et al, 1966; Floris et al, 1968; Vasconetto et al, 1971).  Ishikawa (1968) reported that reduced VEP amplitude recovery in schizophrenics occurred mainly in those whose symptoms included hallucinations.

## P300

Measurements of the P300 wave in schizophrenics have generally shown that it was either absent or markedly reduced in amplitude. This has been demonstrated under active information-processing conditions (Levit et al, 1973), and under conditions of passive attending (Roth and Cannon, 1972).  In our recent study with several modalities of sensory stimuli, the subject is asked to fixate a point on a television monitor and four kinds of stimuli are administered in random order; the conditions seem to favor generation of a small P300, at least in normals.  The P300 in the SEPs of normals can be seen clearly in leads other than Cz in Fig. 1; in Cz it is merged with P180.  Although present, the peak was significantly smaller in the SEPs of schizophrenic patients (Fig. 1). The reduction of P300 amplitude in schizophrenics was seen in EPs of all modalities; this is illustrated in the group means from the vertex (Cz) and other selected leads shown in Fig. 4.

Table 1 provides a summary listing of EP findings in schizophrenic disorders.

## EP FINDINGS IN AFFECTIVE PSYCHOSES

### A. Depression

SEP.  In an early study, patients with depressive psychoses (manic-depressive, psychotic depressive reaction, involutional depression) were found to have greater than normal amplitude across several stimulus intensities (Shagass and Schwartz, 1963a).  Since the intensity-amplitude slopes were high, their results could be interpreted as reflecting an augmenting tendency; this was held in common with all other patient  groups studied, with the exception of "dysthymic" neuroses (anxiety, depression, psychophysiological reactions).  SEPs, recorded within the context of the modified recovery function procedure, were of higher amplitude between 50 and 199 msec, and were less variable between 101 and 200 msec in psychotic depressives than in schizophrenics (Shagass et al, 1974a). The bipolar recording technique used in earlier studies did not favor clear visualization of later SEP events, in contrast with the monopolar montage used in our most recent work.  Although we have so far studied relatively few psychotic depressive patients, the available results demonstrate clear differences in the later SEP events between patients and normals (Fig. 5).  Furthermore, the findings in patients with psychotic depressions also differed

Table 1

## EP Findings in Schizophrenia

1. SEP Amplitude
   (a) before 100 msec
       (i) higher in chronic than in acute, latent or normals
           (Shagass et al, 1974a; Ikuta, 1974)
       (ii) acutes tend to be "reducers" (Shagass et al, 1974a)
       (iii) higher in nondepressed, floridly psychotic
           (Shagass et al, 1974b)
       (iv) greater N60 in chronic (Shagass et al, 1977a)
   (b) after 100 msec:  lower than normal in overt, but not in
       latent (Shagass et al, 1977b)

2. AEP
   (a) amplitude lower than normal (Jones and Callaway, 1970;
       Saletu et al, 1971; Cohen, 1973; Shagass et al, 1977a)
   (b) latency faster than normal (Saletu et al, 1971)

3. VEP
   (a) amplitude results vary; amplitude greater in more chronic
       (Schooler et al, 1976)
   (b) latency faster (Shagass and Schwartz, 1965)
   (c) less after-rhythm (Shagass and Schwartz, 1965)
   (d) "reactives" tend to be "reducers" (Landau et al, 1975)

4. Wave Shape Variability - Temporal
   (a) before 100 msec (SEP) - less in chronics and in nondepressed,
       more floridly psychotic (Shagass et al, 1974b)
   (b) greater in chronics after 100 msec (all modalities) (Callaway
       et al, 1965; Lifshitz, 1969; Cohen, 1973; Shagass et al,
       1974b; Rappaport et al, 1975)

5. Spatial Wave Shape Variability greater than normal (Rodin et al,
   1968)

6. Amplitude Recovery
   (a) reduced from normal (SEP, AEP, VEP) (Shagass and Schwartz,
       1963b; Speck et al, 1966; Floris et al, 1968; Vasconetto
       et al, 1971; Cohen, 1973)
   (b) greater reduction in hallucinated (Ishikawa, 1968)

7. Latency Recovery - faster (Shagass, 1968; Shagass et al, 1974a)

8. P300
   (a) reduced from normal (Roth and Cannon, 1972; Levit et al,
       1973; Shagass et al, 1977a)
   (b) less effect of uncertainty (Levit et al, 1973)

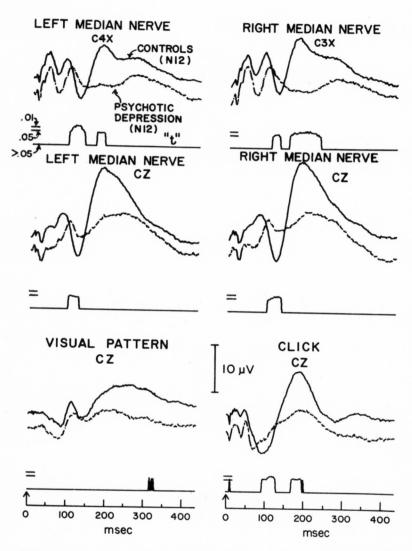

<u>Fig. 5</u> - Comparison of mean EPs of 12 psychotic depressives and 12 nonpatients of same age and sex in selected leads for 4 stimulus modalities.

clearly from those of hospitalized patients with neurotic depressions of the same age and sex (Shagass et al, 1977b); the results
of the neurotic depressives were quite similar to those of non-
patients.  The SEP tracings after 100 msec of the psychotic depressives in Fig. 5 resemble those of the schizophrenic group  in Fig. 3.

SEP recovery function studies have regularly disclosed lower
than normal amplitude recovery of the N20-P30 component and other
peaks before 100 msec in patients with psychotic depressions
(Shagass and Schwartz, 1962a, 1963b, 1966). In contrast to the
reduced amplitude recovery, latency recovery was faster than normal in patients with severe depressions (Shagass, 1968), a finding
recently verified with the modified recovery function procedure
(Shagass et al, 1974a).  Serial studies of SEP recovery in depressive patients receiving treatment showed normalization of the deviant
amplitude recovery findings with clinical improvement (Shagass and
Schwartz, 1962a); this means that reduced recovery is a concomitant
of the depressed state, rather than an enduring trait.  The point
is important, as Wasman and Gluck (1975) found reduced SEP recovery
in slow learners, in whom this might be a trait characteristic.
It should be noted also that, although clearly correlated with the
depressive state, reduced recovery is not specific for severe
depressions.

AEP. Our recent data indicate that AEP amplitudes from about
100 msec to 250 msec post-stimulus are lower than normal in patients
with psychotic depressions (Fig. 5).  There were similar differences
between patients with psychotic and neurotic depressions, the neurotics giving results like normals.  AEP amplitude recovery in
depression was studied by Satterfield (1972).  He found a wide
range of recovery values, but noted that, comparing the extremes
of recovery, patients with reduced AEP recovery had positive family
histories of affective psychoses, whereas those with increased
recovery did not.

VEP. Perris (1975) reported that, the more severe the depression according to a standard scale, the lower the amplitude of VEP
(maximum peak-to-peak excursion over the first three events).
Buchsbaum et al (1973) observed that VEP latencies were shorter
than normal in their depressive patients; the greatest latency
deviations occurred in the unipolar type.  Borge (1973) found that
VEP wave shape variability was greater than normal in patients with
depressive psychoses.

There have been a series of interesting findings in depression
with the VEP test of augmenting-reducing.  Originally, Borge et al
(1971) reported that bipolar depressives were augmenters, whereas
unipolars were reducers; lithium therapy diminished augmenting.
Subsequently, Buchsbaum et al (1973) found that the reducing

tendency in unipolar depressives occurred in male, but not female, patients.  Attempts to distinguish between psychotic and neurotic depressions by means of the VEP intensity-amplitude functions have led to contradictory results (Borge, 1973; von Knorring et al, 1974).

Perris (1974) has obtained VEP findings relating depression to differential hemispheric changes.  VEP to flash were of lower amplitude in left than in right occipital recordings in psychotic depressives; neurotic depressives and schizophrenics did not show the asymmetry.  The relatively attenuated left VEP amplitude returned to normal after effective treatment, indicating that it is a state-related phenomenon.

P300.  Levit et al (1973) found P300 to be of greater ampli-tude in depression than in schizophrenia and that shifts between visual and auditory stimuli increased P300 in depressives as in normals, but reduced it in schizophrenics.

## B. Mania

Relatively few manic patients have been studied because of obvious difficulties in obtaining adequate cooperation for accept-able recordings.  In our current study, even though we have data for only 5 manic or hypomanic patients, some interesting trends have emerged.  Fig. 6 shows the results comparing the EPs of these patients from selected leads with those of nonpatients of the same age and sex.  It will be seen that SEP peaks P100, N130, and P180 tend to be of lower amplitude in the manics, P180 significantly so.  Amplitude of the P200 peak in VEP was lower in manics.  AEP late activity was also reduced in manics, but not to a statistically significant extent.  The findings suggest that the reduced late EP activity found in schizophrenic and depressive psychoses also occurs in mania, although P300 may be less affected in mania.

SEP wave shape variability before 100 msec was greater than normal in manics, as measured within the context of the modified recovery procedure (Shagass, 1975).  The greater early variability in mania contrasts with the lower than normal variability in schizophrenia and a similar tendency toward less early variability in psychotic depressives.

EP findings in affective psychosis are summarized in Table 2.

## EP FINDINGS IN CHRONIC BRAIN SYNDROMES

Table 3 attempts to summarize the EP findings in chronic brain syndromes.  These studies have generally been carried out in

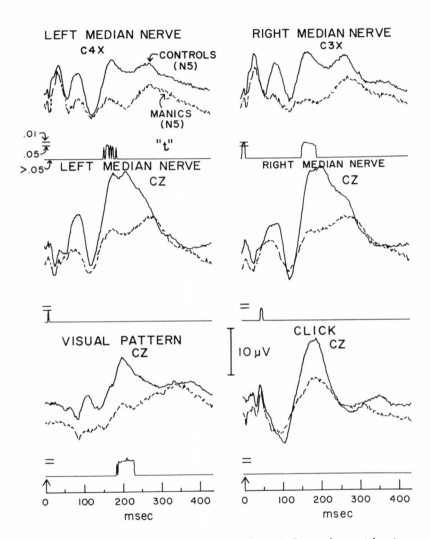

Fig. 6 - Comparison of mean EPs of 5 manic patients and 5 nonpatients of same age and sex in selected leads for 4 stimulus modalities. Note relatively prominent P300 in the manics.

Table 2

EP Findings in Affective Psychoses

A. Depression
   1. SEP
      (a) amplitude of N20-P30 greater, tend to be "augmenters"
          (Shagass and Schwartz, 1963a)
      (b) amplitude after 100 msec reduced (Shagass et al, 1977b)
      (c) amplitude recovery reduced (Shagass and Schwartz, 1962,
          1963b, 1966)
      (d) latency recovery faster (Shagass, 1968; Shagass et al,
          1974a)

   2. AEP
      (a) amplitude reduced after 100 msec (Shagass et al, 1977b)
      (b) less recovery with positive family history (Satterfield,
          1972)

   3. VEP
      (a) amplitude lower in more severe depression (Perris, 1975)
      (b) latency shorter, more in unipolar (Buchsbaum et al, 1973)
      (c) variability greater (Borge, 1973)
      (d) augmenting-reducing
          (i) bipolar are augmenters; male unipolar are reducers
              (Borge et al, 1971; Buchsbaum et al, 1973)
          (ii) psychotic vs neurotic results vary (Borge, 1973;
               von Knorring et al, 1974)
      (e) right VEP > left before treatment (Perris, 1974)

   4. P300 closer to normal than in schizophrenia (Levit et al,
      1973)

B. Mania
   1. Reduced SEP amplitude after 100 msec (Shagass et al, 1977b)

   2. Greater SEP variability before 100 msec (Shagass, 1975)

Table 3

## EP Findings in Chronic Brain Syndromes

1. SEP

    (a) latency prolonged (Levy et al, 1971)
    (b) N100 amplitude reduced (Levy et al, 1971)
    (c) amplitude greater than normal in females, lower than
        normal in males (Straumanis, 1964)
    (d) SEP amplitude (N20-P30) recovery greater (Shagass, 1968)

2. AEP

Greater variability in time and space (Malerstein and Callaway,
    1969; Gerson et al, 1976)

3. VEP

    (a) early VEP amplitude increased (Straumanis et al, 1965;
        Visser et al, 1976)
    (b) latency increased (Straumanis et al, 1965; Visser et al,
        1976)
    (c) less after-rhythm (Cohn, 1964; Straumanis et al, 1965)
    (d) greater spatial variability (Gerson et al, 1976)

patients of advanced age, most of whom have carried diagnoses   of
cerebral arteriosclerosis or senile dementia.


## SEP

Straumanis (1964) recorded SEPs and their recovery functions
in a group of elderly patients with cerebral arteriosclerosis and
matched normals.  The main finding was a large amplitude difference
between sexes in the patient group, females having greater amplitudes than males; no such sex difference was evident in the
controls.  Statistical analysis yielded a significant sex x diagnosis interaction for P30.  Amplitude recovery of N20-P30 was
greater for the brain syndrome patients (Shagass, 1968).

Levy et al (1971) compared patients suffering from senile
dementia with depressed patients of similar age.  They found general prolongation of latencies in the seniles, with the N45 latency
difference achieving statistical significance.  They also found
relative depression of the amplitude of a negative peak at 90 msec
in the seniles, so that the ratio of the N90 to N25 amplitude significantly discriminated the senile from the depressed patients.


## AEP

Malerstein and Callaway (1969) reported that temporal variability of AEP wave shape was greater than normal in patients with
Korsakoff's psychosis.  Gerson et al (1976) obtained a measure
that can be interpreted as spatial wave shape variability between
AEPs recorded from homologous leads over each side of the head.
Spatial variability was significantly lower in a group of elderly
patients with signs of senility than in a group of matched controls.


## VEP

Straumanis et al (1965) found that the amplitude of P45 was
greater than normal in patients with cerebral arteriosclerosis,
and that the latencies of peaks after 100 msec were markedly
increased in the patients.  These findings have been essentially
replicated by Visser et al (1976).  Straumanis et al also found
that the amount of after-rhythm in the VEP was markedly reduced
in brain syndrome patients, as had been noted in a patient  with
Jacob-Creutzfeldt syndrome reported by Cohn (1964).

Gerson et al (1976) recorded VEP as well as AEP in their study
of senile patients.  They found that VEP spatial variability in

the patients was greater than that in controls; there was greater asymmetry between the wave shapes from pairs of homologous leads.

## EEG-SEP RELATIONSHIPS

Since averaging methods are employed to cancel out the EEG in which EP are embedded, EP investigators have tended to focus upon the EP to the exclusion of the EEG. However, the notion that the patterning of EEG and EP events may be clinically relevant seems attractive from a psychiatric viewpoint; psychiatric diagnosis is seldom based upon single behavioral dimensions, but rather on the pattern of relationship between several dimensions. Thus far, the only systematic study in which psychiatric correlates of EEG-EP relationships have been reported is one carried out in our laboratory (Shagass et al, 1975).

SEP data were obtained within the context of the modified recovery function procedure, which yields a number of measurements reflecting amplitude, amplitude recovery, and intensity-amplitude relationships. The EEG measures were mean amplitude, mean frequency, and indices of temporal variability in amplitude and frequency rendered independent of mean level by covariance adjustment. The analysis strategy employed was to test the significance of differences in correlations between EEG and SEP measurements in different clinical groups, comparing psychiatric patients with controls of the same age and sex. The results suggested that each of four major patient groups differed from normal in a specific way with respect to EEG-SEP relationships: chronic schizophrenics; neuroses; personality disorders; manic-depressive, depressed patients.

The main differences from normal for the neuroses occurred in correlations between mean SEP amplitude and mean EEG amplitude; correlations were negative in the patients and positive in the controls. For chronic schizophrenics, the principal differences from normal occurred in correlations between mean SEP amplitude and EEG amplitude variability in time; whereas greater SEP amplitudes were associated with greater EEG variability in the patients, the reverse trend was found in the normals. For personality disorders, the relationships between mean SEP amplitude and mean frequency provided the most common difference; correlations tended to be positive in the patients and negative in the controls. Manic depressive, depressed patients tended to show greater intensity-amplitude slopes (augmenting) when EEG amplitude was higher, whereas the reverse trend was true in the normals; Fig. 7 illustrates one of the correlation differences between these groups.

The findings of this first study obviously require confirmation. However, they do suggest that combinations of EEG and EP variables may provide results unobtainable with either kind of

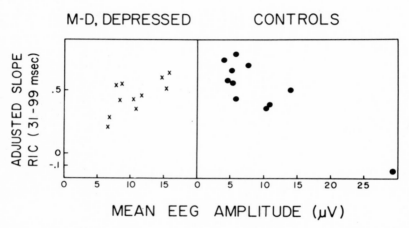

Fig. 7 - Scattergrams for correlations between mean EEG amplitude
and slope relating SEP amplitude from 31-99 msec to stimulus intensity; slope adjusted for variations in mean amplitude level. Positive correlation indicates that augmenting tendency accompanies
high EEG amplitude in patients; reverse trend in controls.

variable alone, and that such combinations may deviate from normal in diagnostically specific patterns.

## DISCUSSION

### Methodological Issues

Few clinical EP investigations do not contain some important methodological flaws. Many studies compare only one patient group in a grossly defined diagnostic category, such as schizophrenia, with a presumably healthy control group. Apart from the possibility that some uncontrolled subject factor other than illness, e.g., nutrition, could be responsible for EP differences, the use of only one patient group makes it impossible to ascertain diagnostic specificity. Also, since it is increasingly recognized that the psychoses are not homogeneous, but are composed of differing subtypes, it may be more productive to compare subtypes within a major group than to compare the main groups. This is suggested by a number of the findings in schizophrenia (Table 1). However, enough studies with adequate numbers of patients have not yet been performed to satisfactorily define the relationships between EP variables and psychopathological characteristics, such as symptoms.

Many interesting EP results have been obtained with patients who were either receiving drugs or had recently been withdrawn from them. In our own studies, patients had been withdrawn from drugs for an average of 10 days before testing. Fortunately, the follow-reasons suggest that many, or perhaps most, of the positive results are not due mainly to drug effects: (1) EP measurements have seldom been found to be correlated with drug dosage in medicated patients when such correlations were attempted. (2) We found only minor SEP changes when we compared the results in schizophrenic patients initially tested when off drugs and retested while receiving phenothiazines. (3) We have also not been able to show that SEP measurements differed in relation to the length of time between drug withdrawal and testing. (4) SEP variability measures have not so far been found to be affected by drugs. (5) Normalization of deviant EP findings has been observed with drugs (Shagass et al, 1962; Heninger and Speck, 1966); this would suggest that initial differences were not the result of drug effects. On the other hand, we know that psychoactive drugs do produce effects (Shagass, 1974), and that such effects may be quite variable depending upon the condition of the patient; this urges caution in accepting evidence that drug effects are absent.

## Diagnostic Discriminations

Given the reservations imposed by methodological problems, it still appears that some EP correlates of psychopathology may be acquiring the status of acceptable fact. This is because of convergent results obtained by different investigators, even though techniques are seldom identical and subject populations are bound to vary from one study to another. This convergence of findings has prompted me to attempt the somewhat hazardous exercise of constructing a schema for differential diagnosis of the psychoses on the basis of EP findings. This schema, presented in Table 4, should be understood as an outline of partially proven possibilities, rather than fully established fact.

I. Psychotic vs nonpsychotic conditions. This distinction could be accomplished by recording several kinds of sensory EP. Low amplitude and highly variable late EP activity, particularly N130 and P180, would favor a psychotic as opposed to a nonpsychotic condition (Figs. 1, 3, 4, 5, 6). Although our recent data suggest that individuals with latent schizophrenia, who are not overtly psychotic, would generally be considered as nonpsychotic by these EP criteria, the fact that they should be readily distinguishable from other schizophrenics could be of value (Shagass et al, 1977b).

II. Brain syndromes vs other psychoses. Having distinguished the psychotic individuals from the nonpsychotic, we could then proceed to separate out the patients with brain syndromes. The two main criteria would be general latency prolongation and greater than normal SEP recovery functions in the brain syndromes. In the other psychotic conditions, latencies would be either within the normal range or faster, taking age into account, and recovery would be generally reduced.

III. Schizophrenia vs affective psychoses. Schizophrenic patients could be distinguished from depressives, and possibly manics, by the reduction of VEP after-rhythm. Recording from the two hemispheres, one would expect amplitude asymmetries in the depressives, but not in the schizophrenics. In a P300 paradigm, P300 would be reduced more in the schizophrenics than in the depressives. A measure of SEP variability in the first 100 msec should show greater than normal variability in manics, normal to low variability in the depressives, and lower than normal variability in the schizophrenics. SEP variability so far appears to be the only sign distinguishing depression and mania.

IV. Chronic vs acute or reactive schizophrenia. Several signs might be used to distinguish chronic from acute or reactive schizophrenia. Early SEP amplitude would be higher and variability lower in chronic schizophrenia, whereas the reverse would be true in the

Table 4

Possible Differential Diagnosis of Psychosis by EP Variables

I

|  | Psychotic | Nonpsychotic |
|---|---|---|
| late EP activity amplitude | low | high |
| late EP variability | high | low |

II

|  | Brain Syndromes | Other Psychoses |
|---|---|---|
| EP latencies | prolonged | normal or fast |
| SEP recovery (early) | augmented | reduced |

III

|  | Schizophrenia | Depression | Mania |
|---|---|---|---|
| VEP after-rhythm | nearly absent | present | present |
| P300 | reduced | near normal |  |
| VEP asymmetry | absent | present |  |
| early SEP | low | normal to low | high |

IV

|  | Chronic Schizophrenia | Acute Schizophrenia |
|---|---|---|
| early SEP amplitude | higher | lower |
| early SEP variability | lower | higher |
| VEP, SEP intensity-amplitude | augmenter | reducer |
| late EP variability | high | not so high |
| late EP amplitude | low | not so low |
| SEP N60 | more posterior | more anterior |

acute or reactive subtypes. The intensity-amplitude curve would tend to be of reducer type in acute or reactive and of augmenter type in the chronic patients. Late EPs of all kinds would tend to be more variable and of lower amplitude in the chronic than in the acute or reactive subtypes. Also, the N60 SEP component would have a higher probability of being maximal in a more posterior location in chronic than in acute patients (Fig. 2).

Although the differential diagnostic schema outlined in Table 4 is undoubtedly premature at present, it would probably meet the criterion of statistical significance if put to empirical test. We hope to provide a partial test soon with data gathered in our laboratory. Clinical significance, in terms of practical utility, would be more important to demonstrate, and is still some way off, because it will be necessary to reduce the number of EP measurements to an acceptable minimum.

## Theoretical Implications

Two kinds of theoretical orientation underlie EP investigations of mental illness; I have elsewhere designated these viewpoints as psychophysiological and pathophysiological (Shagass, 1976). The psychophysiological orientation assumes that there is a one-to-one linkage between psychological and physiological events; consequently, deviant behavior should be accompanied by deviant physiology, e.g., an attention deficit should be accompanied by reduction of brain potentials, such as N130, which reflect attentive activity. The pathophysiological orientation assumes that physiological dysfunction is the primary event; when such dysfunction reaches, or exceeds, the critical level, behavioral symptoms may occur. Consequently, the pathophysiological view does not require a one-to-one linkage between physiological and psychological events. I consider both theoretical orientations to be valid and useful, and I have argued only that investigators be explicit about which orientation is guiding their work.

Many of the possible diagnostic indicators listed in Table 4 involve late EP events; they can be regarded as probably psychophysiological in nature, because the EP phenomena can be manipulated experimentally by altering psychological conditions or instructions. EP data have been marshalled to support a number of theoretical formulations couched in psychological terms. Examples are: segmental set or attention deficits to explain AEP variability in schizophrenia (Callaway et al, 1965), perceptual inconstancy (Ornitz and Ritvo, 1968), self-regulation of stimulus intensity (augmenting-reducing) (Buchsbaum, 1976). These psychophysiological formulations essentially view the EP indicator as a physiological concomitant of one or other psychological dysfunction to be found

in the disorder under investigation.  A more pathophysiological
orientation has been assumed in hypotheses that formulate a deficit
in central regulatory mechanisms (Stevens, 1973; Shagass, 1976).
Although neither kind of hypothesis is etiological in nature, the
pathophysiological formulations attempt to define neural structures
in which malfunctioning may lead to psychopathology.

I have recently attempted a pathophysiological formulation of
impaired perceptual functioning in chronic schizophrenia, based
upon EP findings (Shagass, 1976).  The schematic summary of relevant EP observations distinguishing chronic schizophrenics from
normals and acute or latent schizophrenics is given in Fig. 8.
Essentially, this is a contrast between early and late EP events,
the former being of higher amplitude and showing less temporal
variability in the chronic patients, while the reverse is true of
the later events.  The basic argument is that the high amplitude
and low variability of the early events reflects a deficit of normal modulation or gating, and that this deficit results in impaired
processing of information as reflected in the lower amplitude and
more variable later events.  Evidence was advanced to support the
idea that the deficient gating may result from underactivation of
subcortical structures modulating sensory input, such as septum
or mesencephalic reticular formation.  I drew attention to the
parallel between my formulation, based upon EP observations, and
Stevens' (1973) proposal of a gating deficit, based upon both clinical observations and recent findings concerning neurotransmitters
in neostriatum and limbic striatum.  The changes in distribution
of regional cerebral blood flow observed in chronic schizophrenics
by Ingvar and Franzén (1974) also seemed compatible with the hypothesis, in that they could be interpreted as reflecting overactivity
in posterior brain areas concerned with sensory perception and
underactivity in anterior areas mediating more complex interpretive
activity.

Callaway (1977, personal communication) has recently attempted
to integrate the psychophysiological and pathophysiological orientations with respect to EP studies of schizophrenia.  He considers
schizophrenia to be a "fault in overall regulation", and suggests
that the concept of "excessive responding to normal biases" in
schizophrenia can be considered as a defective gating or ordering
of mental operations.  He argues that defective gating could result
from either a defective neural structure, situational stress, or
faulty early conditioning.  Callaway attempts to integrate phenomena
at different levels, ranging from hypothesized structural abnormalities involving the dopaminergic pathways, to observable motor dis-
coordinations, to behavioral pathology.  He relates these to a
variety of deviant EP findings in schizophrenia and formulates
schizophrenia as a "disordered regulation of responses".  Although
Callaway's formulation attempts to encompass more, it is compatible

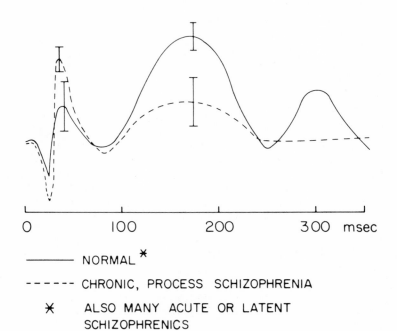

NORMAL *

------ CHRONIC, PROCESS SCHIZOPHRENIA

* ALSO MANY ACUTE OR LATENT
SCHIZOPHRENICS

Fig. 8 - Idealized schematic drawing depicting main EP
differences found between chronic schizophrenics and normals
(also many acute or latent schizophrenics).  Vertical bars depict
wave shape variability.  Note contrast between findings in early
and late events.

with my hypothesis of an impaired filtering mechanism in chronic schizophrenia.  It is also compatible with the clinical effects of antipsychotic drugs, which benefit both excitement and apathy in schizophrenia, i.e., they improve regulation.

It should be apparent that theoretical formulations in this area tend to be broad, and correspondingly vague, because we lack sufficiently specific information about the anatomical sources and functional significance of the EP signals that deviate from normal in the psychoses.  If consistent EP abnormalities were shown to reflect verifiable structural changes in a specified part of the brain in only a subgroup of patients now called schizophrenic, this might lead to more productive theory.  An example of data with this kind of theoretical potential might be our recent finding that the SEP N60 is more posteriorly distributed in chronic schizophrenics.  Goff et al (personal communication) have recently found that high amplitude posteriorly distributed N60 waves occur in the same hemisphere as the lesion in some epileptic patients. This suggests that abnormal N60 may result from a structural abnormality, or at least a fundamental alteration of functional organization.  More important perhaps, since N60 is the last SEP component in the specific (i.e., contralateral) cortical response, it offers the possibility of an animal model for experimental manipulation of underlying mechanisms.

It seems likely that satisfactory theory will not be developed until the data base of correlations between EP characteristics and psychopathology contains enough clearly established and replicable findings.  I believe that the present review of EP findings in psychosis suggests that the needed data base is emerging.

## REFERENCES

Borge, G. F.  Perceptual modulation and variability in psychiatric patients.  Arch. Gen. Psychiatry, 29:760-763, 1973.

Borge, G. F., Buchsbaum, M., Goodwin, F., Murphy, D. and Silverman, J.  Neuropsychological correlates of affective disorders. Arch. Gen. Psychiatry, 24:501-504, 1971.

Buchsbaum, M.  Self-regulation of stimulus intensity:  Augmenting-reducing and the average evoked response.  In:  G. E. Schwartz and D. Shapiro (Eds.) Consciousness and Self-Regulation, Vol. 1.  Plenum Publishing Corp., New York, 1976. pp. 101-135.

Buchsbaum, M., Landau, S., Murphy, D. and Goodwin, F.  Average evoked responses in bipolar and unipolar affective disorders: Relationship to sex, age of onset and monoamine oxidase.  Biol. Psychiatry, 7:199-212, 1973.

Buchsbaum, M. and Silverman, J. Stimulus intensity control and the cortical evoked response. Psychosom. Med., 30:12-22, 1968.

Callaway, E., Jones, R. T. and Layne, R. S. Evoked responses and segmental set of schizophrenia. Arch. Gen. Psychiatry, 12: 83-89, 1965.

Cohen, R. The influence of task-irrelevant stimulus varia- tions on the reliability of auditory evoked responses in schizo- phrenia. In: A. Fessard and G. Lelord (Eds.) Human Neurophysiol- ogy, Psychology, Psychiatry: Average Evoked Responses and Their Conditioning in Normal Subjects and Psychiatric Patients. Inserm, Paris, 1973. pp. 373-388.

Cohn, R. Rhythmic after-activity in visual evoked responses. Ann. N.Y. Acad. Sci., 112:281-291, 1964.

Dawson, G. D. Cerebral responses to electrical stimulation of peripheral nerve in man. J. Neurol. Neurosurg, Psychiatry, 10:134-140, 1947.

Floris, V., Morocutti, C., Amabile, G., Bernardi, G. and Rizzo, P. A. Recovery cycle of visual evoked potentials in normal, schizophrenic and neurotic patients. In: N. S. Kline and E. Laska (Eds.) Computers and Electronic Devices in Psychiatry. Grune and Stratton, New York, 1968. pp. 194-205.

Gerson, I. M., John, E. R., Bartlett, F. and Koenig, V. Average evoked response (AER) in the electroencephalographic diag- nosis of the normally aging brain: A practical application. Clin. Electroencephalography, 7:77-91, 1976.

Heninger, G. and Speck, L. Visual evoked responses and mental status of schizophrenics. Arch. Gen. Psychiatry, 15:419-426, 1966.

Ikuta, T. Somatosensory evoked potentials (SEP) in normal subjects, schizophrenics and epileptics. Fukuoka Acta Medica, 65: 1010-1019, 1974.

Ingvar, D. H. and Franzèn, G. Distribution of cerebral activ- ity in chronic schizophrenia. Lancet, ii:1484, 1974.

Ishikawa, K. Studies on the visual evoked responses to paired light flashes in schizophrenics. Kurume Medical Journal, 15:153- 167, 1968.

Jones, R. T. and Callaway, E. Auditory evoked responses in schizophrenia. A reassessment. Biol. Psychiatry, 2:291-298, 1970.

Landau, S. G., Buchsbaum, M. S., Carpenter, W., Strauss, J. and Sacks, M.  Schizophrenia and stimulus intensity control.  Arch. Gen. Psychiatry, 32:1239-1245, 1975.

Levit, A. L., Sutton, S. and Zubin, J.  Evoked potential correlates of information processing in psychiatric patients. Psychol. Med., 3:487-494, 1973.

Levy, R., Isaacs, A. and Behrman, J.  Neurophysiological correlates of senile dementia:  II. The somatosensory evoked response.  Psychol. Med., 1:159-165, 1971.

Lifshitz, K.  An examination of evoked potentials as indicators of information processing in normal and schizophrenic subjects. In:  E. Donchin and D.  B. Lindsley (Eds.)  Average Evoked Potentials:  Methods, Results and Evaluations.  National Aeronautics and Space Administration, Washington, D.C., 1969.  pp. 318-319 and 357-362.

Malerstein, A. J. and Callaway, E.  Two-tone average responses in Korsakoff patients.  J. Psychiat.Res., 6:253-260, 1969.

Ornitz, E. M. and Ritvo, E. R.  Neurophysiologic mechanisms underlying perceptual inconstancy in autistic and schizophrenic children.  Arch Gen. Psychiatry, 19:22-27, 1968.

Perris, C.  Averaged evoked responses (AER) in patients with affective disorders.  Acta Psychiat. Scand., 1974 suppl., pp.89-98.

Perris, C.  EEG techniques in the measurement of the severity of depressive syndromes.  Neuropsychobiology, 1:16-25, 1975.

Petrie, A.  Individuality in Pain and Suffering.  University of Chicago Press, 1967.

Rappaport, M., Hopkins, H. K., Hall, K., Belleza, T. and Hall, R. A.  Schizophrenia and evoked potentials:  Maximum amplitude, frequency of peaks, variability, and phenothiazine effects. Psychophysiology, 12:196-207, 1975.

Rodin, E., Grisell, J. and Gottlieb, J.  Some electrographic differences between chronic schizophrenic patients and normal subjects.  In:  J. Wortis (Ed.)  Recent Advances in Biological Psychiatry, Vol. X.  Plenum Press, New York, 1968.  pp. 194-204.

Roth, W. T. and Cannon, E. H.  Some features of the auditory evoked response in schizophrenics.  Arch. Gen. Psychiatry, 27:466-471, 1972.

Saletu, B., Itil, T. M. and Saletu, M.  Auditory evoked

response, EEG, and thought process in schizophrenics.  Amer. J. Psychiatry, 128:336-344, 1971.

Saletu, B., Saletu, M. and Itil, T. M.  The relationships between psychopathology and evoked responses before, during and after psychotropic drug treatment.  Biol. Psychiatry, 6:45-74, 1973.

Satterfield, J. H.  Auditory evoked cortical response studies in depressed patients and normal control subjects.  In.  T. A. Williams, M. M. Katz and J. A. Shields, Jr. (Eds.)  Recent Advances in the Psychobiology of the Depressive Illnesses.  U. S. Government Printing Office, DHEW Publication No. (HSM) 70-9053, 1972. pp. 87-98.

Schooler, C., Buchsbaum, M. and Carpenter, W. T.  Evoked response and kinesthetic measures of augmenting-reducing in schizophrenics:  Replications and extensions.  J. Nerv. Ment. Dis., 163: 221-232, 1976.

Shagass, C.  Averaged somatosensory evoked responses in various psychiatric disorders.  In:  J. Wortis (Ed.)  Recent Advances in Biological Psychiatry, Vol. X.  Plenum Press, New York, 1968. pp. 205-219.

Shagass, C.  Evoked Brain Potentials in Psychiatry.  Plenum Press, New York, 1972.

Shagass, C.  Effects of psychotropic drugs on human evoked potentials.  In:  T. Itil (Ed.)  Psychotropic Drugs and the Human EEG.  S. Karger, Basel, 1974.  pp. 238-257.

Shagass, C.  EEG and evoked potentials in the psychoses.  In: D. X. Freedman (Ed.)  Biology of the Major Psychoses.  A Comparative Analysis.  Raven Press, New York, 1975.  pp. 101-127.

Shagass, C.  An electrophysiological view of schizophrenia. Biol. Psychiatry, 11:3-30, 1976.

Shagass, C., Overton, D. A. and Straumanis, J. J.  Evoked potential studies in schizophrenia.  In:  H. Mitsuda and T. Fukuda (Eds.)  Biological Mechanisms of Schizophrenia and Schizophrenia-like Psychoses.  Igaku-Shoin Co., Ltd., Tokyo, 1974a.  pp. 214-234.

Shagass, C., Roemer, R. A., Straumanis, J. J. and Amadeo, M. Evoked potential correlates of psychosis.  Presented at annual meeting of Society of Biological Psychiatry, Toronto, Canada, 1977b.

Shagass, C. and Schwartz, M.  Reactivity cycle of somatosensory cortex in humans with and without psychiatric disorder. Science, 134:1757-1759, 1961.

Shagass, C. and Schwartz, M.  Cerebral cortical reactivity in psychotic depressions.  Arch. Gen. Psychiatry, 6:235-242, 1962.

Shagass, C. and Schwartz, M.  Psychiatric disorder and deviant cerebral responsiveness to sensory stimulation.  In:  J. Wortis (Ed.) Recent Advances in Biological Psychiatry, Vol. V.  Plenum Press, New York, 1963a.  pp. 321-330.

Shagass, C. and Schwartz, M.  Psychiatric correlates of evoked cerebral cortical potentials.  Amer. J. Psychiatry, 119: 1055-1061, 1963b.

Shagass, C. and Schwartz, M.  Visual cerebral evoked response characteristics in a psychiatric population.  Amer. J. Psychiatry, 121:979-987, 1965.

Shagass, C. and Schwartz, M.  Somatosensory cerebral evoked responses in psychotic depression.  Brit. J. Psychiatry, 112:799-807, 1966.

Shagass, C., Schwartz, M. and Amadeo, M.  Some drug effects on evoked cerebral potentials in man.  J. Neuropsychiatry, 3:S49-S58, 1962.

Shagass, C., Soskis, D.A., Straumanis, J.J. and Overton, D.A. Symptom patterns related to somatosensory evoked response differences within a schizophrenic population.  Biol. Psychiatry, 9:25-43, 1974b.

Shagass, C., Straumanis, J.J. and Overton, D.A.  Psychiatric diagnosis and EEG-evoked response relationships.  Neuropsychobiology, 1:1-15, 1975.

Shagass, C., Straumanis, J.J., Jr., Roemer, R.A. and Amadeo, M.  Evoked potentials of schizophrenics in several sensory modalities.  Biol. Psychiatry, 12:221-235, 1977a.

Speck, L. B., Dim, B. and Mercer, M.  Visual evoked responses of psychiatric patients.  Arch Gen. Psychiatry, 15:59-63, 1966.

Spitzer, R.L., Endicott, J., Cohen, J. and Fleiss, J.L. Constraints on the validity of computer diagnosis.  Arch. Gen. Psychiatry, 31:197-203, 1974.

Stevens, J.R.  An  anatomy of schizophrenia?  Arch. Gen. Psychiatry, 29:177-189, 1973.

Straumanis, J.J.  Somatosensory and visual cerebral evoked response changes associated with chronic brain syndrome and aging. Unpublished M.S. thesis in Psychiatry, Univ. of Iowa, 1964.

Straumanis, J., Shagass, C. and Schwartz, M.  Visually evoked cerebral response changes associated with chronic brain syndrome and aging.  J. Gerontology, 20:498-506, 1965.

Vasconetto, C., Floris, V. and Morocutti, C.  Visual evoked responses in normal and psychiatric subjects.  Electroenceph. clin. Neurophysiol., 31:77-83, 1971.

Visser, S.L., Stam, F.C., van Tilburg, W., op den Vedle, W., Blom, J.L. and deRijke, W.  Visual evoked response in senile and presenile dementia.  Electroenceph. clin. Neurophysiol., 40:385-392, 1976.

von Knorring, L., Espvall, M. and Perris, C.  Average evoked responses, pain measures, and personality variables in patients with depressive disorders.  Acta Psychiat. Scand., 1974 suppl. 255, pp. 99-108.

Wasman, M. and Gluck, H.  Recovery functions of somatosensory evoked responses in slow learners.  Psychophysiology, 12:371-376, 1975.

## ACKNOWLEDGEMENTS

Author's research supported (in part) by a grant, MH12507, from the U. S. Public Health Service.  Professional collaborators in the research are Drs. M. Amadeo, D.A. Overton, R.A. Roemer, J.J. Straumanis.  Thanks are due to I.C. Hung, A. McLean, T. McLean, J. Pressman, W. Nixon, and S. Slepner for computer, engineering, and technical assistance.

# LATE EVENT-RELATED POTENTIALS AND SCHIZOPHRENIA

Walton T. Roth
Thomas B. Horvath
Adolf Pfefferbaum
Jared R. Tinklenberg
Juan Mezzich
Bert S. Kopell

Department of Psychiatry and Behavioral Sciences
Stanford University School of Medicine
Stanford, California
and
Veterans Administration Hospital
Palo Alto, California

Event-related potential (ERP) correlates of schizophrenia have recently been reviewed in a series of articles in the Schizophrenia Bulletin [Buchsbaum, 1977; Roth, 1977; Shagass, 1977]. Differences between patients and controls have been found for ERP components of various latencies and topographic distribution although generally only single ERP paradigms have been applied at one time. This paper reports the results of a pilot study designed to investigate schizophrenic patients in a multiple ERP paradigm design. We tested subjects on three paradigms, each of which emphasized different late ERPs. Components with latencies over 50 msec are generally more sensitive than earlier components to psychological variables, such as attention and expectancy, and for that reason might be more sensitive to psychological alterations commonly reported in schizophrenia. By eliciting different ERP components in the same subjects we hoped to get an idea of the relative sensitivity of these components to schizophrenic illness.

The first paradigm elicited a contingent negative variation (CNV) and allowed measurement of CNV amplitude, CNV return to baseline

NOTE: This work was supported by the Veterans Administration. The authors wish to thank M.J. Rosenbloom, P.L. Krainz, C.M. Doyle, P.A. Berger and his staff, J.P. Tubbs, and E. Courchesne who helped in various phases of this project.

or resolution, and reaction time.  Reduction in CNV amplitude has
often been reported for schizophrenics [Abraham, 1973; Abraham et
al., 1976; McCallum & Abraham, 1973; Timsit-Berthier et al., 1973]
and in some cases schizophrenics show an amplitude reduction of as
much as 50% [McCallum & Abraham, 1973].  In addition, there have
been several reports of slower CNV resolution in schizophrenics
(e.g., Dubrovsky & Dongier, 1976; Timsit-Berthier, 1973].

The second paradigm elicited auditory ERPs with negative (N1)
and positive (P2) components to stimuli at three interstimulus
intervals (ISI).   The relationship of the ERP amplitude and ISI can
be expressed as a temporal recovery function.  Recovery of ERP components earlier than N1 and P2 has been shown to differ in psychiatric
populations for somatosensory stimuli [e.g., Shagass, 1972] and
visual stimuli [Floris et al., 1968;  Speck et al., 1966].  Recovery
of N1 and P2 components of the auditory ERP in depressed patients
has been studied by Satterfield [1972].  In schizophrenic patients
one might expect impaired temporal recovery in the auditory modality
since such patients often experience hallucinatory stimuli which
might act in the same way as exogenous stimuli and decrease the
effective ISI.

The third paradigm presented unpredictable and infrequently
occurring stimuli which elicit a late positive wave (LPW).  Such
waves have been found to be significantly attenuated in schizophrenic patients [Levit et al., 1973;  Roth & Cannon, 1972;
Shagass et al., 1977].

METHODS

Subjects

Male patients were recruited from the Psychiatry Service of the
Palo Alto Veterans Administration Hospital.  A project psychiatrist
selected candidates who met the diagnostic criteria for schizophrenia
established by Spitzer et al. [1975].  These criteria were designed
to screen out borderline conditions, brief hysterical or situational
psychoses, and paranoid states.  The study was described to the
patient, and his informed consent was obtained.  After initial
screening, a thorough clinical assessment of the patient was made
using the Present State Examination [Wing et al., 1974];  Within 24
hours of the time of testing, the subject was rated on a modified
version of the Brief Psychiatric Rating Scale [Overall & Gorham,
1962].  On the basis of these assessments, each patient was classified as paranoid or undifferentiated and hallucinatory or non-hallucinatory.   Patients were considered hallucinatory if they had
reported hallucinations within a month of testing.  Descriptive
information regarding the 25 patients used in the study is summarized

Table 1

Description of subjects

Schizophrenics: (n = 25)        Male        Age:  24-46 (mean = 32.4)

Research classifications

|  |  |  |  |
|---|---|---|---|
| Paranoid | 13 | Undifferentiated | 12 |
| Hallucinatory | 14 | Non-hallucinatory | 11 |
| Medicated | 15 | Drug-free | 10 |

(mean chlorpromazine
equivalent dose = 761.3 mg)

Controls:        (n = 20)        Male        Age:  25-52 (mean = 33.6)

in Table 1.    The large proportion of drug-free patients was a
result of referrals from a research ward where medication was
withheld in connection with biochemical studies.

Controls were men of approximately the same ages as the
patients.  They were recruited from the local office of the State
Employment Development Agency, and were screened to exclude those
with a history of or current symptoms of psychopathology.  This
decision was made on the basis of the Symptom Check List [Derogatis
et al., 1973], rated for the last year period and on the basis of
an interview by a psychiatrist.  Controls were also scored on the
modified Brief Psychiatric Rating Scale before testing.    Two of 22
controls subjects interviewed were rejected.

General Procedures

Subjects were tested in a sound-attenuated electrically shielded
booth.   The three paradigms described below were given over 1½ to 2
hours.   Between runs, subjects received various cognitive tests.

The EEG was recorded with subdermal pin electrodes from Fz, Cz,
and Pz referred to linked disc electrodes attached to the earlobes.
The EOG was recorded from disc electrodes 3 cm above and 2.5 cm below
the right eye.  Pin electrodes had a resistance below 100 kilohms,
and disc electrode resistance was below 5 kilohms.  For the Recovery
Function and Unexpected Stimulus Paradigms, amplifiers were set to
a bandpass of 0.03 to 100 c/sec (3 dB points of 6 dB octave rolloff
curves).    For the CNV paradigm, the amplifiers were set to have the
same high frequency response and a time constant of 10 sec.    Amplifiers were AC coupled for all paradigms and had an input impedance

of 100 megohms.  The use of pin electrodes on the scalp minimizes
the possibility of electrodermal artifacts in the EEG signal [Corby
et al., 1974] without a loss of low frequency response in amplifiers
of adequate input impedance [Cooper, 1976].

Each subject performed a series of eye movement maneuvers prior
to stimulus presentation that allow estimation of the contribution
of both blink and shift of gaze artifacts at the various EEG leads
[Roth, 1973].  Subjects were told to keep their eyes open during
stimulus presentation.

Auditory stimuli were tone pips shaped to have a rise and fall
time of 2.5 msec and were given binaurally through earphones.
Visual stimuli in the CNV paradigm were presented binocularly
through a tachistoscope.

## CNV Paradigm

The CNV paradigm was a simple reaction time (RT) paradigm in
which a warning tone (S1) was followed 1 sec later by a series of
light flashes (S2) to which the subjects pressed a button as quickly
as possible.  This button was such that a 670 gm weight would close
the circuit after a 2.4 mm depression.  S1 was a 50 msec 1000 c/sec
65 dB tone pip.  S2 was a square of light with a $1.4°$ visual arc and
a brightness of 1.3 log foot lamberts.  The square flashed on and
off at 100 msec intervals until the button was pressed.  A dim star-
shaped pattern was illuminated throughout the run and served as a
fixation point which the subject was told to watch.   Inter-trial
intervals ranged randomly from 33 to 58 sec.  A total of 20 trials
were given over the 15 min run.  The 1 sec S1-S2 interval was chosen
as the one used by McCallum & Abraham [1973], and the long inter-
trial intervals followed the work of Timsit-Berthier [1973].  These
inter-trial intervals would presumably allow time for CNV resolution
to be complete by the time a new trial began.

Much care was taken to exclude any artifacts that might influence
the results.  First, individual trials were edited on the basis of
a computer display of the 5500 msec of EEG and EOG from each trial.
Those trials in which any of the EEG leads were contaminated by slow
eye movement artifact, amplifier blocking, or noise due to muscle or
body movement artifact were rejected.  In addition, any trials in
which the RT was less than 5 msec or greater than 5500 msec were
excluded.  Subjects for whom less than 7 trials remained after this
editing were excluded from further analysis.  In this way, 6 patients
and 2 controls were excluded.  For the remaining subjects, the mean
number of usable trials was 11.8 among the controls and 11.2 among
the patients.  These trials were used to create ERP averages.
Second, eye blink artifacts were removed by subtracting fractions of

the EOG lead from each EEG lead.    The fraction differed for each subject and lead, and was based on eye blinks during the eye maneuvers performed previously.  The use of eye blink fractions was necessary because blinks and vertical eye movements contributed differently to the EEG [Corby & Kopell, 1972].   The procedure of rejecting eye-blink contaminated trials was not feasible for our data, because the number of trials in which no blink occurred within 5.5 sec of S1 was too small for adequate averaging.

The CNV and its resolution were measured in terms of the difference between a baseline derived from mean voltage 40 msec prior to S1 onset and the mean voltages in the following latency ranges: 800-1000 msec post S1 (CNV);   350-1500 msec post S2 (Resolution 1); 1500-3500 msec post S2 (Resolution 2);   and 3500-5500 msec post S2 (Resolution 3).

## Recovery Function Paradigm

This paradigm was a shorter version of one that we had studied previously in normal subjects [Roth et al., 1976b].    The 4 min stimulus sequence consisted of 156 tone pips (50 msec, 65 dB SPL, 1000 Hz) occurring in a pseudorandom sequence with ISI of 0.75, 1.5, and 3.0 sec.  Subjects were told that they would hear a sequence of tones, but that they should not pay any special attention to them.

Three separate stimulus-synchronized averages for stimuli preceded by different ISI were computed for each lead.  One patient was excluded from further data analysis because of gross muscle artifact, but the data from the other subjects were adequate.  Averages of the EOG leads were quite flat.  A peak measurement program calculated the latency of the minimum voltage between 50 and 150 msec (N1), and the maximum voltage between N1 and 250 msec (P2).  N1 and P2 amplitudes were calculated as the difference between these peak voltages and a baseline derived from mean voltage 20 msec prior to stimulus onset.

## Unexpected Stimulus Paradigm

This paradigm was based on one we have studied in normal subjects [Roth et al., 1976a].  Background tones, 50 msec long, 65 dB SPL, and 800 c/sec, were delivered at a rate of 1/sec.  At random intervals, the sequence was interrupted by substituting a 1 sec 80 dB chord consisting of 800 c/sec and 1200 c/sec tones.  Half of the chords, randomly selected, were preceded by a warning tone identical to the background tones in duration, intensity, and timing, but higher in pitch (1200 c/sec).  A total of 60 chords occurred in the sequence, of which 30 were preceded by a warning tone.  The proportion of stimulus types was such that the probability of the warning tone and the unwarned chord were both 0.1.  Thus, the background tones

and the warned chords were probable expected events, while the
warning tone and the unwarned chords were improbable and unexpected
events. Subjects were told that they would hear a sequence of
different kinds of tones, but that they should not pay any particular attention to them.

Averages were calculated for warning tones, background tones
preceding chords, warned chords, and unwarned chords. The presence
of eye-blink artifact in the EEG leads made it necessary to apply
the same subtraction procedure that was used for the CNV paradigm
data. Five of the patients were excluded because of technical
difficulties or artifacts other than eye blinks. A number of waves
appear in the various averages, but here we will only be concerned
with the LPW to the two types of improbable events. In order to
conform with previous studies, this LPW was measured in two ways:
a wide latency measurement as in Roth & Cannon [1972], which we will
refer to simply as P3, and a narrower later measurement based on
the work of N. Squires et al.[1975], which they have called P3b.
P3 is defined as the maximum voltage between 200 and 422 msec, and
P3b as the maximum between 280 and 422. Amplitudes of these peaks
were calculated as the difference between peak voltage and a baseline
derived from mean voltage 80 msec prior to the eliciting stimulus.

These three paradigms were given to the subjects in the following order so that ERPs more susceptible to habituation were elicited
first: Unexpected Stimulus, Recovery Function, and CNV.


Statistical Analysis

Event-related potential measures from each paradigm were subjected to analysis of variance. Factors in the analysis were group
(schizophrenic or control) and lead (Fz, Cz, and Pz). For the Recovery Function paradigm ERPs, ISI (0.75 sec, 1.5 sec, and 3 sec)
was also a factor. Additional analysis was performed on data for
schizophrenics to determine differences between three dichotomous
classifications within the schizophrenic group: paranoid vs. undifferentiated; hallucinatory vs. non-hallucinatory; medicated vs.
drug-free (patients were considered drug-free if they had not taken
anti-psychotic medication in the last 14 days and no sedatives in
the last 7 days). These three dichotomies were relatively independent. The coefficient of association between paranoid-undifferentiated and hallucinatory-non-hallucinatory was 0.22 (p >.1);
between hallucinatory-non-hallucinatory and medicated-non-medicated
was 0.22 (p >.1), and between paranoid-undifferentiated and medicated-
non-medicated was 0.29 (p >.1).

Product moment correlations were calculated for the schizo-
phenic group between certain ERP measures and drug dose, age, and 3
measures of thought process disorder. One of the thought disorder

measures was derived from the Brief Psychiatric Rating Scale and the others were the Intensity and Consistency scores on the Bannister-Fransella Grid Test of Psychiatric Disorder [Bannister & Fransella, 1967] which was administered to subjects following ERP testing.  Anti-psychotic drug dose was expressed in terms of equivalent chlorpromazine dose according to the table of Davis [1974]. A product moment correlation was also calculated separately for the control group between RT and CNV measures.

ERP measures chosen to be both representative and uncontaminated by other components were selected from each paradigm for the correlations.  (1) CNV paradigm:  CNV and CNV resolution measures from the Cz lead were used.  (2) Recovery Function paradigm:  the slope of N1 amplitude (collapsed over leads) vs. ISI, N1 and P2 amplitudes (collapsed over leads and intervals), and N1 and P2 latency (collapsed over intervals from the Cz lead only) were used.  (3) Unexpected Stimulus paradigm:  P3 and P3a amplitude and latency from Cz lead were used.

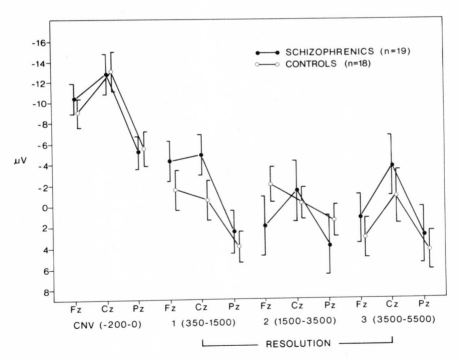

Figure 1:  Means and standard errors of CNV and CNV resolution measurements for schizophrenics and controls.

Table 2

RT and ERP correlations in the CNV paradigm

| | | CNV | RESOLUTION 1 | RESOLUTION 2 | RESOLUTION 3 |
|---|---|---|---|---|---|
| RT | C | .11 | .16 | .17 | .27 |
| | S | -.77+ | -.74+ | -.50* | -.32 |
| CNV | C | | .74 | .60 | .62 |
| | S | | .60 | .40 | .41 |
| RESOLUTION 1 | C | | | .68** | .70+ |
| | S | | | .78+ | .51* |
| RESOLUTION 2 | C | | | | .89+ |
| | S | | | | .83+ |

C = control     Significance levels:    *   p <.05

                                                **   p <.01

S = schizophrenic                             +   p <.001

## RESULTS

### CNV Paradigm

    Figure 1 shows the means and standard errors of the ERP measures for the schizophrenics and controls. Mean CNV amplitudes for each group are almost identical. Mean CNV resolutions at Cz for each post S2 epoch are greater for controls than for schizophrenics, although these differences did not reach statistical significance due to the large degree of variability in each group. Among schizophrenics, there was a group × lead interaction for the hallucinatory-non-hallucinatory dichotomy, indicating that patients with hallucinations had smaller CNVs than patients without hallucinations at Cz and Pz leads. Table 2 lists correlations between RT and ERP variables for schizophrenics, indicating that schizophrenics with shorter RTs had larger CNVs, but there were no correlations for controls. There were

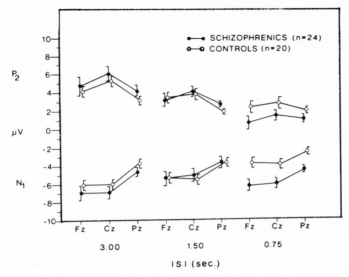

Figure 2: Means and standard errors of N1 and P2 amplitude in the Recovery Function Paradigm for schizophrenics and controls.

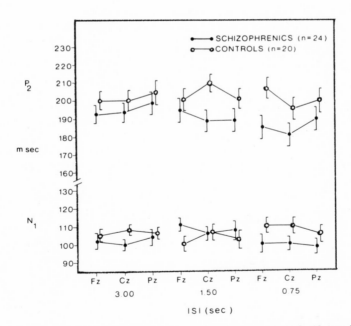

Figure 3: Means and standard errors of N1 and P2 latencies in the Recovery Function Paradigm for schizophrenics and controls.

a number of significant correlations between CNV amplitude and CNV resolution variables for both groups. While RTs were larger and more variable for schizophrenics (mean 528 ± 392) than for controls (mean 355 ± 169), this difference did not reach statistical significance (t = 1.83, p >.05). Among the schizophrenic subgroups, mean RTs and standard deviations were as follows: paranoid 423 ± 202, undifferentiated 642 ± 509; hallucinators 599 ± 447, non-hallucinators 427 ± 276; medicated 416 ± 330, drug-free 649 ± 476.

## Recovery Function Paradigm

Figure 2 shows the mean and standard errors of N1 and P2 amplitudes and Figure 3 the means and standard errors of N1 and P2 latency for schizophrenics and controls. Amplitude differences were insignificant, while P2 latency is shorter for schizophrenics than for controls (p <.05). Within the schizophrenic groups, N1 amplitude showed a medication group × interval interaction (p <.05). At a 3 sec interval, N1 was larger for medicated than for drug-free patients. P2 amplitude showed a diagnostic group × interval × lead interaction (p <.05) that was apparently due to smaller amplitudes at Fz and Cz for a 3 sec interval for paranoids. Although amplitudes were not different between hallucinators and non-hallucinators, there were latency differences. Hallucinators had shorter N1 latencies than non-hallucinators (p <.05). Hallucinators had shorter P2 latencies for all intervals at Cz and for the 0.75 and 3.0 sec in intervals at Fz and Pz (group × interval × lead interaction : p <.01).

Three significant correlations emerged from this paradigm. N1 latency and age had a correlation of -.45 (p <.05). This negative correlation is contrary to findings of stable auditory peak latencies from adolescence to old age [Schenkenberg, 1970], so it is relevant to note that in our sample hallucinators (who had shorter latencies) were slightly older (35.9 ± 7.4) than non-hallucinators (28.2 ± 6.6). Drug dose and N1 slope had a correlation of -0.49 (p <.05), which is consistent with the analysis of variance results for medicated and drug-free patients. In addition, N1 amplitude and P2 latency had a correlation of -.48 (p <.05).

## Unexpected Stimulus Paradigm

Figure 4 shows the means and standard errors of P3b amplitude and latency for the schizophrenics and controls. Because of the large standard errors in both groups, the considerable differences in mean P3b amplitude were not significant. The latency of P3b to the warning tone was longer for schizophrenics than for controls (p <.01). The broader latency P3 measure did not show significant amplitude or latency effects. Mean P3 latencies were about 40 msec less than mean P3b latencies. It is possible that the P3 latency range overlaps with P2 latencies and the peak location program was selecting

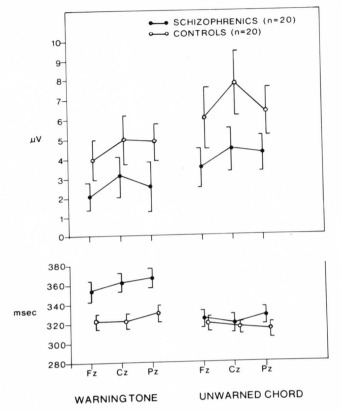

Figure 4: Means and standard errors of the amplitude of P3b to the warning tone and to the unwarned chord for schizophrenics and controls.

P2s instead of the late positive wave associated with unexpected stimuli. Probably the P3 measure is less valid as a measure of that late positive wave than is P3b. Within the schizophrenic group there were no significant differences between any pair of the three dichotomous classifications. There was, however, a tendency for medicated schizophrenics to have larger P3s to the unwarned chord than drug-free schizophrenics.

Correlations were high between P3 and P3b amplitude measures (.47 to .89) but were much lower for latency measures (.03 to .43). The amplitude of P3 to the chord and the Brief Psychiatric Rating Scale thought disorder score had a correlation of -.54 (p <.05), but for P3b amplitude this correlation (-.34) was not significant. Neither P3 nor P3b correlated significantly with either of the Bannister-Fransella grid scores. Although these grid score correlated highly with each other (.67), they had insignificant negative correlations (-.38 and -.39) with the Brief Psychiatric Rating Scale thought disorder score.

## DISCUSSION

This pilot study enabled us to focus on several issues in ERP studies of schizophrenia. While the failure to replicate some earlier findings was disappointing, the study did provide some evidence of the psychophysiological manifestations of schizophrenia. A marked feature of our data was high individual variability. Some of this variability probably stems from individual differences which have nothing to do with psychological states or traits, but come from anatomical variations in the geometry of brain structures and skull thicknesses. Such variability poses less of a problem in experimental designs where ERPs are compared within a subject under various conditions than in designs where one group of subjects is compared with another. Another source of variability is uncontrolled differences in psychological state during testing that are nonspecific to schizophrenia or normalcy. For example, in paradigms which make no task requirements, subjects have freedom to pass the time as they desire. Some may listen to the stimulus sounds to detect patterns, while others may ignore them and be preoccupied with other thoughts. Passive paradigms have been favored because they capitalize on the capacity of the ERP technique to assess even nonverbal uncooperative subjects and also assess individual differences in the non-task-involved or "idling" brain [Callaway, 1975; see, for example, the discussion on pp 62 and 138], but these advantages are obtained at the cost of increased variability to which between-subject designs are particularly vulnerable.

These nonspecific sources of variability affect all ERP studies. ERP studies of schizophrenia are additionally vulnerable to the wide range of symptom type and symptom severity included within even stringent diagnostic criteria of schizophrenia. In our study, we attempted to investigate this intra-group variability by dichotomizing our group of schizophrenic patients along three variables (paranoid-non-paranoid; hallucinatory-non-hallucinatory; medicated-drug-free). The size of our pilot patient sample, however, was inadequate to fully exploit intra-group variability and future studies will employ larger samples and more specific internal subgroupings.

Several earlier studies have reported reduced CNV amplitudes and delayed CNV resolution in schizophrenic patients,and a start has been made in relating CNV differences to symptom differences [McCallum & Abraham , 1973]. The CNV is basically a reaction time task, and alterations in RT behavior have long been observed in schizophrenics. It is unfortunate that few ERP investigators have

reported the RTs of patients engaged in CNV tasks.  In our study,
we found that although mean RT tended to be slower and more variable
among schizophrenics than controls (the expected findings), mean CNV
amplitude was virtually identical in the two groups (an unexpected
finding).  We also found that among schizophrenics there was an
association between RT and CNV amplitude such that patients with
longer RTs had smaller CNVs.  Among the controls, on the other hand,
we found a lack of correlation between CNV and RT;  this lack of
association has been reported by other investigators [Näätänen &
Gaillard, 1974;  Rebert & Tecce, 1973].  Our failure to replicate
earlier findings of reduced CNV amplitude in schizophrenics could be
due to a number of factors including differences in diagnostic
criteria for selection of schizophrenic patients, standards for
exclusion of trials contaminated by artifacts produced by eye and
body movement, and the instability of CNVs derived from a small
number of trials selected from a 15 min recording session.  In our
study, CNV resolution correlated with RT among the schizophrenics;
it also generally tended to be slower for schizophrenics than
controls, corroborating earlier reports [Timsit-Berthier, 1973].
We found this CNV resolution to be highly correlated with CNV amplitudes, as has Abraham [personal communication, 1976].  Perhaps it is
in the relationship between CNV amplitude, CNV resolution, and RT
that more satisfactory group discriminators can be discovered.  Many
technical difficulties, however, lie in the path of researchers using
CNV paradigms requiring long averaging epochs.  When averaging epochs
last more than 5 sec, restless schizophrenic patients render many
trials unusable due to artifacts and blocking of amplifiers that
occurs after high amplitude EMG signals.  We are not the only investigators who have encountered this problem.  Dongier et al. [1977]
reported that from a similar paradigm 53% of patient recordings and
23% of control recordings were unusable.

Our hypothesis that hallucinations would result in smaller N1s
and P2s in the Recovery Function Paradigm was not sustained.  Either
endogenous hallucinatory stimulation does not take place at the
neurological level represented by the auditory recovery function, or
our criterion of hallucinations within the past month was too coarse.
Ideally, one should compare patients who were hallucinating during
the recording session with those who were not, but in our series few
patients were able to report the timing of their hallucinations very
precisely, and inference of hallucinations from the patients' behavior
seemed unreliable.  The relationship between hallucinations and CNV
amplitude is not strong enough to be conclusive although it is in
line with the report of Abraham [1973], who found lower CNVs in
patients who hallucinate even though there was no evidence of their
experiencing hallucations during the recording session.

Latency differences found between schizophrenics and controls
in the Recovery Function Paradigm are consistent with the thesis
that schizophrenics, particularly those who hallucinate, pay less

attention to external task-irrelevant stimuli.   Earlier we found
that, in normals, P2 latencies are shorter when subjects are engrossed
in a book than when they must pay attention to auditory stimuli
[Roth et al., 1976b].   Shorter N1-P2 latencies in schizophrenics
have also been reported by Saletu et al. [1973].   Similarly, the
later P3b to the warning tone in the Unexpected Stimulus Paradigm
could be a consequence of less stimulus processing.   Unexpected
stimuli elicit LPWs of longer latency when such stimuli are less
confidently or less easily detected [Ford et al., 1976; Squires,
K.C., et al., 1973].   Perhaps the reason that this effect did not
appear for the unwarned chord was that the loud 85 dB chord was
always quickly detected whereas the 65 dB warning tone was more like
the background tones and was noticed later by the schizophrenics who
were less engaged in stimulus processing.

      Inter-subject variability apparently prevented the mean group
differences observed for P3 amplitudes in the Unexpected Stimulus
Paradigm from attaining statistical significance.   The differences
were in the expected direction, however, providing additional ERP
evidence that schizophrenics pay less attention to task-irrelevant
stimuli than normal subjects.

      Some of the advantages and disadvantages of studying late rather
than early ERPs in pathological groups are manifest in this study.
The chief disadvantage of late ERPs is that they can be sensitive to
psychological variables that are unlikely to be basic to psychiatric
diagnostic categories.   For example, inattention to task-irrelevant
stimuli might be found in a schizophrenic attending to internal
voices,   in a neurotic compulsively preoccupied about personal
problems, or in a control subject fighting to stay awake in the
testing booth.

      The chief advantage of late ERPs is that they have been rather
thoroughly studied by psychologically-oriented investigators who
have elucidated many of the parameters that determine their amplitudes
and latencies.   Thus, group differences are less likely to be
erroneously interpreted as a basic neurophysiological aberration
when attentional differences are the real explanation.   In this way,
we can hope to avoid some of the less profitable detours on the path
to understanding of mental disease.


                              REFERENCES

Abraham, P.  An approach to standardizing clinical assessments in
     CNV studies of psychiatric patients.  Proceedings of the INSERM
     Colloquium on Average Evoked Responses and Conditioning in Normal
     Subjects and Psychiatric Patients.   Paris:  Editions INSERM, 1973,
     394-404.

Abraham, P., McCallum, W.C., & Gourlay, J.    The CNV and its relation
    to specific psychiatric syndromes.    In W.C. McCallum & J.R. Knott
    (Eds.), The Responsive Brain.    Bristol:  John Wright, 1976,
    144-149.

Bannister, D., & Fransella, F.    A grid test of thought disorder:
    A standard clinical test.  Barnstaple:  Psychological Test
    Publications, 1967.

Buchsbaum, M.    The middle evoked response components in schizo-
    phrenia.    Schiz. Bull., 1977, 3, 93-104.

Callaway, E.    Brain electrical potentials and individual psycho-
    logical differences.  New York:  Grune & Stratton, 1975.

Cooper, R.    Chairman's Opening remarks on present state of methodo-
    logy of slow potential changes.    In W.C. McCallum & J.R. Knott
    (Eds.), The Responsive Brain.    Bristol:  John Wright, 1976, 1-4.

Corby, J.C., & Kopell, B.S.    Differential contributions of blinks
    and vertical eye movements as artifacts in EEG recording.
    Psychophysiology, 1972, 9, 640-644.

Corby, J.C., Roth, W.T., and Kopell, B.S.    Prevalence and methods
    of control of the cephalic skin potential EEG artifact.
    Psychophysiology, 1974, 11, 350-360.

Davis, J.M.    Dose equivalence of the anti-psychotic drugs.    J.
    Psychiat. Res., 1974, 11, 65-69.

Derogatis, L.R., Lipman, R.S., & Covi, L.    SCL-90:  An outpatient
    psychiatric rating scale--preliminary report.    Psychopharmacol.
    Bull., 1973, 9, 13.

Dongier, M., Dubrovsky, B., & Engelsmann, F.    ERSP in psychiatry:
    Problems of methodology and symptom evaluation.    In D. Otto (Ed.),
    Multidisciplinary Perspectives in Event-Related Brain Potential
    Research.    Washington, DC:  US Government Printing Office,
    (in press, 1977).

Dubrovsky, B., & Dongier, M.    Evaluation of event-related potentials
    in selected groups of psychiatric patients.  In W.C. McCallum &
    J.R. Knott (Eds.), The Responsive Brain.    Bristol:  John Wright,
    1976, 150-153.

Floris, V., Morocutti, G., Amabile, G., Bernardi, G., & Rizzo, P. Recovery cycle of visual evoked potentials in normal, schizophrenic and neurotic patients. In N.S. Kline & E. Laska (Eds.), Computers and Electronic Devices in Psychiatry. New York: Grune & Stratton, 1968, 194-205.

Ford, J.M., Roth, W.T., & Kopell, B.S. Auditory evoked potentials to unpredictable shifts in pitch. Psychophysiology, 1976, 13, 32-39.

Levit, A.L., Sutton, S., & Zubin, J. Evoked potential correlates of information processing in psychiatric patients. Psychol. Med., 1973, 3, 487-494.

McCallum, W.C., & Abraham, P. The contingent negative variation in psychosis. Electroenceph. & clin. Neurophys., 1973, Supp. 33, 329-335.

Näätänen, R., & Gaillard, A.W. The relationship between the contingent negative variation and the reaction time under prolonged experimental conditions. Biol. Psychol., 1974, 1, 277-291.

Overall, J.E., & Gorham, D.R. The Brief Psychiatric Rating Scale Psychol. Rep., 1962, 10, 799-812.

Rebert, C.S., & Tecce, J.J. A summary of CNV and reaction time. Electroenceph. & clin. Neurophys., 1973, Supp. 33, 173-178.

Roth, W.T. Auditory evoked response to unpredictable stimuli. Psychophysiology, 1973, 10, 125-137.

Roth, W.T. Late event-related potentials and psychopathology. Schiz. Bull., 1977, 3, 105-120.

Roth, W.T., & Cannon, E.H. Some features of the auditory evoked response in schizophrenics. Arch. Gen. Psychiat., 1972, 27, 466-471.

Roth, W.T., Ford, J.M., Lewis, S.J., & Kopell, B.S. Effects of stimulus probability and task-relevance on event-related potentials. Psychophysiology, 1976a, 13, 311-317.

Roth, W.T., Krainz, P.L., Ford, J.M., Tinklenberg, J.R., Rothbart, R.M., & Kopell, B.S. Parameters of temporal recovery of the human auditory evoked potential. Electroenceph. & clin. Neurophys., 1976b, 40, 623-632.

Saletu, B., Saletu, M., & Itil, T.M. The relationship between psychopathology and evoked responses before, during and after psychiatric treatment. Biol. Psychiat., 1973, 6, 45-74.

Satterfield, J.   Auditory evoked cortical response studies in de-
    pressed patients and normal control subjects.   In T.A. Williams
    & M.M. Katz (Eds.), Recent Advances in the Psychobiology of the
    Depressive Illnesses.   Washington, DC:   US Government Printing
    Office, 1972.

Schenkenberg, T.   Visual, auditory and somatosensory evoked responses
    of normal subjects from childhood to senescence.   Unpublished
    doctoral dissertation.   University of Utah, Salt Lake City, 1970.

Shagass, C.   Evoked Brain Potentials in Psychiatry.   New York:
    Plenum Publishing, 1972.

Shagass, C.   Early evoked potentials.   Schiz. Bull., 1977, 3, 80-92.

Shagass, C., Straumanis, J.J., Roemer, R.A., & Amadeo, M.   Evoked
    potentials of schiophrenics in several sensory modalities.
    Biol. Psychiat., 1977 (in press).

Speck, L., Dim, B., & Mercer, M.   Visual evoked responses of psychi-
    atric patients.   Arch. Gen. Psychiat., 1966, 15, 59-63.

Spitzer, R.L., Endicott, J., & Robins, E.   Research diagnostic
    criteria (RDS) for a selected group of functional disorders.
    New York:   New York State Department of Mental Hygiene, 1975.

Squires, K.C., Hillyard, S.A., & Lindsay, P.H.   Vertex potentials
    evoked during auditory signal detection:   Relation to decision
    criteria.   Percept. & Psychophys., 1973, 14, 265-272.

Squires, N.K., Squires, K.C., & Hillyard, S.A.   Two varieties of
    long-latency positive waves evoked by unpredictable auditory
    stimuli in man.   Electroenceph. & clin. Neurophys., 1975, 38,
    387-401.

Timsit-Berthier, M.   Étude de la VCN, des potentiels lents évoqués
    et du Potentiel Moteur chez un groupe de sujets normaux et un
    groupe de malades psychiatriques.   [Study of the CNV, evoked slow
    potentials, and motor potential in a group of normal subjects and
    a group of psychiatric patients].   Proceedings of the INSERM
    Colloquium on Average Evoked Responses and their Conditioning in
    Normal Subjects and Psychiatric Patients. Tours, 1972.   Paris:
    Editions INSERM, 1973, 327-366.

Timsit-Berthier, M., Delaunoy, J., Koninckx, N., & Rousseau, J.C.
    Slow potential changes in psychiatry.   I. Contingent Negative
    Variation.   Electroenceph. & clin. Neurophysiol., 1973, 35, 355-361.

Wing, J.K., Cooper, J.E., & Sartorius, N.   The Measurement and
    Classification of Psychiatric Symptoms.   London:   Cambridge
    University Press, 1974.

# SCHIZOPHRENIA AND EVOKED POTENTIALS

Enoch Callaway, M.D.

Langley Porter Neuropsychiatric Institute
401 Parnassus Avenue
San Francisco, California 94143

For the purposes of discussion, let me suggest that we have been approaching the problem of evoked potentials in schizophrenia completely the wrong way around. I can say such an outrageous thing, because all of us on this section of the program are members of the same family in more ways than one. If we hold to the biblical injunction that only who is without sin should cast the first stone, then I would be paralyzed. However, there is a new and different way of looking at this matter. I am not responsible for this new viewpoint, and while I am afraid I cannot give exact citations as to its origins, I can give an outline of what seems a more appropriate approach.

To begin with, the search for correlations between diagnosis and evoked potentials (EP) is a very poor approach, not because the EP are weak, but because psychiatric diagnosis is such a shoddy thing. From this it follows that one should attempt to make classification on the basis of EP and then study these psychophysiologically defined subtypes. This might allow us to make more effective use of EP, and in addition, to clean up the mess that passes for a psychiatric nosology. To illustrate this, I first will offer an alternative model for schizophrenia and then suggest how EP defined classifications might be used to bring a new approach to the study of this syndrome.

For a long time, many of us had been studying correlations between EPs and schizophrenia. There have been some statistical successes, but by and large, it has been very disappointing. Some time back, for practical reasons, I began to look at healthy Navy recruits. We discovered that EPs could classify them according to their performance on standard pencil and paper IQ type tests. The correlations were not impressive, but encouraging; we could correctly classify about 64% if we used the upper one-third and lower one-third of Navy recruits ranked according to IQ. Of course, performance on an IQ test is not a much better criterion than the clinical diagnosis of schizophrenia, since so many different things can affect the outcome. We also looked at a group of low IQ recruits who could also not read at an acceptable level, and we attempted to predict their success in a remedial reading program. Here, we did a little better and batted about 68%. Most recently Greg Lewis and Bernie Rimland have used this same EP battery to predict the performance of selected radar school candidates on radar simulation tasks. Here, the ability of EP to classify the subjects was an even more impressive 80%. In other words, the more homogeneous our group and the better our behavioral criteria for classifying our groups, then the better the EPs seemed to perform.

In the meantime, other investigators were reporting similar findings. Roy John has been able to make very elegant discriminations between various subgroups. His most recent data on discriminating between various forms of learning disabilities are quite impressive. Peter Tanguay, in unpublished studies from UCLA, has equally impressive discrimination between diseidetic and disphonetic reading disability cases.

Can our data be trying to tell us something? If we listen carefully, I think we can hear them say that the EP can make excellent discriminations between well defined groups, so we should suspect that it is the psychiatric diagnoses that account for the poor EP/diagnostic correlations. Let us consider schizophrenia as a diagnosis in point. Looked at from an etiological standpoint, schizophrenia is a bizarre diagnosis. We know very well that phenomenologically we cannot distinguish between schizophrenia and a variety of organic diseases. If we have hypothyroidism, temporal epilepsy, porphuria, a black widow spider bite, amphetamine intoxication, pelagra, encephalitis, etc., we do not make the diagnosis of schizophrenia, although the symptoms may be indistinguishable from those of patients for whom a panel of blueribbon psychiatrists would find easy consensus in the diagnosis of schizophrenia.

Looked at from the standpoint of treatment, this situation is no more appetizing. Even excluding those cases that can be confidently expected to respond to things as diverse as thyroid, niacin or anti-inflamatory steroids, we are left with a bewildering array of responses and non-responses. Some schizophrenics respond to phenothiazines; others get well spontaneously; a few respond to lithium, and as a result may get rediagnosed as manics.

Instead of looking at schizophrenia as a disease in the more conventional sense, we can consider it as simply a syndrome of disregulation. This is not a novel idea, but it seems to be one that slips through the mental fingers rather easily. So, let me use the absurdly simple diagram in Figure 1 to try to pin it down. When a cognitive operation, labeled Process A, is in action, then this action is sensed by the Regulator which, in turn, tends to maintain Process A until it is completed, and in the meantime, the Regulator inhibits competing Process B. Matthysse has drawn an analogy between a cognitive regulator involving mesencephalic nuclei and nucleus acumbens and a motor regulator identified as the nigrostriatal system. Over-activity of this motor regulator tends to cause difficulty in initiating new acts, as seen in Parkensonianism. Underactivity of this system means defective inhibition and the excessive release of new, competing responses, leading to the disjointed, interrupted movements of the distonias and choreas.

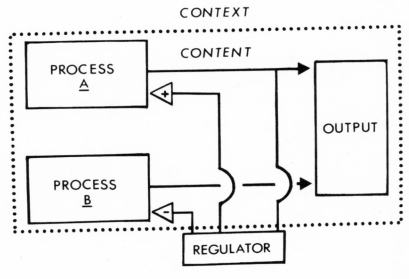

Figure 1

Cognitively, the release of interfering processes results in what Chapman and Chapman refer to as excessive responding to normal biases. That is, to Chapman and Chapman, the central disorder in schizophrenia. Excessive action in this system leads to the kind of thick-headedness and difficulty in initiating thought that some of our patients complain of when we give them phenothiazines.

I do not, however, wish to identify the Regulator in my diagram solely with the mesencephalic nucleus acumbens system, but rather to suggest that it is a manifestation of a much larger set of operations which I have labeled "context". Our thoughts and actions are content; they make up the game. The rules of the game are part of the context in which the game is played. This idea of context has also been talked about as epistemology, or self-system, or even as point-of-view. The syndrome of disregulation (or schizophrenia) is then a disturbance in context, or in self-system, or in epistemology, or of the Regulator, and the disturbance in content is secondary.

The notion of a contrast between content and context, or epistemology, is troublesome. Bateson's Steps Toward an Ecology of Mind is a good reference source. Let me, instead, remind you of the joke about the guard at the construction site who was troubled by a worker who took home a wheelbarrow of straw every night. Every night the guard went through the straw, but never found anything. Later, in another state, the guard saw the workman in a bar. "Now that I can't do anything to you, " said the guard, "would you please tell me what you were stealing that you had hidden in the straw?" "Nothing." replied the workman, "I was stealing wheelbarrows." Any more elaborate treatment of how regulation is related to point of view or how context defines what is admitted as data would take us too far afield, so let us return to our overly-simple Figure 1.

Now, with a disturbance in the Regulator we might tend to see two general classes of results. One class is primarily a result of disturbance in the Regulator, and the other is a class of responses which represent secondary attempts at compensation. These are shown in Table 1. Let us take the primary effects of the disregulation first. These fall into two classes. The first would be a defect in the lateral inhibitory action that tends to hold back competing processes. The other would be a defect in the excitatory action, or positive feedback, on ongoing operations.

Now, let us turn to the evoked potential studies and see how this might fit such a scheme. Early components of the evoked response would reflect the activity of inhibition that was residual from previous ongoing operations. When any process first starts, it must overcome some lingering inhibition from a previous process.  A defect in this inhibition would show up early in the evoked potential as short latency, high amplitude, and low variability responses.  This, of course, is exactly what has been reported.

Later in the evoked response, however, we would have the results of an established and ongoing process, and we would see the combined effect of the positive feedback maintaining this process and of the lateral inhibition on competing operations. For relatively simple sensory responses, such as those preceding the P300, we would continue to expect short latencies, because if the action was started early, it would still be manifested early in these later, but more or less locked-in, operations. However, if we are looking at the results of more complex processes which might be interrupted, then we would expect longer latencies, lower amplitudes, and higher variability.  This is also exactly what is reported for the later components of the evoked response.

## TABLE 1

### ERP FINDINGS IN SCHIZOPHRENIA

A.  Reflecting Regulator Defect.

    1.  Failure to inhibit "B" = unhibited initiation of new processes with;

        a.  Short latency components up to 300 msec.
        b.  High amplitude components up to 100 msec.
        c.  Low variability early components up to 100 msec.

    2.  Failure to excite "A" relative to "B" (may also include failure to inhibit "B"s) = interrupted completion of ongoing process with:

        a.  Low amplitude after 100 msec.
        b.  High variability after 100 msec.
        c.  Long latency after 300 msec.

B.  Reflecting Compensatory Effort.

    1.  Reducing.

?.  SEP Reduced Amplitude Recovery.

   After an action has been completed and the old process fin-
ished, it should be inhibited by the new process and a late post-
response activity such as the post-imperative negative potential,
might again reflect failure to inhibit competing responses.

   Finally, if this Regulator was malfunctioning, we might
expect some compensatory action.  So far, I only know one measure
that seems to fit into this group, and that is Augmenting/Reduc-
ing.  Reducing can be induced in a non-reducer by overloading the
individual.  This gives us reason to suspect that reducing in a
schizophrenic may indicate compensatory and protective reactions.
The fact that it occurs in good prognosis schizophrenics suggests
that it may, indeed, reflect a restorative process.

   Based on the arguments I have given, I will assert that it is
time we looked at patients with psychotic disorders using an
evoked response battery, classify them according to their EPs and
then study these EP syndromes to see if they give us better indications for treatment and prognosis.  With that in mind, we can
look again at the EP data and see if they suggest which measures
we should include in our battery.  What we find is a strong hint
that the measures that correlate with diagnosis are precisely the
ones we should not study.

   Most EP correlates of a schizophrenia diagnosis, I suggest,
are simply correlates of the failure of regulatory operations to
properly manage content that can be assessed in a wide variety of
other ways, many of which are just as good as EPs.  Put another
way, if the EP changes I have attributed to disregulation are
just that, then they tell us little more than an interview, which
could also reveal instability in the rules the patient is following.  It would be better to examine measures which show only weak
relationships to diagnosis, but that might better indicate which,
out of the many possible factors, are disturbing the regulator.

   I would make one exception.  We should include the Augment-
ing/Reducing measure, because I suspect Reducing reflects a compensatory activity.  I would also consider allowing very short
latency SEP recovery functions into my new battery on condition
that Shagass take a challenge which I will make.  Some time ago
I asserted that I could take any evoked potential correlate of
schizophrenia and set up appropriate situations so that normals
would respond like schizophrenics or so that schizophrenics would
respond like normals. Shagass asserted that this would not be true
for the short latency somato-sensory recovery function.  My challenge is that he, at least, give it a good try and see if, indeed,
his measures are immune to changes in the way the subject per-
ceives the test situation. That is to say, if they are, indeed,
not a function of the subject's frame of reference, or Regulator
(as we call it here), then I would allow his measures in our

battery too.

Now, to conclude:  I hope it is apparent that I have over-stated a point for emphasis.  Studies of correlations between EPs and diagnosis have, indeed, taught us a lot.  From these we have learned more about EPs and more about schizophrenia.  The papers we have heard today, of course, stand on their own merits.  But the issue I raise is, nevertheless, a serious one.  We should look more for measures that are not simply measures of disregula-tion, for they will only tell us what we already know.  We should, instead, look for ERP measures that may single out sub-groups whose disregulation arise from different sources, just as thyroid function tests can single out a schizophrenic subgroup that is reclassed as myxedematous madness.  Perhaps it is time for us to admit to ourselves that we are on more solid ground when we talk about evoked potentials than the psychiatrist is when he talks about diagnosis.  Perhaps we should at least con-consider putting the cart behind the horse.

## Bibliography

Bateson, G., Steps Toward an Ecology of Mind, Ballantine: New
    York, 1972.

Chapman, L.J. and Chapman, J.P., Disordered Thought in Schizophre-
    nia, Prentice-Hall: Englewood Cliffs, N.J., 1973.

Matthysse, S., Schizophrenia: Relationships to dopamine transmis-
    sion, motor control and feature extraction. Schmitt, F.O.
    and Worden, F.G. (Eds.), The Neurosciences: Third Study Pro-
    gram, MIT Press: Cambridge, Mass., 1974.

Section IV

# DATA ANALYSIS

# NEUROPHYSIOLOGICAL CORRELATES OF CENTRAL MASKING

M. L. Lester, M. J. Kitzman, B. Z. Karmel and G. J. Crowe

Psychology Department, University of Connecticut

Vincent Giambalvo

Mathematics Department, University of Connecticut

Robert D. Sidman

Mathematics Department, Southwestern Louisiana University

Visual backward masking is an experimental paradigm used to study information processing in the visual system (Kahneman, 1968). Using this paradigm, minor changes in the temporal intervals between two tachistoscopically presented stimuli produce major changes in the accuracy of perceiving the first (or target) stimulus. In dichoptic masking the target stimulus is presented to one eye and a contoured stimulus (or mask) is presented to the other eye. In monoptic masking the target and mask stimuli are presented to the same eye. Monoptic masking is considered to be primarily related to peripheral interactions, while dichoptic masking, because is involves integration beyond the optic chiasm, is considered to be more centrally mediated.

Although most theories of dichoptic masking have assumed a central neurophysiological basis for this perceptual phenomenon (Turvey, 1973, Breitmeyer and Ganz, 1976), to our knowledge, there have been no evoked potential (EP) studies that have used humans as subjects to test such theoretical propositions. Furthermore, an analysis of the paradigm suggests that visual masking in conjunction with electroencephalographic procedures may provide the empirical base for a detailed understanding of neuropsychological processes involved in perception.

525

Masking is a paragon of procedural simplicity and precise stimulation control--on each trial two stimuli are presented, the intensity, duration and configuration of each and the temporal relation
between them exactly specifiable by the experimenter.  Consequently,
the stimulation parameters of the task can be titrated to the limits
of a subject's perceptual processing capabilities., Near these limits,
constrained by the spatial-temporal stimulation requirements of the
task, the set of internal operations necessary for perception are
maximally challenged.  Under these circumstances, the subject per-
ceives the target on some trials but not on others.  With experience,
however, the subject's performance in the dichoptic masking task improves (Schiller and Wiener, 1963; Schiller, 1965).

     Thus, across masking trials of invariant stimulation conditions,
perceptual performance is variable and improves with subject experience in the task.  The subject apparently is able to do something on
certain masking trials which optimizes his perceptual ability and to
learn with practice in the task how to more reliably perform well.

     Another important aspect of the masking paradigm is that it
probes a complex psychological phenomenon.  The subject must not only
detect a signal in the presence of noise, but in addition, correctly
identify it.  In masking studies the target stimuli are usually symbolic (e.g. letters, numerals, consonant trigrams or words) which are
presumed to require for perception the utilization of high level
mental functions as well as basic sensory capacities (Haber and
Hershenson, 1973).

     If individual symbols are used as target stimuli, then on each
masking trial a subject's performance can be unambigucusly classified
as accurate or inaccurate based upon target report.  When a target is
correctly reported, one may assume that the operations critical for
perception have occurred.  However, when a target is masked, a failure in one or more of these operations can be assumed.  If surface
recorded brain electrical activity indexes the neurophysiological
support for these perceptual operations, then the masking paradigm
may offer a means of concretely specifying the sequence of neuropsychological events basic to perception.

     The principle idea motivating the study reported here is that a
comparison of EP data recorded during successful and unsuccessful attempts to perceive under identical stimulation conditions might reveal those processes most critical for accurate perception in the
masking task.


PROCEDURES

     A 3-field tachistoscope was used to present individual trials of
stimuli consisting of a target followed by a mask.  The target stimuli were single letters of the alphabet while the mask stimulus was

a compact group of abnormally oriented letters.  Target and mask
stimuli were each 50 msec in duration.  Each target letter subtended
0.79 degrees of arc while the mask subtended 1.73 x 3.89 degrees.
The luminance of the target field was 6.72 cd/m$^2$ while that of the
masking field measured 7.88 cd/m$^2$; the luminance of the fixation
field upon which both target and mask were superimposed was 3.56
cd/m$^2$.

Prior to each trial onset, an experimenter changed the target
letter and then initiated the trial with a verbal "ready" command.
Within one second after the "ready" signal, a fixation-point field
was displayed to both eyes and remained on for 1000 msec.  At 300
msec after fixation field onset, the target letter was superimposed
on the field of the subject's non-dominant eye.  The mask was presented to the subject's dominant eye simultaneous with target presentation or at a specific time point after target onset.  These are
standard procedures for obtaining dichoptic masking (cf. Turvey,
1973).

Eye dominance was defined as the eye which controlled perception
when the subject was instructed to binocularly sight a near object in
line with a more distal fixation point.  The temporal separation between target and mask onsets is termed the stimulus onset asynchrony
(SOA) period.  Subjects were tested under four SOA conditions.  These
conditions which spanned the full range of task performance were:
(1) 0-SOA (approximately 15% correct report), (2) 25-SOA, (3) 50-SOA,
and (4) 75-SOA (approximately) 80% correct report.

During masking trials, we recorded event related potentials from
a 6-lead monopolar occipital-parietal montage.  The lead sites were
$O_1$, $O_2$, $O_z$, $P_3$, $P_4$, and $P_z$ referenced to linked mastoids.  Eye movements were recorded from a transorbital pair of electrodes across the
right eye to detect eye-movement artifacts in the analyses of EP effects.  All electrode impedances were between 15-20 K   Data were amplified 12,500x by a Beckman Dynograph model 411R with EEG bandpass
down 3 db at .35 Hz and 30 Hz.  All data and stimulus protocols were
stored on a Vetter Model 'A' FM-tape recorder and analyzed off-line
using a minicomputer system (PDP-8I) outputing data onto paper tape
for further analyses on an IBM-370 computer system.


RESULTS


Dipole Source Localization Analysis

To index the moment-to-moment neurophysiological functioning
associated with perception during masking, we submitted the scalp-
recorded data to a dipole localization method of analysis (DLM).
The analysis describes the location, orientation and energy character-

istics of generator sources in the brain which would best replicate
the observed EP data.  Each of these neural generators is represented
in the analysis as a dipole point source.  Any focal region of polar-
ized tissue can be modeled with good approximation by a dipole point
(Geisler and Gerstein, 1961; Henderson, Butler, and Glass, 1975).

A point source dipole and the equipotential voltage lines of the
electric field generated by the dipole are illustrated in Figure 1
(cf. Brazier, 1949).  The figure also shows the voltage distributions
expected from a line of recording electrodes for two special cases of
dipole source orientation:  (1) when the polarization axis of the dipole is oriented vertically to the recording surface, and (2) when
the dipole axis is oriented horizontally to the surface recording
plane.

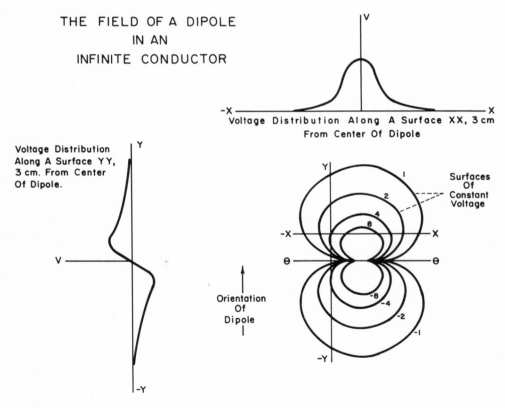

Figure 1.  Voltage distribution for planes parallel and at right
angles to a dipole.

Figure 1 indicates those characteristics expected of voltage distribution measurements taken from recording sites oriented in a straight line parallel or perpendicular to the dipole axis for a dipole source within an infinitely conductive medium. The model that DLM utilizes is more sophisticated in that it takes into account the following: (1) that the dipole occurs within a conductive medium that is bounded by an approximately spherically shaped head and that the voltage field generated by this dipole is measured from recording sites along this curved surface and, (2) that specific systematic changes in such recorded voltages will be observed for any subset of recording sites depending on the dipole's location, orientation, and moment (Henderson, et. al., 1975). Using six recording sites, no four of which are co-planar, one can calculate a unique single equivalent dipole "best solution" for any observed voltage distribution measured at those recording sites (Sidman, Giambalvo, Allison, and Bergey, 1977).

For the DLM analysis, the scalp-recorded brain electrical activity was digitized at a 6 msec sampling rate for 900 msec after the beginning of fixation field onset. Thus, a 300 msec period prior to target onset and a 600 msec period after target onset and mask presentation was included in the analyses reported here.

The dipole source localization analysis determined the degree to which these surface voltages simultaneously observed at different scalp locations were accounted for by an idealized coherent dipole source within the brain. An IBM-370 machine language program developed by V. Giambalvo compared the observed voltage values at each time point across a set of leads to an expected distribution of voltage values at those recording sites assuming a single equivalent dipole source of a specific magnitude, orientation and location within the brain. A least squares criterion of goodness-of-fit was applied to this comparison. The program systematically altered the idealized dipole until a minimum of unaccounted variance between real data and idealized data was achieved. Once the minimum solution was obtained, the program printed the dipole parameters and the goodness-of-fit estimate, rho.

Several important differences between DLM and the component peak-to-peak analysis of most EP studies should be summarized: (1) DLM uses a six lead montage at a minimum rather than one or two leads to measure surface voltage fluctuations; (2) the instantaneous voltage distribution over the six lead sites is taken as the primary date unit and each voltage distribution is analyzed independently over the experimental trial epoch for each sampled instant of time, (3) the data distributions are evaluated in reference to an explicit physical model of the electrical conductance properties of the brain and its protective coverings, and (4) both single data trials and averaged data trials can provide the raw datum for the analyses. Thus, DLM produces estimates of the changing configuration of electrical activity within

the brain over time to be related to task and stimulation variables;
whereas, more conventional EP analyses use voltage amplitudes measured at one or more scalp surface sites for this purpose. The approach of the former is to describe the surface electrical activity
in terms of generator sources within the brain's three-dimensional
volume; the latter accepts the two-dimensional surface representation
as the primary descriptive language for analysis. More importantly,
the two approaches look to different sets of scientific principles,
different models, for guiding the evaluation and interpretation of
surface recorded data. In a dipole analysis the first level of formal evaluation is predicated upon how well the structure of the data
conforms to a biophysical model. This contrasts markedly with the
adoption of a statistical model as the primary basis for the formal
evaluation of EP data. Whereas the language of the dipole analysis
may be directly informative of the moment-to-moment flow of events in
the central nervous system (CNS), statistical descriptions of EP data,
such as mean voltage levels, factor analysis waveforms (Donchin, 1969;
Squires and Donchin, 1976; Thatcher and Maisel, 1978) or multivariate
voltage vectors (Karmel, Hoffmann and Fegy, 1974; Lieb and Karmel,
1974), in principle can not specify the momentary locus of activity
in the brain.

## DLM Applied to the Masking EP Data

Trials on which a subject correctly reported the target were designated 'hits'; all others were labelled 'miss' trials. Figures 2 and
3 are representative samples for single hit and miss trial comparisons
respectively. Six channels of EP data and accompanying eye movement
data are shown in the lower portion of each figure. The single trial
data were analyzed by DLM. In the upper portion of each figure the
goodness-of-fit parameter, rho, is graphed on an inverse log (base 10)
scale.

Rho is the fraction of total data variance that is unaccounted
for by the dipole solution. Consequently, the rho parameter indicates
the degree to which the observed data conforms to the model's best representation of a single generator source for the data. If the DLM
dipole source poorly describes the surface-recorded data, then further
evaluation of the dipole solution is not warranted. We will concentrate on these rho values in order to evaluate the adequacy of the dipole model at this most general level. Other parameters of the model
such as dipole location and moment will not be discussed in this paper
in detail.

A visual inspection of Figures 2 and 3 reveals that a dipole model accounts very well for the observed data on each of these trials.
Points above the line on the rho parameter graphs indicate that over
99% of the raw data variance can be accounted for by the single equivalent dipole source specified by the analysis at that time instant.

In addition, the dipole model simulates the data at some time points better than at others.  Most importantly though, the temporal pattern of dipole best-fit appears to be different for the brain data preceding accurate report as compared to that preceding inaccurate report.

To test for the consistency of this observation, we performed the following numerical analysis:  First, the time points during which the dipole model fit the EP data at better than a 95% variance-accounted-for criterion, log (1/rho) 1.30, were determined for each trial.  We then calculated the proportion of time points the model fit the data during each successive 30 msec interval using this proportion to determine the average behavior of the model for hit and miss trials

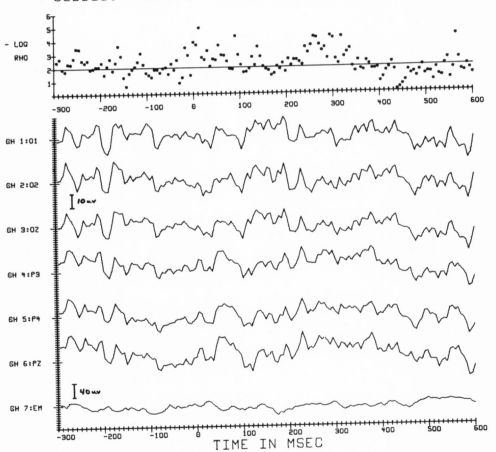

Figure 2.  EP data and rho values plotted for a single hit trial. Time in msec is referenced to target onset.  Positive voltage is up.

separately.  We could then compare the behavior of the model across
time for each type of perceptual experience.

The bar graph in Figure 4 describes such differences in performance of the model.  Upward deflection of the bars indicate better fit
for hits, downward deflections indicate better fit for misses.

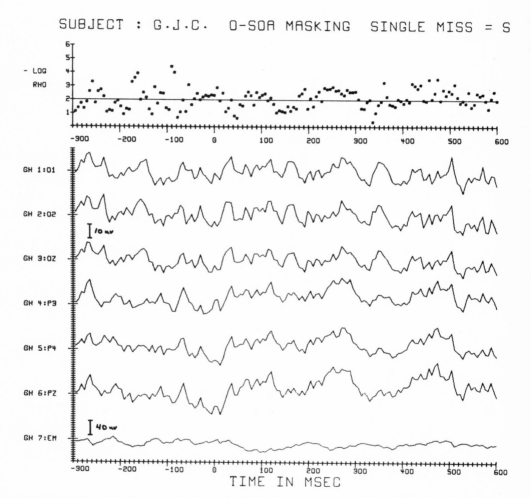

Figure 3.  EP data and rho values plotted for a single miss trial.
Time in msec is referenced to target onset.  Positive voltage is up.

The model appears to fit the hit trial data better than the missed trial data when the fixation field comes on, and still better just prior to target onset. We interpret these differences to indicate that attentional mechanisms which ready the information reception and response organization systems of the subject are contributing factors determining subject performance in the dichoptic masking task. The relationship between what seem to be dipole analysis correlates of attention and the expectancy and attentional correlates derived from averaged surface recorded data require further investigation. This would seem a promising inquiry especially in light of the fact that dipole analysis differences occur not only prior to the onset of significant information as with the contingent negative variation (Walter, 1967; Tecce, 1973) but are also apparent around 300 msec after target onset (cf. Donchin, Kubovy, Kutas, Johnson and Herning, 1973).

In the EP literature a consistent finding is that component amplitudes at latencies around 100 and 160–180 msec correlate with the spatial frequency or contour density of the stimulus that is viewed (Spehlmann, 1965; Harter and White, 1970; Karmel, Hoffmann and Fegy, 1974; White, 1974). Apparently, CNS mechanisms involved in stimulus contour processing are active during these post-stimulus time regions.

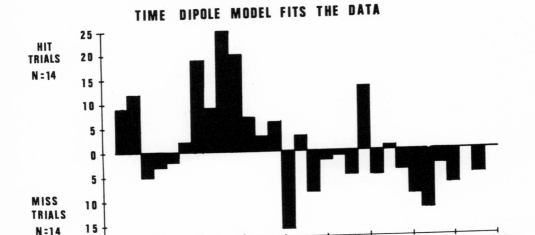

Figure 4. Bar graph showing the relative degree that the DLM solution accounts for the brain activity data for hit and miss trials in 30 msec time blocks.

Brain activity data exhibits greater coherence, in terms of the dipole model, the more a single dipole source adequately describes that set of data.  Figure 4 reveals that a dipole model describes the miss trial data better than the hit data at post-target onset latencies of 100 and 160 msec.  These data suggest that if the mask is capable of producing greater coherence in the CNS than the target, the mask will dominate the system forcing the contour target information below a sufficient signal level for perception of the target to occur. This hypothesis is especially compelling when one considers that the mask, in terms of physical properties and presentation technique, is the favored stimulus in this type of study--the mask has greater energy  than the target, is more contoured than the target and is presented to the subject's dominant eye (Flom, Heath and Takahashi, 1963).  It follows from this argument, however, that if the interfering effects of the mask are to be avoided, the subject's perceptual system might have to organize prior to target and mask onset to ensure a biasing of signal levels of the incoming information at an early stage of neurophysiological transduction.

Finally, differences between hit and miss trials also appeared very late after target onset in the 360-500 msec latency range.  These long latency dipole coherence differences might be related to CNS activity during semantic information processing as suggested by Thatcher and Maisel (1978) in this volume.

In summary, the dipole analysis results suggest that multiple psychophysiological processes--attention, expectancy, contour and semantic dependent operations--are involved in perception during the dichoptic masking task.  A major advantage of DLM is that it uses evoked information on single trials and requires no previous information to discriminate effects in the single trial events, whereas more tradition EP analysis techniques require averaged trials followed by statistical manipulation (Donchin, 1969; Thatcher and John, 1977; John, 1977; Squires and Donchin, 1976).  The experimental results indicate that DLM might afford us the opportunity to more closely analyze the mechanisms of perception in that the model appears to efficiently index the dynamics of information flow in the brain without having to average across trials.  The obvious advantage of this increased efficiency for future research with hard-to-test subjects such as infants and hyperactive children is anticipated.

## Eye Control and Attention Variables in Masking

Paradigms such as masking which use fixation fields followed by rapidly displayed discrete presentations have been assumed by experimenters to be free of confounding eye-movement variables (Averbach and Coriel, 1965; Kahneman, 1968).  However, in reviewing the eye movement

records of this study, we found that on many masking trials micro-
saccades, saccadic movements or eye tremor did occur.  Approximately
25% of the records showed some form of eye movement in time regions
close to target and mask onset.  Furthermore, on these trials the eye
movement patterns preceding accurate target report appeared to be different from those preceding incorrect report.

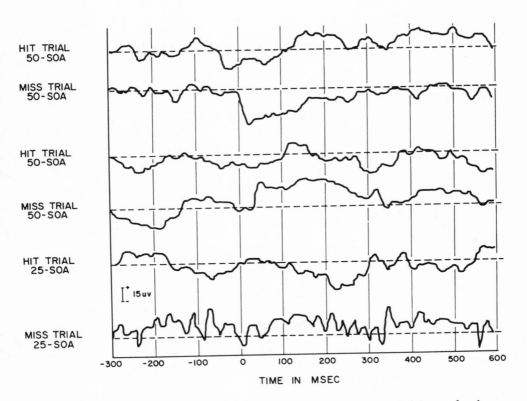

Figure 5.   Eye movement records for selected pairs of hit and miss
trials.

Figure 5 displays eye movement data for several hit and miss trial sets. For hit trials saccadic movements, if present, usually occurred before and/or after target and mask presentation; however, for miss trials eye movements occurred most often during the presentation of the target stimulus. The eye tremor (Goren and Komada, 1972) shown in the last trace in Figure 5 was observed on 2 of the 28 data samples of this report--both miss trials. These data emphasize the importance for perception of eye control and attentional mechanisms.

In order to optimize perceptual performance (Fowler and Turvey, 1978), a subject in the masking experiment must foveate prior to target onset the point in the visual field where the target is to be presented (Vaughan and Silverstein, 1968; Bouma, 1971). Kurtzberg and Vaughan (1977) have used an analysis similar to DLM and have observed consistently the occurrence of coherent dipole sources in the preoccipital and posterior parietal regions prior to the initiation of a directed eye saccade to a point in the contralateral visual field. For an attentive subject, a fixation saccade is easily accomplished within 250 msec (Ditchburn, 1973). However, from trial to trial a subject's attention-motivational state may be presumed to fluctuate resulting in delayed fixation reaction times on some trials. If the center of the visual field is fixated close to or during target onset then saccadic suppression effects would attenuate the transmission of target information through the visual system (Stark, Michael and Zuber, 1969; Singer and Bedworth, 1974). This sequence of events would be expected to lead to incorrect target report (cf. miss trial eye movements of Figure 5).

On most masking trials, however, the eye that we recorded from (and presumably the other, also) is fixated prior to target onset; nevertheless, on some of these trials the target is seen and on others it is not. We believe that the variable functioning of neurophysiological mechanisms of directed visual attention may account for some of the performance variability in these cases also. Mountcastle and his colleagues have identified and studied several classes of parietal neurons which appear to be active in modulating visual attention (Mountcastle, Lynch, Georgopoulos, Sakata, and Acuna, 1975; Lynch, Mountcastle, Talbot, and Yin, 1977). Two classes of neurons are of particular interest: (a) saccade neurons and (b) fixation neurons. Saccade neurons are active prior to an eye movement to fixate a visual object of learned importance to the subject. Fixation neurons are active during fixations of visual objects or regions of the visual field which previously have been associated with important events for the subject and they cease activity shortly after the occurrence of the anticipated significant visual event. Experience appears to shape the firing patterns of these neurons. Their activity pattern becomes selectively tuned in terms of a particular area of the visual field and the content of the information within that area.

These parietal area 7 neurons are enmeshed in a complex central network of connections in which the parietal cortex is reciprocally linked with other cortical and subcortical structures which have been identified as neural substrates of importence for motivation, attention, eye control and visual perception (Petras, 1971; Pandya and Kuypers, 1969; Wurtz and Mohler, 1974; Kievit and Kuypers, 1975; Wilson, 1978). The structural-temporal neural activity relations within this extended system most likely define focal attention in functional terms prescribing where in visual space to search for information, when in reference to an external signal to initiate, and perhaps end, the search, what type of information, if knowable beforehand, to search for, and for what purpose the sought after information is being obtained.


## DISCUSSION

Several previous studies have emphasized the attention-dependent nature of masking. For example, Erdelyi and Blumenthal (1973) demonstrated that a mask stimulus of strong emotional meaning produces more masking than does a more neutral stimulus. Other research has shown that pretuning a subject to specific target stimuli dramatically improves perceptual ability in the task (Eriksen and Collins, 1969; Bachmann and Allik, 1976).

Perception may be conceptualized as a cyclic phenomenon mutually dependent upon the information of environmental events and the information seeking activity of the perceiver (Gibson, 1966; Neisser, 1976). From this theoretical perspective, a perceiver would attempt to optimize perceptual performance under very restrictive stimulus information circumstances by tightly constraining activities which enhance perceptual sensitivity for incoming information.

In the masking paradigm, a subject is required to perceive under conditions marginally sufficient in terms of stimulus information. Under these circumstances, the dipole analysis indicates that just prior to target onset is a period of greatest difference in brain activity between trials on which a target is perceived and those on which it is misperceived. During this period the location of the dipole source appears to shift back and forth regularly between posterior cortical areas and midbrain regions. These shifts may describe the spatio-temporal order of CNS activity during highly constrained attention focussing.

We conclude from this study that perceptual performance in the dichoptic backward masking paradigm is predicated upon multiple CNS mechanisms. The most critical of these central operations occur prior to target onset and are theorized to be related to the perceiver's attention focussing capabilities.

APPENDIX

The localization of sources of electrical activity generated within the human body is a fundamental problem in electroencephalo-graphy. Brazier (1949) stated the problem succinctly: "Most of our work in human electroencephalography is a study of the voltage dis-tribution on the surface of a volume conductor--the brain. We would like to know what kind of generators inside this volume conductor could give us the voltage distributions which we find experimentally."

In this connection a mathematical treatment has proved useful. Basically the physiological data is organized into a simplified model about which strictly mathematical questions are posed and answered. These answers can hopefully be reinterpreted in a physically meaning-ful way. The competing requirements are simplicity and relevance.

The particular model that we have used has several components. The head is simulated by three concentric spheres of differing con-ductivities representing the brain, skull, and scalp. At a particu-lar time instant potentials observed at recording sites on the outer-most sphere (scalp) are assumed to be generated by a single current dipole in the innermost sphere (brain). The mathematical problem is to find an inverse solution, to construct a theoretical dipole which, if actually present, would produce the known surface potentials, at least in the sense of minimizing the variance between the theoretical and observed potentials. This variance is a function of the six vari-ables that describe the location and moments of the theoretical source. The function is minimized numerically to produce the "best fit" dipole. This method has been referred to as the Dipole Localization Method (DLM).

Previous work suggests that the simplifying assumptions concern-ing the symmetry and homogeneity of the head are reasonable as a first approximation (Gabor and Nelson, 1954; Rush and Driscoll, 1968, 1969; Schneider, 1972; Vaughan, 1974; Henderson et al., 1975). The assump-tion of a single dipole source introduces some problems. For some EP components generated in primary sensory cortex the active region is a small area of tissue lying in a plane, the best-case condition. For most components, however, the extent and geometry of the active area are unknown and a generator model with several sources should perhaps be used, (Regan, 1972).

The numerical results that are produced by DLM include the mini-mum value of the variance and the location and direction of the theo-retical source. If this minimum is small then there is a strong evi-dence that the underlying source of scalp potentials is synchronous. Then the theoretical source can be examined to see if it does, in fact, coincide with a physiological one.

In order to validate the method and define its utility DLM has been applied to human EP components of known origin. It has been used to localize the source of some early somatic EP components evoked by right medial nerve stimulation (Sidman et al., 1977). Additionally, Henderson et al., (1975) employed a simplified version of DLM to locate the sources of eye-blink potentials.

Schneider (1972), Smith et al., (1973) and Henderson et al., (1975) have used this mathematical method with a 1-sphere model of the head for EEG and EP analysis. Assume that the head is a homogeneous sphere of radius 1 and conductivity $o_1$. If a retangular coordinate system with origin at the center of the sphere has been introduced and $A(\delta_1,\delta_2,\delta_3)$ is a point on the surface, then a current dipole D at location $(p_1,p_2,p_3)$, with moments $m_1,m_2,m_3$, will produced at A the potential

$$V(A,D) = \frac{1}{4\pi o_1} \sum_{i=1}^{3} \frac{m_i}{q_0} \left[ \frac{2(\delta_i - p_i)}{q_0^2} + \delta_i + \frac{\delta_i s - p_i}{q_0 + 1 - s} \right]$$

where

$$q_0 = \left[ \sum_{j=1}^{3} (\delta_j - p_j)^2 \right]^{\frac{1}{2}} \quad \text{and} \quad s = \sum_{j=1}^{3} \delta_j p_j .$$

This formula, due to Brody et al., (1973), is preferable to the classical formula of Wilson-Bayley (1950) which is used in the first and third references above since it is not indeterminant when the dipole D is centric or radial.

The inverse problem for the one sphere model is stated and solved as follows. If voltages $V(A_k)$ are recorded at the surface sites $A_k$, $k=1,\ldots,n$ respectively (with respect to a reference electrode, presumably at zero potential) then the dipolar source D which best reproduces the surface potentials can be found by minimizing.

$$\text{rho}(p_1,p_2,p_3,m_1,m_2,m_3) = \frac{\sum_{k=1}^{n} [V(A_k,D) - V(A_k)]^2}{\sum_{k=1}^{n} [V(A_k)]^2}$$

where $V(A_k)$ is the empirical potential recorded at electrode $A_k$, $V(A_k,D)$ has the form above, and n is the number of electrodes. It will be seen that rho is a residual sum of squares. Its

minimization thus provides a least-squares best fit between the calculated and empirical potentials.

The head is not a single homogeneous sphere and it would be
better simulated by three concentric spheres. Although this 3-sphere
model still invokes geometric symmetry and homogeneity, a great simplification of the true physiology of the head, it does account for
the attenuation of cortical and subcortical potentials caused by the
presence of the highly resistive skull (middle shell). Unfortunately
the quantities $V(A_k,D)$ no longer have the simple closed Brody form
and it is difficult to minimize rho directly. However, a mathematical argument can show that this 3-sphere optimal dipole can be constructed from the 1-sphere dipole; it produces the same value of **rho**
and has the same direction as the 1-sphere dipole but lies closer to
the surface by a factor of 1.28.

## ACKNOWLEDGEMENTS

This research was supported in part by NIMH Predoctoral Research
Award #1 F31 MH07373-01 BLS to the first author and a University of
Connecticut Research Foundation Grant to the third author.

Appreciation is extended to Steven J. Roy for his computer programming and technical assistance and to Alice Gangaway for her help
in preparing the manuscript.

## BIBLIOGRAPHY

Averbach, E., and Coriell, A. S. Short-term memory in vision.
    Bell System Technical Journal, 1961, 40, 309-328.
Bachmann, T. and Allik, J. Integration and interruption in the
    masking of form by form. Perception, 1976, 5, 79-97.
Bouma, H. Visual recognition of isolated lower-case letters.
    Vision Research, 1971, 11, 459-474.
Brazier, M. A. B. The electrical fields at the surface of the head
    during sleep. Electroencephalogy and Clinical Neurophysiology,
    1949, 1, 195-204.
Breitmeyer, B. and Ganz, L. Implications of Sustained and Transient
    Channels for Theories of Visual Pattern Masking, Saccadic
    Supression, and Information Processing. Psychological Review,
    1976, 83, 1-35.
Brody, D. A., Terry, F. H., and Ideker, R. E. Eccentric dipole in
    a spherical medium; generalized expression for surface potentials.
    IEEE Transactions on Biomedical Engineering, 1973, BME-20,
    141-143.
Coren, S. and Komada, M. Eye Movement Control in Voluntary
    Nystagmus. American Journal of Ophthalmology, 1972, 74, 1161-1165.

Ditchburn, R. W. Eye-Movement and Visual Perception. Oxford: Clarendon Press, 1973.

Donchin, E. Data analysis techniques in average evoked potential research, in: Average evoked potentials: Methods, results and evaluations, E. Conchin and D. B. Lindsley (Eds.), Washington, D. C., U.S. Government Printing Office, 1969, NASA SP-191, 199-236.

Donchin, E., Kubovy, M., Kutes, M., Johnson, R., and Herning, R. I. Graded changes in evoked response (P300) amplitude as a function of cognitive activity. Perception and Psychophysics, 1973, 14, 324-419.

Erdelyi, M. H. and Blumenthal, D. G. Cognitive masking in rapid sequential processing: The effect of an emotional picture on preceding and succeeding pictures. Memory and Cognition, 1973, 1, 201-204.

Eriksen, C. W. and Collins, J. F. Visual perceptual rate under two conditions of search. Journal of Experimental Psychology, 1969, 80, 489-492.

Flom, C., Heath, C. G. and Takahashi, E. Contour interaction and visual resolution: Contralateral effects. Science, 1963, 142, 979-980.

Fowler, C. A. and Turvey, M. T. Skill acquisition: An event approach with special reference to searching for the optimum of a function of several variables, in: Information processing in motor control and learning, G. Stelmach (Ed.), New York: Academic Press, in press 1978.

Gabor, D. and Nelson, C. V. Determination of the resultant dipole of the heart from measurements on the body surface. Journal of Applied Physics, 1954, 25, 413-416.

Geisler, C. D. and Gerstein, G. L. The surface EEG in relation to its sources. Electroencephalogy and Clinical Neurophysiology, 1961, 13, 927-934.

Gibson, J. J. The Senses Considered as Perceptual Systems. Boston: Houghton Mifflin Co., 1966.

Haber, R. N. and Hershenson, M. The Psychology of Visual Perception. New York: Holt, Rinehart and Winston, Inc., 1973.

Harter, M. R. and White, C. T. Evoked cortical responses to checkerboard patterns: effect of check size as a function of visual acuity. Electroencephalography and Clinical Neurophysiology, 1970, 28, 48-54.

Henderson, C. J., Butler, S. R. and Glass, A. The localization of equivalent dipoles of EEG sources by the application of electrical field theory. Electroencephalogy and Clinical Neurophysiology, 1975, 39, 117-130.

John, E. R. Functional Neuroscience Volume 2 Neurometrics: Clinical Applications of Quantitative Electrophysiology. John Wiley & Sons, New York, 1977.

Kahneman, D. Method, findings, and theory in studies of visual masking. Psychological Bulletin, 1968, 70, 404-425.

Karmel, B. Z., Hoffmann, R. F. and Fegy, M. J. Processing of contour information by human infants evidenced by pattern-dependent evoked potentials. Child Development, 1974, 45, 39-48.

Karmel, B. Z. and Maisel, E. B. A neuronal activity model of infant visual attention, in: Infant Perception: From Sensation to Cognition. Part I: Basic Visual Processes. Volume I. L. B. Cohen and P. Salapatek (Eds.), New York, Academic Press, 1975, 77-131.

Kievit, J. and Kuypers, H. G. J. M. Basal forebrain and hypothalamic connections to frontal and parietal cortex in the rhesus monkey. Science, 1975, 187, 660-662.

Kurtzberg, D. and Vaughan, H. G., Jr. Electrophysiologic observations on the visuo-motor system and visual sensorium, in: Visual Evoked Potentials in Man: New Developments, J. E. Desmedt (Ed.), London: Oxford Univ. Press, 1977.

Lieb, J. P. and Karmel, B. Z. The processing of edge information in visual areas of the cortex as evidenced by evoked potentials. Brain Research, 1974, 76, 503-519.

Lynch, J. C., Mountcastle, V. B., Talbot, W. H. and Yin, T. C. T. Parietal lobe mechanisms for directed visual attention. Journal of Neurophysiology, 1977, 40, 362-389.

Mountcastle, V. B., Lynch, J. C., Georgopoulos, A., Sakata, H., and Acuna, C. Posterior parietal association cortex of the monkey: Command functions for operations within extrapersonal space. Journal of Neurophysiology, 1975, 38, 871-908.

Neisser, U. Cognition and Reality. San Francisco: W. H. Freeman & Co., 1976.

Pandya, D. N. and Kuypers, H. G. J. M. Cortico-cortical connections in the rhesus monkey. Brain Research, 1969, 13, 13-36.

Petras, J. M. Connections of the parietal lobe. Journal of Psychiatric Research, 1971, 8, 189-201.

Regan, D. Evoked Potentials in Psychology, Sensory Physiology and Clinical Medicine, John Wiley & Sons, New York, 1972.

Rush, S. and Driscoll, D. A. Current distribution in the brain from surface electrodes. Anesthesia and Analgesia. Current Researches, 1968, 47, 717-723.

Rush, S. and Driscoll, D. A. EEG electrode sensitivity--an application of reciprocity. IEEE Transactions on Biomedical Engineering, 1969, BME-16, 15-22.

Schiller, P. H. Monoptic and dichoptic visual masking by patterns and flashes. Journal of Experimental Psychology, 1965, 61, 193-199.

Schiller, P. H. and Wiener, M. Monoptic and dichoptic visual masking. Journal of Experimental Psychology. 1963, 66, 386-393.

Schneider, M. R. A multistage process for computing virtual dipolar sources of EEG discharges from surface information. IEEE Transactions on Biomedical Engineering, 1972, BME-19, 1-12.

Sidman, R. D., Giambalvo, V., Allison, T. and Bergey, P. A dipole localization method for determination of sources of human cerebral evoked potentials. 31st annual meeting of the American EEG Society, Miami, Florida, June 22-24, 1977.

Singer, W. and Bedworth, N. Correlation between the effects of brain stem stimulation and saccadic eye movements on transmission in the cat lateral geniculate nucleus. Brain Research, 1974, 72, 185-202.

Smith, D. B., Lell, M. E., Sidman, R. D. and Mavor, H. Nasopharyngeal phase reversal of cerebral evoked potentials and theroetical dipole implications. Electroencephalography and Clinical Neurophysiology, 1973, 34, 654-658.

Spehlmann, R. The averaged electrical response to diffuse and to patterned light in the human. Electroencephalography and Clinical Neurophysiology, 1965, 19, 560-576.

Squires, K. C. and Donchin, E. Beyond averaging: The use of discriminant functions to recognize event related potentials elicited by single auditory stimuli. Electroencephalography and Clinical Neurophysiology, 1976, 41, 449-459.

Stark, L., Michael, J. A. and Zuber, B. L. Saccadic suppression: A Product of the saccadic anticipatory signal, in: Attention in Neurophysiology, C. R. Evans and T. B. Mulholland (Eds.), London, Butterworth & Co., 1969, 281-303.

Tecce, J. J. Contingent negative variation (CNV) and psychological processes in man. Psychological Bulletin, 1972, 77, 73-108.

Thatcher, R. W. and John, E. R. Functional Neuroscience Volume 1: Foundations of Cognitive Processes, John Wiley & Sons, New York, 1977.

Thatcher, R. W. and Maisel, E. B. Functional Landscapes of the brain: An Electrotopographic Perspective, in: Evoked Brain Potentials and Behavior, Henri Begleiter (Ed.), Plenum Press, New York, in press, 1978.

Turvey, M. T. On peripheral and central processes in vision: Inferences from an information-processing analysis of masking with patterned stimuli. Psychological Review, 1973, 80, 1-52.

Vaughan, H. G., Jr. The analysis of scalp-recorded brain potentials, in: Bioelectric Recording Techniques. Part B. Electroencephalography and Human Brain Potentials, R. F. Thompson and M. M. Patterson (Eds.), Academic Press, New York, 1974, 157-207.

Vaughan, H. G., Jr. and Silverstein, L. Metacontrast and Evoked Potentials: A Reappraisal, Science, 1968, 160, 207-208.

Walter, W. G. Slow potential changes in the human brain associated with expectancy, decision and intention. Electroencephalography and Clinical Neurophysiology, Supplement, 1967, 26, 123-130.

White, Carroll T. The visual evoked responses and patterned stimuli, in: Advances in Psychobiology. Volume Two, G. Newton and A. H. Riesen (Eds.), John Wiley & Sons, New York, 1974, 267-295.

Wilson, F. N. and Bayley, R. H. The electric field of an eccentric dipole in a homogeneous spherical conducting medium. Circulation, 1950, 1, 84-92.

Wilson, M.  Visual function:  Pulvinar-extrastriate system, in:
    Handbook of Behavioral Neurobiology, Vol. 1:  Sensory Integration,
    R. B. Masterton (Ed.), Plenum Press, New York, in press 1978.
Wurtz, R. H. and Mohler, C. W.  Selection of visual targets for the
    initiation of saccadic eye movements.  Brain Research, 1974,
    71, 209-214.

# BASIS FUNCTIONS IN THE ANALYSIS OF EVOKED POTENTIALS[1]

Donald C. Martin, David Borg-Breen, Veronica Buffington

Departments of Biostatistics and Psychiatry

SC-32, University of Washington, Seattle WA 98195

## 1.1. ABSTRACT

ER data may be reduced to a more compact form by approximating the original responses by a linear combination of functions. Two main classes of approximating functions are discussed. The first of these are fixed basis functions. These are functions that do not depend upon the data. These are sine-cosine (Fourier), Walsh-Hadamard (square waves), Haar functions (square wave impulse functions), and polynomials. The other functions are random in that they depend upon the data. These arise from various multivariate statistical procedures. The procedures discussed are principal components, factor analysis, union-intersection tests, and canonical correlation.

Some of the relative advantages of each of the methods are discussed. The fixed basis function methods are relatively fast and simple to compute. The multivariate methods are difficult to compute but tend to be better approximations because they depend upon the sample to select the functions. The multivariate test statistics based upon the union-intersection principle may be interesting because, in some cases, they both generate test statistics and characteristic waveforms. Most of these methods have not been used enough to offer any concrete recommendations.

[1]This study was supported by Public Health Service Grant 5 R01 MB 00184-03, Grant 63-0625 from the Alcoholism and Drug Abuse Institute at the University of Washington, and AA01881 from the National Institute on Alcohol Abuse and Alcoholism.

Fourier, polynomial, Walsh-Hadamard, Haar, principal components and factor analysis are compared in a least squares sense for
goodness of fit for average evoked responses for 43 subjects.  The
principal components procedure will always result in a best fit.
Factor analysis was the next best approximation with Fourier approximation next best and sometimes better.  The Walsh-Hadamard and
Haar were not as good but might well be satisfactory for some types
of analysis, especially in view of their computational efficiency.
Polynomial approximations are poor for low degree polynomials but
improve more rapidly than the Walsh-Hadamard and the Haar approximations.  Polynomial approximations are not as good as Fourier for
these data and they are slower to compute.

The direct use of multivariate methods may be impractical due
to the large matrices involved.  However, hybrid methods that use
Fourier, Walsh-Hadamard or Haar functions to reduce the dimensions
and then use principal components or union-intersection tests may
prove useful.

## 1.2 MEASUREMENT PROBLEMS

The usual measurements of AERs are the maximum amplitudes and
latencies of selected peaks.  These measurements have been a source
of a number of problems due mostly to variations in the shapes of
waveforms both between and within individuals.  These variations
may lead to variations between experimenters in the selection of
peaks to measure.  Attempts to program computers to recognize standard peaks have not been very successful.  The usual peak measurements also result in several statistical problems.  The addition of
random variation or noise will result in an upwards bias in measuring positive peaks and a downward bias in negative peaks.  This effect is more pronounced when the peak has a relatively flat top.
The latter situation also results in a poor measure of latency.

## 1.3 BASIS FUNCTIONS

One useful way of compressing data is to fit the observations
with some function and then use the function in further analyses
instead of the original data.  The most frequently used approximations are of the form:

$$A(t) = a_1 f_1(t) + a_2 f_2(t) + \ldots + a_k f_k(t)$$

As an example, the $f_k(.)$ functions are sines and cosines in a
Fourier approximation.  It will be useful to discuss approximations
to a set of AERs or ERs.  Let $Y_n(t)$ denote the t-th time point in
the AER for the n-th subject.  The same methods may be used for

individual ERs within a subject as well as for more than one AER per subject but there is little to be gained by defining a more complicated notation at this point.  Now the approximation for the AER of the n-th subject is

$$A_n(t) = \sum_{k=1}^{K} a_{nk} f_k(t)$$

where $a_{nk}$ is the coefficient for the k-th term and the n-th subject. Thus, the coefficients of the approximation can vary from one subject to the next.  One common measure of the adequacy of an approximation is the sums of squares of deviations

$$\sum_{t=1}^{T} (Y_n(t) - A_n(t))^2$$

for the subject n and

$$\sum_{n=1}^{N} \sum_{t=1}^{T} (y_n(t) - A_n(t))^2$$

for a group of N subjects.  Approximations that minimize this measure of poorness of fit are called least squares approximations.  While these may be computed by the usual method of least squares, the resulting approximation may not have the usual statistical properties associated with least squares methods because the original AERs do not follow the statistical assumptions used in deriving these properties.  Thus, an approximation that is best in the least squares sense may not be the optimal choice for a given analysis and data set.  Relatively little information is available about the statistical properties of AERs that can be used to select approximations at this time.  Perhaps the safest procedure is to plot the approximations and the original observations for a large number of cases. The approximation should be selected so that it retains the features of the AER that the experimenter assumes are relevant.

The usual least squares calculations involve solving a set of K simultaneous equations for each subject.  While this is feasible even on a moderate minicomputer for most situations, a clever choice of the functions can avoid this calculation.  If

$$\sum_{t=1}^{T} f_k(t) f_p(t) = 0, \text{ if } p =/= k$$

then the functions are said to be orthogonal.  The choice of

orthogonal functions greatly simplifies the mathematics and reduces
the complexity of calculations.  Hence, orthogonal functions are
preferred.  It has been assumed that there are T equally spaced
time observations in each response.  The basis functions may be
represented by a table of values rather than a mathematical formula.  This allows factor analytic methods and principal components
to be viewed as simply alternate methods for finding basis functions.
This also justifies the term basis in the usual algebraic sense because if T=K, i.e., there are as many approximating terms as there
are observations in an AER, then the set of basis functions is an
orthogonal basis in the usual matrix algebra sense.

## 2.1 BLOCK FUNCTIONS

The simplest choice of basis functions is to let $f_k(t)=1$ for
$A_k$ to $B_k$ and zero otherwise.  Then, $a_{nk}$ is the average amplitude
in the time interval determined by $A_k$ and $B_k$.  As an example, we
might choose five intervals of 100 milliseconds for a half second
ER.  A plot of the approximation usually looks discouraging but
the approach has been used with some success by  a number of researchers.  Shagass (1972, p.43) mentions this method.  This approach does not extend to a general set of functions and the block
functions are orthogonal only if the intervals do not overlap.  Unlike the other functions discussed in this note, block functions
do not form an orthogonal basis function set.  However, Haar functions are extensions of block functions.

## 2.2 FOURIER APPROXIMATIONS

If sine and cosine basis functions are used with an integer
multiple of the length of the AER for the period, a truncated
Fourier series for the approximation results.  This choice of functions has a number of advantages:  i) the mathematical properties
of the Fourier series have been extensively studied and are widely
known, ii) the recent rediscovery of a group of algorithms called
the fast Fourier transform, FFT, make the calculation very efficient, iii) Fourier methods have been widely used in physics and
engineering and frequency interpretations of the coefficients are
well known.  Experience with Fourier approximations to AERs shows
that a 500 millisecond AER can usually be approximated very well
by 10 to 24 coefficients.  For some analyses, a smaller number of
terms might be adequate.

There are numerous references on Fourier series.  A recent book
by Brigham (1974) is probably a good starting point.  The two Alden
House FFT Conference Proceedings published in Vol. 15, 1967 and

Vol. 17, 1969, of the IEEE Transactions on Audio and Electroacoustics are also very useful.

## 2.3 WALSH-HADAMARD FUNCTIONS

Walsh functions are usually developed from the standpoint of
using square waves instead of sine waves in an analog to Fourier
methods. This leads to an extension of frequency that is called
sequency. The sequency is simply the number of sign changes in the
basis function over the interval of approximation. An orthogonal
matrix discovered by Hadamard also generates all of the discrete
Walsh functions but not in the usual sequency order.

The major advantage of the Walsh-Hadamard functions is simplicity. The functions only take on two values, +1 and -1. Table
1 shows the discrete Walsh functions for T=8.

These functions have advantages:

i) The computations are very fast on small computers because
they only require additions and subtractions and seldom require
multiplications and divisions.

ii) No tables of sines or equivalent algorithms are needed.

iii) These functions are very well adapted for the very efficient special purpose hardware for bit manipulations in a computer.

iv) An algorithm similar to the fast Fourier transform is available and the computation is extremely fast.

v) For many digital processing problems, the Walsh-Hadamard
is more natural or direct than Fourier methods.

## 2.4 HAAR FUNCTIONS

Haar functions consist of a single cycle of a square wave.
Thus, they take on only three values +1, 0 and -1. This leads to
many of the same computational advantages of Walsh functions. The
Haar functions for 8 points are shown in Table 2.

There is very little literature on Haar functions. They are
briefly described by Bremerman (1968) and in a text by Collatz
(1966). Several image coding papers by Andrews and associates
(1971) have a plot that refers to Haar transforms but no references.

TABLE 1

WALSH–HADAMARD FUNCTION FOR 8 POINTS

|          | t   |     |     |     |     |     |     |     |
|----------|-----|-----|-----|-----|-----|-----|-----|-----|
|          | 1   | 2   | 3   | 4   | 5   | 6   | 7   | 8   |
| $f_1(t)$ | 1   | 1   | 1   | 1   | 1   | 1   | 1   | 1   |
| $f_2(t)$ | 1   | 1   | 1   | 1   | -1  | -1  | -1  | -1  |
| $f_3(t)$ | 1   | 1   | -1  | -1  | -1  | -1  | 1   | 1   |
| $f_4(t)$ | 1   | 1   | -1  | -1  | 1   | 1   | -1  | -1  |
| $f_5(t)$ | 1   | -1  | -1  | 1   | 1   | -1  | -1  | 1   |
| $f_6(t)$ | 1   | -1  | -1  | 1   | -1  | 1   | 1   | -1  |
| $f_7(t)$ | 1   | -1  | 1   | -1  | -1  | 1   | -1  | 1   |
| $f_8(t)$ | 1   | -1  | 1   | -1  | 1   | -1  | 1   | -1  |

The Walsh–Hadamard functions were originally developed over fifty years ago but the major interest in applications has been in the last eight years. A recent article by Jacoby (1977) is a good introduction. The primary references are three conference proceedings:

i) Bass, C.A. (Ed.) Application of Walsh functions. Symposium, Springfield: National Technical Information Service, 1970, document AD 707 431.

ii) Zeek, R.W. & Showalter, A.E. (Eds.) Applications of Walsh functions, Springfield: National Technical Information Service, 1971, document AD 727 000.

iii) Zeek, R.W. & Showalter, A.E. (Eds.) Applications of Walsh functions, Springfield: National Technical Information Service, 1972, document AD 744 650.

TABLE 2

HAAR FUNCTIONS FOR 8 POINTS

| | 1 | 2 | 3 | t 4 | 5 | 6 | 7 | 8 |
|---|---|---|---|---|---|---|---|---|
| $f_1(t)$ | 1 | 1 | 1 | 1 | 1 | 1 | 1 | 1 |
| $f_2(t)$ | 1 | 1 | 1 | 1 | -1 | -1 | -1 | -1 |
| $f_3(t)$ | 1 | 1 | -1 | -1 | 0 | 0 | 0 | 0 |
| $f_4(t)$ | 0 | 0 | 0 | 0 | 1 | 1 | -1 | -1 |
| $f_5(t)$ | 1 | -1 | 0 | 0 | 0 | 0 | 0 | 0 |
| $f_6(t)$ | 0 | 0 | 1 | -1 | 0 | 0 | 0 | 0 |
| $f_7(t)$ | 0 | 0 | 0 | 0 | 1 | -1 | 0 | 0 |
| $f_8(t)$ | 0 | 0 | 0 | 0 | 0 | 0 | 1 | -1 |

These functions differ from both the Fourier and Walsh in that there is not an obvious natural order. The advantage of Haar functions lies in their similarity to the block average functions. They describe local amplitude changes rather than behavior of the entire sample period. Thus, by choosing among these functions, it is possible to represent some parts of the AER with greater accuracy than others. Also, the coefficients are tied to specific time intervals. Hence, a significant difference can be related to an interval for interpretation.

A fast Haar transform is very simple to devise. The basic procedure, shown in table 3, is to difference alternate values for the coefficients and then to sum the adjacent values to generate an array of half of the numbers of points. The same algorithm is then repeatedly applied to the array of sums.

## 2.5 ORTHOGONAL POLYNOMIALS

The usual mathematical approximation methods rely very strongly on polynomials. Numerous programs are available to fit polynomials such as BMD 5 R (Dixon, 1974). Thus, at first glance, polynomial approximations would seem to be a good starting point for the approximation of AER data. This is not the case. High degree poly-

TABLE 3

8 POINT FAST HAAR TRANSFORM
SAMPLE CALCULATION

| t | Y(t) | ÷2 | ÷4 | ÷8 | $a_t$ |
|---|------|----|----|----|----|
| 1 | 1 | 3 | −1 | 8 | 1 |
| 2 | 2 | −4 | 9 | −10 | −10/8 |
| 3 | −4 | 7 | 7 | | 7/4 |
| 4 | 0 | 2 | 5 | | 5/4 |
| 5 | 4 | −1 | | | −1/2 |
| 6 | 3 | −4 | | | −4/2 |
| 7 | 1 | 1 | | | 1/2 |
| 8 | 1 | 0 | | | 0 |

The sums and differences are computed for pairs of points. The differences are then divided by a power of two to obtain the coefficients. The same operation is then repeated on the sum column until only two terms remain. In the above example, the differences are underlined.

nomials, 15 to 25 terms for 500 msec, are usually required to approximate an AER. The usual least squares program tends to become very inaccurate for high degree polynomials. A 32 bit real number representation will usually fail in fitting a degree 5 polynomial and a 64 bit number will enable the program to get to about degree 8 before failing. Wampler (1970) illustrates failures of many of the major statistical programs. These computational failures can be avoided by fitting Chebychev polynomials in a linear regression program. The Chebychev polynomials can be defined with the transformation part of the package. Any medium level numerical analysis text such as Ralston (1965) has a section on Chebychev polynomials.

Orthogonal polynomials tend to eliminate the computational problems involved with ordinary polynomials. The only problem is computing adequate tables of orthogonal polynomials. The standard

tables do not go to high enough degree or have enough points.  If
care is exercised to avoid inaccuracies due to subtractions, the
formulas given by Milne (1949, pp.259-260) can be used.  Be sure
to carefully check the polynomials.  Rounding errors are tricky
and can be hard to pick up.  An alternate method is to apply a modified Grahm-Schmidt orthogonalization algorithm to Chebychev polynomials.  This procedure seems to avoid most of the problems.

## 3.1 DISCRIMINANT METHODS

The union-intersection multivariate tests associated with
linear discriminant functions produce basis functions.  These are
discussed in a later section.

Donchin (1969) proposed the use of stepwise discriminant procedures for the analysis of ER data.  This approach is discussed by
Glasser and Ruchkin (1976) and has been used by several authors.
This is a useful technique in exploratory data analysis but some
caution is required if further analyses are to be based upon these
results.  Stepwise procedures are empirical methods and have several
problems.  Numerous examples are known where stepwise procedures do
not find the best function.  An even more serious problem is that
the associated significance tests are biased towards false significant results.  The bias is more serious for small samples and large
numbers of observations in a sweep.  These are common in ER data.
This problem is discussed by Lachin and Schachter (1974).

## 3.2 PRINCIPAL COMPONENTS

Hotelling (1933) developed many of the ideas of principal components.  The basic procedure is to find a set of orthogonal basis
functions such that the first function minimizes the sum of squares
of the residuals for a single function.  The second function is then
chosen such that it achieves the maximum reduction when added to the
first function.  This procedure is continued until all of the variation is accounted for.  The resultant sequence of basis functions
are optimal in the least squares sense; that is, no other approximation based upon the same number of basis functions can have
smaller sum of squares of residuals.  Marriot (1974) has a very
good discussion of this method.

There are several important features of this method that need
to be considered.  The major difficulty in most applications is
that the variables are not measured in the same units.  An example
could be weight, height and age.  Thus a variance that pools these
sums of squares is not meaningful.  This problem should not occur
in ER applications where all of the measurements should be proportional to voltages.  In fact, this probably makes principal

components a better choice than factor analysis for ER data.

The second problem with principal components is that it is essentially a single sample procedure. It is difficult to apply this method to experimental data where some of the sources of variability have been controlled or manipulated. The basic problem is that the principal components and factor analysis usually assume a homogeneous sample and thus mix the sources of variation in this type of analysis. This may not be too serious because both regression and ANOVA methods can then be used to attempt to separate the sources of variability of the reduced variables. However, the effect of combining the different analysis is unknown and distribution of the usual test statistics could be affected. This is probably a minor effect in large samples.

The computation of the principal components is difficult for large numbers of variables. This calculation is not well suited to minicomputers and even large computers have accuracy problems unless care is used in selection and programming of the algorithm.

The resulting basis functions are subject to sampling variations. These are largely unknown and difficult to treat in the analysis. Thus it is important to translate the analysis back into the original time and voltage plots so that the results may be compared across studies.

Principal components is sometimes referred to as a Karhoumen-Loeve transformation or filter in the engineering literature. The latter method is for continuous functions rather than discrete sample values but the distinction is not critical in applications. Principal components is often confused with factor analysis. The major difference is that principal components is a variance-covariance based method while factor analysis is a correlation based method. Marriot (1974) discusses these differences in detail.


### 3.3 FACTOR ANALYSIS

Factor analysis differs from principal components analysis in that the procedure accounts for correlations observed between points instead of the variances. The maximum likelihood method proposed by Lawley is described in most multivariate statistics texts (Morrison, 1976, pp.304-314; Harmon, 1976, pp.197-216). This procedure is based upon a set of assumptions that appear hard to justify for ER data and applications of this method to ER data are rare.

Principal factor methods are the most frequently used method and perhaps the most useful for ER data. Marriot (1974) has a good discussion of both maximum likelihood and principal factor

factor methods.  Principal factor methods estimate the commonalities and then usually use a rotational procedure such as the varimax to simplify the interpretation.  This method is frequently confused with the method of principal components.  The major advantages of principal components factor analysis are: i) This method
is more data analysis oriented than the maximum likelihood factor
methods.  The principal components method has been used successfully
on a wide variety of data from different fields.  ii) Computer programs are widely available for this method,  although some care
should be exercised.  Some programs do not have good eigenvalue
calculations and these may fail for the large matrices involved in
evoked responses.  iii) Many researchers, particularly psychologists,
have some experience in interpreting the results of this calculation
and find it a useful data analysis tool.

Factor analysis methods lead to several problems.  The between
subject variances may not be very homogeneous across times in the
ER.  This can be misleading because the correlation based procedure
standardizes the variances.  Thus, time points that show little
variation are given a large weight.  As an example, the sample data
used in this paper has a large variance at about 160 milliseconds
that is about 30 times the smaller variances.  Thus, a factor analyses of these data is much less sensitive to between subject variation in the N140-P200 area than the method of principal components.
Factor analysis methods are also hard to use or interpret when the
data are from an experimental design or have several sources of
variation.

### 3.4 UNION-INTERSECTION STATISTICS

Principal components and factor analysis techniques are difficult to apply when there are groups of subjects.  If the covariance
for matrices groups are pooled, the techniques do not reflect the
between group variation, which is probably the most important part
of the data in a multi-group experimental design.  On the other
hand, if a common covariance matrix is computed across all groups
with a common mean vector, then the between subject and between
group variances are confounded.

One way to approach this problem is through the use of multivariate analysis of variance.  These methods follow the usual univariate procedures in partitioning the total variance into components.  Roy (1957) has proposed a multivariate test statistic that
is the multivariate analog of the univariate F tests.  This statistic is usually called the union-intersection statistic or the
largest root statistic because it is the largest root (or eigenvalue) of the characteristic function of a matrix.  Morrison (1977)
uses the largest root tests in an introductory multivariate

analysis text.  Several of the common MANOVA computer programs print
the largest root and any further roots that exceed some test value.

The interesting point in the analysis of ER data is that each
of these roots is associated with an eigenvector and the sequence
of eigenvectors form an orthogonal basis for the evoked responses.
Thus, a plot of the eigenvectors associated with the larger roots
should be interpretable in terms of the shape changes across responses associated with the union-intersection test statistics.
In some cases, for example, a two group MANOVA, the associated
eigenvector may be the discriminant function.  Some programs may
label the eigenvectors as discriminant functions even when this is
not the usual terminology.

This technique has the advantage of associating the set of
basis functions with a test statistic.  In addition, it follows
from analysis of variance techniques that have proved useful in a
wide variety of situations.  It has several disadvantages.  It is
untried, the computation is difficult, the procedure is based upon
complex statistical methodology, and the results may be difficult
to interpret.

### 3.5 CANONICAL CORRELATION ANALYSIS

Factor analysis can be described as a method that attempts to
clarify the correlational structure within a single set of variables
by developing a smaller number of uncorrelated variables that account for most of the observed correlation.  Canonical correlation
analysis is an attempt to clarify the correlations between two sets
of variables by developing two smaller sets of variables that account
for the correlations between the sets while each set of the new variables are uncorrelated within each set.

An obvious approach in ER data is to use ER measurements as
one set of variables and the second set of variables as some potentially related measures.  Examples could be intelligence tests,
personality tests, neurological "soft" signs, performance tests,
etc.  Evaluation batteries are frequently found in studies of schizophrenia, affective disorders, minimal brain disfunction, learning
disabilities, reading disabilities, hyperkinesis, etc., to mention
a few areas where ER methods have been used or proposed.

Canonical correlation methods are not scale dependent as are
the principal components.  Nor do they have the rotational indeter-
minacy of some of the factor analytic methods.  The distribution
theory is poorly developed and only a few large sample approximate
tests are available.  Less theory, as well as less informal lore,
are available on applications than the other multivariate methods

discussed in this paper.

## 4.1 COMPARISON OF METHODS

The computational problems of the multivariate methods will probably tend to limit their direct application. These methods require the calculation of both large covariance matrices and eigenvalues of large matrices. The union-interaction statistics are also of limited use when the number of samples in the sweep are not small relative to the sample size.

A two stage procedure may prove useful. The approach would be to use a fixed basis method such as a Fourier transform to replace the original observations with an approximation vector of much smaller dimensionality. Then the multivariate methods can be applied to this vector. This loses some of the information in the original data but this loss is not likely to be important if the truncated Fourier series is a good fit.

Factor analysis is commonly used as a data reduction technique. Further analyses are then performed on the factor loadings. The same procedure has been proposed for principal components. The effect on subsequent analyses of this two stage procedure is not known but the method is probably reasonable if the sample sizes are large.

A small empirical study was performed on the data from Martin, Becker, and Buffington (1977). The intensity 16 average VERs for 43 subjects were used. Averaging four adjacent points reduced 128 points to 32 points over a half second sweep. All baseline (DC components) had been previously removed so that the observations in each sweep summed to zero. The 32 by 32 covariance matrix was computed across all 43 subjects. A principal components analyses and a principle components factor analysis were both compoted for these data. The proportion of the total sum of squares accounted for by the first 16 terms of each of these methods are shown in the first two columns of Table 4. The same proportion of variance is shown for the Fourier approximation. Only even numbers of terms were used because the coefficients were computed for sine-cosine pairs. Orthogonal polynomials were computed for degree 1 to 15 and the percentage variance was found. The first 16 Walsh functions were also computed. Haar functions do not have a natural order as found in the previous functions. The first Haar function column is based upon the order used in the example. The major order is based upon the length of the positive part and the minor order is from left to right in the interval. One of the advantages of Haar functions is that they can be selected to improve the approximation. The last column is the best order Haar function for these data. This is somewhat overly optimistic but it is an upper bound. It is impossible for any other ordering of Haar functions to do any better.

If all of the variances (the diagonal of the 32 by 32 covariance matrix) were equal then the factor analysis would also be
optimal. The relatively poor performance of the factor analysis
is due to a large between subject variance increase near 150
milliseconds after the flash. This is probably due to latency
variation between subjects. The major advantage of principal components over factor analysis is its relative insensitivity to large
variances.

The Fourier approximation performs quite well after about 8
terms are used while the two multivariate methods are better for
small numbers of terms. Polynomials, Walsh, and Haar are generally

TABLE 4

PROPORTION OF VARIANCE ACCOUNTED FOR BY
DIFFERENT NUMBERS OF TERMS IN APPROXIMATIONS
GENERATED BY PRINCIPAL COMPONENTS, FACTOR ANALYSIS,
FOURIER, POLYNOMIAL, WALSH-HADAMARD, HAAR, AND BEST ORDER HAAR

| NO. TERMS | PRIN. COMP. | FACT. ANAL. | FOUR- IER | POLY- NOMIAL | WALSH | HAAR 1 | HAAR 2 |
|---|---|---|---|---|---|---|---|
| 1 | .375 | .218 | | .099 | .135 | .203 | .134 |
| 2 | .547 | .472 | .278 | .209 | .271 | .383 | .337 |
| 3 | .679 | .575 | | .304 | .382 | .517 | .381 |
| 4 | .754 | .644 | .506 | .356 | .483 | .572 | .436 |
| 5 | .800 | .706 | | .454 | .534 | .627 | .615 |
| 6 | .837 | .757 | .677 | .556 | .617 | .681 | .650 |
| 7 | .867 | .781 | | .595 | .668 | .725 | .667 |
| 8 | .891 | .814 | .778 | .667 | .702 | .760 | .688 |
| 9 | .913 | .843 | | .713 | .748 | .783 | .742 |
| 10 | .933 | .868 | .864 | .767 | .782 | .804 | .796 |
| 11 | .948 | .885 | | .813 | .812 | .825 | .820 |
| 12 | .960 | .900 | .925 | .832 | .834 | .843 | .837 |
| 13 | .969 | .911 | | .866 | .853 | .861 | .850 |
| 14 | .975 | .919 | .945 | .895 | .865 | .878 | .864 |
| 15 | .979 | .926 | | .916 | .874 | .891 | .872 |
| 16 | .983 | .932 | .958 | - | .878 | .904 | .879 |

It is known mathematically that principal components is the best
approximation in the least squares sense.

as good as the Fourier approximation for up to 8 terms but worse for higher numbers of terms.

An alternative presentation of the same information is shown in Table 5.

The Fourier approximation appears to be the best choice of the fixed basis methods if more than 10 terms are used. However, the computational advantage of the Walsh and Haar may outweigh the reduced error in some applications. This is particularly true on mini or microcomputers that have poor floating point computation speeds. Haar approximations seem to be as good or better than Fourier for smaller numbers of term. Shanks gives the details of the fast Walsh transform.

TABLE 5

PROPORTION OF VARIANCE ACCOUNTED FOR BY
THE NUMBER OF TERMS REQUIRED TO ACCOUNT
FOR VARIOUS PERCENTAGES OF THE VARIANCE
OF VERS FOR A SAMPLE OF 43 SUBJECTS

| % VAR. | PRIN. COMP. | FACT. ANAL. | FOUR- IER | POLY- NOMIAL | WALSH | HAAR 1 | HAAR 2 |
|--------|-------------|-------------|-----------|--------------|-------|--------|--------|
| 50 | 2 | 3 | 4 | 6 | 5 | 3 | 5 |
| 60 | 3 | 4 | 6 | 8 | 6 | 5 | 5 |
| 70 | 4 | 5 | 8 | 9 | 8 | 7 | 9 |
| 80 | 5 | 8 | 10 | 11 | 11 | 10 | 11 |
| 90 | 9 | 12 | 14 | 15 | 18 | 16 | 18 |

The smallest number of terms that can account for a fixed percentage of the variance are shown.

BIBLIOGRAPHY

Andrews, H.C.  Multidimensional rotations in feature selection.
    IEEE Transactions, 1971, C-20(9), 1045-1051.

Bass, C.A. (ed.).  Application of Walsh functions symposium.
    Springfield:  National Tehcnical Information Service, 1970.

Biemerman, H.J.  Pattern recognition, functionals, and entropy.
    Transactions on Biomedical Engineering, 1968, BME-15, 201-207.

Brigham, E.O.  The fast Fourier transform.  New Jersey;
    Prentice-Hall, 1974.

Collatz, L.  Functional analysis and numerical mathematics,
    New York:  Academic Press, 1966.

Dixon, W.J. (Ed.).  Biomedical computer programs.  Berkeley:
    University of California Press, 1974.

Donchin, E.  Discriminant analysis in average evoked response
    studies:  The study of single trial data.  Electroencephalo-
    graphy and Clinical Neurophysiology, 1969, 27, 311-314.

Glasser, E.M., & Ruchkin, D.S.  Principles of neurobiological
    signal analysis.  New York:  Academic Press, 1976.

Harmon, H.H.  Modern factor analysis.  Chicago:  University of
    Chicago Press, 1976.

Hotelling, H.  Analysis of a complex of statistical variables into
    principal components.  Journal of Educational Psychology
    1933, 24, 417-441, 498-520.

IEEE Transactions on audio and electroacoustics.  1969, AU-17,
    66-76.

IEEE Transactions on audio and electroacoustics.  1967, AU-15,
    45-55.

Jacoby, B.F.  Walsh functions.  Byte, 1977, 2(9), 190-198.

Lachin, J.M., & Schachter, J.  On stepwise discriminant analyses
    applied to physiologic data.  Psychophysiology, 1974, 11,
    703-709.

Marriot, F.H.C.  The interpretation of multiple observations.
    New York:  Academic Press, 1974.

Martin, D.C., Becker, J. & Buffington, V.  An evoked potential
    study of endogenous affective disorders in alcoholics.
    Printed in this volume, Begleiter, H. (Ed.), 1977.

Milne, W.E. Numerical calculus.  Princeton:  Princeton University
    Press, 1949.

Morrison, D.F.  Multivariate statistical methods. New York:
    McGraw-Hill, 1976.

Ralston, A.A.  A first course in numerical analysis.  New York:
    McGraw-Hill, 1965.

Shagass, C.  Evoked brain potentials in psychiatry.  New York:
    Plenum Press, 1972, 43.

Shanks, J.L.  Computation of the fast Walsh-Fourier transform.
    IEEE Transactions on Computers, 1969, May, 457-459.

Wampler, R.H.  A report on the accuracy of some widely used least
    squares computer programs.  Journal of the American Statistical
    Association, 1970, 65(330), 549-565.

Zeek, R.W., & Showalter, A.E.  Applications of Walsh functions.
    Springfield:  National Technical Information Service, 1971.

Zeek, R.W., & Showalter, A.E.  Applications of Walsh functions.
    Springfield:  National Technical Information Service, 1972.